Fundamentals of Anaesthesia and Acute Medicine

Neuromuscular Transmission

Fundamentals of Anaesthesia and Acute Medicine

Neuromuscular Transmission

Edited by
Leo HDJ Booij
Professor, Institute for Anesthesiology, University of Nijmegen, The Netherlands

Series editors
Ronald M Jones
Professor of Anaesthetics, St Mary's Hospital Medical School, London

Alan R Aitkenhead
Professor of Anaesthesia, University of Nottingham

and

Pierre Foëx
Nuffield Professor of Anaesthetics, University of Oxford

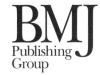

© BMJ Publishing Group 1996

All rights reserved. No part of this publication may be reproduced,
stored in a retrieval system, or transmitted, in any form or by any
means, electronic, mechanical, photocopying, recording and/or
otherwise, without the prior written permission of the publishers.

First published in 1996
by the BMJ Publishing Group, BMA House, Tavistock Square,
London WC1H 9JR

British Library Cataloguing in Publication Data

A catalogue record for this book is available from the British Library

ISBN 0–7279–0929–0

Typeset by Apek Typesetters Ltd, Nailsea, Bristol
Printed and bound in Great Britain by Latimer Trend Ltd, Plymouth

Contents

Contributors

David R Bevan, MB, MRCP, FFARCA
Professor and Chairman, University of British Columbia and Vancouver Hospital, British Columbia, Canada

Leo HDJ Booij, MD, PhD, FRCA
Professor, Institute for Anesthesiology, University of Nijmegen, The Netherlands

WC Bowman, PhD, DSc, FRSE, HonFRCA
Professor of Pharmacology, Department of Physiology and Pharmacology, University of Strathclyde, Glasgow, UK

François Donati, PhD, MD, FRCPC
Professor and Chairman, Department of Anaesthesia, Université de Montréal and Hôtel-Dieu Hospital, Montréal, Québec, Canada

Kent S Pearson, MD
Associate Professor, University of Iowa School of Medicine, Iowa City, Iowa, USA

IM Ramzan, PhD
Senior Lecturer in Pharmaceutics, Department of Pharmacy, University of Sydney, Australia

Eric N Robertson, FRCA
Senior Clinical and Research Associate, Institute for Anesthesiology, University of Nijmegen, The Netherlands

CA Shanks, MD, ChB
Professor of Anesthesia, Northwestern University, Chicago, Illinois, USA

Martin Sokoll, MD
Professor, University of Iowa School of Medicine, Iowa City, Iowa, USA

Edward S Wegrzynowicz, MD
Associate Professor, University of Iowa School of Medicine, Iowa City, Iowa, USA

Foreword

The pace of change within the biological sciences continues to increase and nowhere is this more apparent than in the specialties of anaesthesia, acute medicine, and intensive care. Although many practitioners continue to rely on comprehensive but bulky texts for reference, the accelerating rate of biomedical advances makes this source of information increasingly likely to be dated, even if the latest edition is used. The series *Fundamentals of anaesthesia and acute medicine* aims to bring the reader up to date and authoritative reviews of the principal clinical topics which make up the specialties. Each volume will cover the fundamentals of the topic in a comprehensive manner but will also emphasise recent developments or controversial issues.

International differences in the practice of anaesthesia and intensive care are now much less than in the past, and the editors of each volume have commissioned chapters from acknowledged authorities throughout the world to assemble contributions of the highest possible calibre. Three volumes will appear annually and, as the pace and extent of clinically significant advances varies among the individual topics, new editions will be commissioned to ensure that practitioners will be in a position to keep abreast of the important developments within the specialties.

Not only does the pace of advance in biomedical science serve to justify the appearance of an international series of this nature but the current awareness of the need for more formal continuing education also underlines the timeliness of its appearance. The editors would welcome feedback from readers about the series, which is aimed at both established practitioners and trainees preparing for degrees and diplomas in anaesthesia and intensive care.

RONALD M JONES
ALAN R AITKENHEAD
PIERRE FOËX

Preface

Over the past decade knowledge about neuromuscular transmission and the clinical use of neuromuscular blocking agents has increased tremendously. This has resulted in the refinement of the use of relaxants both in the operating room and in the intensive care unit, and the introduction of a variety of new agents. The aim of this book is to update readers with respect to the recent developments in the field. All the contributors have wide experience in both research and the clinical application of relaxants, and thus are capable of judging these developments. The first few chapters give a mainly mechanistic view, while the later chapters deal principally with the individual agents.

I would like to thank all the authors for their excellent contributions, produced in a very short time under the mounting pressure of deadlines. I am also grateful to the staff of the BMJ Publishing Group books division, without whose efforts the book would not have appeared.

I hope you enjoy reading this book.

Leo H D J Booij
November 1995

1: Prejunctional mechanisms involved in neuromuscular transmission

WC BOWMAN

Introduction

Skeletal muscles are innervated by somatic efferent nerve fibres which are fast conducting, myelinated, group Aα axons with cell bodies in the motor nuclei of the cranial nerves in the brain stem, or in the anterior horns of grey matter in the spinal cord. The axons of these motoneurons pass without interruption from the central nervous system to the muscles, where each axon branches extensively, the branching occurring at nodes of Ranvier. Through its extensive branching, a single axon innervates many muscle fibres. With few exceptions, in mammals most muscle fibres are focally innervated, that is, the fibre receives its innervation at a single focus, somewhere near its middle. The axon, together with the muscle fibres that it innervates, is called a motor unit. The whole nerve–muscle system consists of thousands of motor units. As it approaches a muscle fibre, the terminal branch of an axon loses its myelin sheath and, where it makes contact with the muscle fibre, it breaks up into a number of short twigs (telodendria) that lie in gutters, the junctional clefts, in the muscle fibre membrane. The surface of the junctional cleft in apposition to the nerve ending is thrown into folds, the junctional folds, forming so called secondary clefts. At its narrowest, the junctional gap between the plasma membranes of nerve ending (axolemma) and muscle fibre (sarcolemma) is about 60 nm wide. The gap, including the secondary clefts, is filled with an ill defined material that looks, under the electron microscope, rather like barbed wire. This is the so called basement membrane, a material rich in mucopolysaccharides and with some of the characteristics of collagen. The basement membrane contains much of the junctional acetylcholinesterase embedded within it. Electron micrographs and diagrams of the innervation of skeletal muscles may be found in reviews.[1 2]

The terminal Schwann cells (teloglia) of the axon twigs form "lids" to the junctional clefts so that the neuromuscular junctions are enclosed. The space enclosed by the axon, the terminal Schwann cells, and the postjunctional face of the muscle fibre membrane may be regarded as the biophase or effect compartment. Diffusion of drugs into it must be restricted to some extent by the terminal Schwann cells. Diffusion presumably occurs between these Schwann cells (rather than through them) which are probably held in position by desmosomes. Diffusion inside the effect compartment may be restricted by the basement membrane, to which some drugs (for example, tubocurarine) actually bind, and, if the drug interacts reversibly with receptors, by the process of buffered diffusion during which the drug molecules "bounce" their way across the receptor region before escaping. Transmitter acetylcholine molecules are small enough to diffuse rapidly through the basement membrane, but they do have to traverse the hurdle of the acetylcholinesterase embedded there, and some of the acetylcholine is in fact destroyed before it reaches the receptors. Transmitter that does reach the receptors survives long enough, generally, to interact only with one receptor before it too is hydrolysed.

The process of neuromuscular transmission is conceptually simple, the main basic events having been established and widely accepted for more than 40 years. The neurotransmitter acetylcholine is synthesised within the nerve endings and stored in vesicles. A small, ineffective amount is continuously released spontaneously, mainly from the axoplasm but also from the vesicles. Vesicular release (but not axoplasmic release) is abruptly and greatly accelerated, through a Ca^{2+} dependent mechanism, by the arrival of a nerve impulse at the nerve endings. The released acetylcholine diffuses across the narrow junctional cleft and combines fleetingly with the nicotinic acetylcholine receptors on the postjunctional membrane of the motor endplate. The consequence is a localised depolarisation, the endplate potential, which initiates a propagating action potential that passes around the muscle fibre membrane to trigger the contractile mechansim. Although these basic tenets of the transmission process have been accepted for many years, important advances in detailed knowledge continue to be made through the accelerating developments of new skills and techniques, especially in the fields of molecular biology and electrophysiology. This chapter is concerned only with the prejunctional events in this process. It therefore deals with the electrical changes and ionic fluxes in the terminals, with the synthesis, storage, release, and destruction of the main transmitter (acetylcholine), with the possible release and functions of additional co-transmitters, and with the roles and types of receptors that are located on the nerve terminals.

Nerve action potentials

Gated potassium channels are absent from mammalian nodes of Ranvier,[3] so that the falling phase of the action potential arises simply from dissipation of the Na^+ after rapid inactivation of the sodium channels. Hence, drugs that block the delayed rectifier type of potassium channels (for example, 4-aminopyridine) have no effect on the duration of the action potential in the myelinated parts of the axon. Although absent from the nodes of mammalian myelinated axons, potassium channels are actually present in the axon membrane beneath the myelin. Repetitive nerve activity causes temporary swelling and loosening of the myelin sheath immediately next to the nodes (the paranodal region) and this exposes potassium channels in the axon membrane, which then contribute to the nodal action potential by hastening repolarisation and thereby reducing spike duration. The physiological importance of this phenomenon is not understood, nor is the function of the K^+ channels beneath the myelin in the internodal region. There are no Na^+ channels in the axolemma of the internodal region.

Potassium channels operated by voltage are present in the peripheral non-myelinated terminals of the motoneurons. Brigant and Mallart[4] developed an elegant technique for recording the extracellular action currents from non-myelinated nerve endings, and they used this technique to study the nature of the ion channels in the terminals of rat motor nerve fibres. According to these workers, Na^+ channels cease to be present after the last node of Ranvier so that the action potential propagation stops there. They propose that the action potential at the last node of Ranvier depolarises the terminal axolemma simply by decremental spread. This causes the opening, in the terminals, of the voltage operated calcium channels which have an essential role in transmitter release as described below. Influx of Ca^{2+} causes further depolarisation, but voltage operated gated K^+ channels are also opened and K^+ efflux restores the membrane potential to the resting value.

Figure 1.1 illustrates experiments based on the techniques of Brigant and Mallart[4] but recorded from the motor nerve terminals of a mouse muscle by Dr E Rowan. The recording electrode is placed near the last node of Ranvier and, as the nerve impulse reaches it, it records the voltage change consequent upon Na^+ influx at that point. The reversal in potential at the last node causes the opening of peripherally located K^+ channels as described above. The *efflux* of K^+ at the more peripheral site is "seen" by the recording electrode as an *influx* of local circuit currents. Hence, the two spikes that reflect adjacent Na^+ influx (I_{Na}) and more distant K^+ efflux (I_K) both occur in the same direction (downward in fig 1.1a). The I_K actually masks an inward Ca^{2+} current which can be seen only if I_K is blocked. I_K may be blocked by an aminopyridine (3,4-diaminopyridine in the experiment of fig 1.1a) when the upward deflection, known[5] to be a consequence of Ca^{2+} influx (I_{Ca}) is seen. As the I_K would normally repolarise the membrane and tend to close the calcium channels, the I_{Ca} seen in fig 1.1 is presumably greater than normal, because I_K has been blocked. Excess intracellular Ca^{2+} is cytotoxic and it appears that the large Ca^{2+} influx quickly gives rise to a calcium activated K^+ efflux (I_{KCa}) that prevents

3

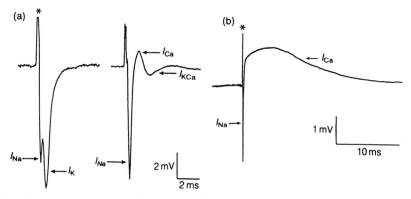

Fig 1.1 Presynaptic waveforms recorded by placing an electrode inside the perineural sheath of a motor nerve innervating a mouse triangularis sterni nerve–muscle preparation. (a) Left shows the average of 20–25 control waveforms (*stimulus artefact); and the right is in the presence of 3,4-diaminopyridine 400 μmol/l. I_{Na} is the waveform corresponding to the inward sodium current, I_K to the outward potassium current, I_{Ca} to the inward calcium current, and I_{KCa} to the outward calcium activated potassium current. (b) Recordings from a similar experiment in which both 3,4-diaminopyridine and tetraethylammonium (4 mmol/l) were applied. The I_{KCa} is blocked by the tetraethylammonium and the I_{Ca} greatly augmented. All recordings were made in the presence of μ-conotoxin (0·1 μmol/l) which selectively prevents muscle contraction. (Reproduced with permission from Braga MFM, Rowan EG, Harvey AL, Bowman WC. Interactions between suxamethonium and non depolarizing neuromuscular blocking drugs. *Br J Anaesth* 1994;72:198–204)

further Ca^{2+} entry.[6] Drugs that block calcium activated K^+ channels, such as tetraethylammonium (fig 1.1b) or the scorpion toxin known as charybdotoxin, greatly enhance the inward Ca^{2+} current.[6]

Acetylcholine

Synthesis of acetylcholine

Acetylcholine is synthesised in the terminal axoplasm from choline and acetyl coenzyme A, under the influence of the enzyme choline acetyltransferase. Most of the enzyme is dissolved in the axoplasm, but some is attached to the membranes of vesicles. The enzyme reaction is reversible. This enzyme, which is synthesised in the cell bodies and transported to the terminals by axoplasmic flow involving the neurofilaments, is virtually exclusively located in cholinergic nerves. The enzyme has been purified from several species and copy DNAs have been cloned. Acetyl coenzyme A is probably generated from mitochondrial pyruvate, although some uncertainty remains as to whether pyruvate is the only precursor.[2] Choline is mainly obtained from the extracellular fluid which contains about 10 μmol/l of free choline, derived both from the diet and from synthesis in the liver. Choline, being a cation, would not normally penetrate lipid membranes. A high affinity, Na^+ dependent, choline carrier mechanism (Michaelis constant or K_m of 1–5 μmol/l) is, however, present in cholinergic nerve endings.[7] This carrier transports choline into the axoplasm for acetylcholine synthesis. Some of the choline that is transported comes from the breakdown of transmitter acetylcholine. In fact about half of the choline derived from acetylcholine hydrolysis is taken up again into the nerve endings by the choline carrier.[8][9]

Another choline carrier mechanism, although of lower affinity (K_m 50–200 μmol/l), is present in all cell membranes. This system is concerned with the transport of choline for the synthesis of phosphatidylcholine for membrane phospholipids. Membrane phosphatidylcholine can act as a source of choline for acetylcholine synthesis under certain conditions. The uptake of choline and the synthesis of acetylcholine in cholinergic nerve terminals are geared to its release,[9–11] so that under normal physiological conditions the amount of acetylcholine stored within the nerve endings remains constant at around 30 mmol/l, even during intense activity. The precise mechanisms through which uptake, release, and synthesis are coupled is not yet understood, although influx of Na^+ and Ca^{2+} during activity appear to be involved.[10][12] It has been shown that, in a sympathetic ganglion, acetylcholine synthesis is stimulated by adenosine derived from breakdown of ATP.[13][14] It is probable that a similar mechanism exists at the neuromuscular junction. ATP is released from motor nerve terminals along with acetylcholine, as referred to below. ATP is quickly broken down to adenosine and, assuming that the mechanism resembles that in sympathetic ganglia, the adenosine is then taken up, by a special nucleoside transporter, to an intracellular site where it stimulates the synthesis of acetylcholine which is subsequently loaded into vesicles for release. Co-release of ATP with acetylcholine may thus provide a nice mechanism for coupling release to synthesis and availability.[15]

The enzyme choline acetyltransferase may be inhibited in vitro by a number of compounds, of which certain naphthylvinylpyridines are examples. None of the compounds is, however, selective for choline acetyltransferase, and in any case acetylcholine is synthesised, intracellularly, at so many sites in the body, including the brain, that even if selectivity for the enzyme could be achieved the actions of an inhibitor would probably be too widespread for any therapeutic use to which it could conceivably be put.

Choline transport, by both the low and the high affinity systems, may be inhibited by a range of drugs, the first and still the most effective of which is called hemicholinium-3.[16][17] The high affinity system is generally the more sensitive. The transport inhibitors combine with the choline carrier in the membrane, thereby preventing its combination with choline. The interaction is competitive, so the inhibition is overcome by an excess of choline. It is therefore characteristic of the neuromuscular transmission failure, produced by this type of inhibitor, that it is reversed by choline. Some inhibitors may be transported across the membrane, released from the carrier, acetylated by choline acetyltransferase, and then released by nerve impulses in place of acetylcholine. The properties of compounds that may be synthesised into so called cholinergic false transmitters in this way have been reviewed.[18]

About 70% of the acetylcholine located at the neuromuscular junction is present in the motor nerve terminals, about 20–25% is located in the muscle fibres,[19 20] and the remainder is in the terminal Schwann cells. Muscle fibres and Schwann cells are devoid of choline acetyltransferase, but they contain another enzyme, carnitine acetyltransferase. This enzyme can accept choline as a substrate and is thought to be responsible for the non-neuronal acetylcholine synthesis.[21] Acetylcholine present in muscle and Schwann cells persists after denervation of the muscle. Schwann cell acetylcholine may be spontaneously released, and is detectable by electrophysiological techniques after chronic denervation of the muscle.[22] The physiological functions of muscle and Schwann cell acetylcholine, if any, are not yet known.

Choline uptake into muscle occurs mainly at the postjunctional motor endplate membrane.[23] Most of this choline is incorporated into membrane phosphatidylcholine which is present throughout the membrane. The breakdown of phosphatidylcholine with release of choline also occurs most actively in the motor endplate region. The fact that both uptake and release of muscle choline occur most prominently at the motor endplate suggests that this choline is in some unknown way involved in the transmission process, an observation that has been discussed by Wessler.[24]

Storage of acetylcholine

Motor nerve terminals, like other presynaptic terminals that release non-protein transmitters, contain many thousands of small spherical vesicles, each about 50 nm in diameter. A motor nerve terminal at a frog neuromuscular junction, for example, may contain as many as a million such vesicles. The vesicles are formed in the cell body by budding off from the Golgi apparatus, and they pass to the terminals by microtubule transport. Once in the terminals, the vesicles are repeatedly recycled. About half of the acetylcholine present in each nerve terminal is contained in the vesicles. The rest is dissolved in the axoplasm where its concentration is controlled by the soluble form of acetylcholinesterase.

Each vesicle contains about 12 000 molecules of acetylcholine when full. This gives a concentration that is hypertonic with respect to the axoplasm so that an active transport mechanism for loading acetylcholine into vesicles against its concentration gradient is necessary. All synaptic vesicle membranes contain a V type proton pumping ATPase, which is similar to that in lyosomes and Golgi membranes. The first stage of vesicular acetylcholine uptake depends on the active transport of hydrogen ions into the vesicle with hydrolysis of ATP. The second stage involves the exchange of the intravesicular protons for acetylcholine cations by means of a transport protein, the acetylcholine transporter. For further details, a review by Parsons et al[25] may be consulted.

Certain drugs, the most important of which is (−)-vesamicol, inhibit the acetylcholine transporter and thereby deprive the vesicles of acetylcholine. The consequence is a slowly developing failure in neuromuscular transmission, occurring as the previously filled vesicles are used up. Vesamicol is proving of value as an experimental tool for studying the processes involved in mobilisation of acetylcholine within the nerve endings.[26] It is possible that, in the future, drugs of this type might find therapeutic use in the control of some forms of muscle spasticity. Most physiologists believe that it is the acetylcholine present in the vesicles that is responsible for the transmission event, and indeed the ability of vesamicol to cause transmission failure forms part of the evidence for this view.[27]

Some of the nerve terminal vesicles (about 1%) are lined up at specialised release sites, the active zones, of the axon terminal membrane. This is the so called immediately available or readily releasable store. The remaining vesicles are distributed throughout the terminal axoplasm as a large reserve store. They are anchored to the actin strands and the microtubules of the cytoskeleton, and sometimes to each other. Freshly synthesised acetylcholine is preferentially loaded into the vesicles of the immediately available store, and these vesicles seem to be mainly responsible for the maintenance of transmitter release when nerve activity is relatively low. The contents of about 100 vesicles are released by a single nerve impulse. This number of vesicles is called the quantal content of the endplate potential. It is only when heavy demands are placed upon the system that *mobilisation* of the reserve store becomes necessary. Some physiologists are of the opinion that the acetylcholine of the mobilised reserve vesicles is transferred to the vesicles of the immediately available store before being released.

Release of acetylcholine

Acetylcholine is continually released spontaneously from the nerve endings in the absence of nerve impulses. By far the greatest proportion of the spontaneous release (>99%) occurs as a Ca^{2+} independent continuous leakage, so called molecular leakage, apparently through the terminal membrane; possibly some of it comes from the muscle fibres. The leakage is sufficient to produce a steady concentration of about 0·01 μmol/l in the junctional cleft, resulting in a small endplate depolarisation. The depolarisation is far too small to activate the process of muscle contraction, but is clearly blocked by tubocurarine, which, consequently, appears to produce a small endplate hyperpolarisation. Surprisingly, the molecular leakage is blocked by vesamicol[28] implying that an acetylcholine transporter is involved, and leading to the suggestion that the leakage may arise because vesicular membranes, and therefore acetylcholine transporter proteins (albeit working in the reverse direction), are transiently incorporated into the terminal axonal membrane.

A small amount of acetylcholine (<1% of the spontaneous leakage) is released randomly in a quantal, Ca^{2+} dependent manner, presumably from vesicles. The frequency of the release of quanta differs in different muscles and in different species, but is around 1/s. It is widely, though not unanimously, believed that each small quantum is that contained within a single vesicle. Vesicles, probably not from the readily releasable pool, are thought to release their contents into the junctional cleft whenever they randomly collide in an appropriate way with a release site. Sufficient Ca^{2+} to support spontaneous quantal release is already present in the axoplasm. Extracellular Ca^{2+} is not necessary. The released acetylcholine produces a small (0·5–1·0 mV) depolarisation of the postjunctional motor endplate membrane, a so called miniature endplate potential (MEPP), which is much too small to excite the muscle fibre to contract.

A small proportion of MEPPs are smaller in amplitude than the rest (subminiature MEPPs), and a few are five to ten times larger (giant MEPPs) although still too small to excite the muscle fibre to contract (reviewed in Bowman[2]). The functions of spontaneously released acetylcholine are not known; possibly it exerts some trophic influence on the muscle fibre.

When acetylcholine is released by a nerve impulse, the contents of some 100 vesicles or so are ejected simultaneously from the nerve endings to produce the full sized endplate potential (EPP). This process is strongly dependent on extracellular Ca^{2+} which enters through voltage operated Ca^{2+} channels in the axon terminal membrane. The main Ca^{2+} channels involved are not affected by the therapeutically useful calcium channel blocking drugs (for example, verapamil, nifedipine, diltiazem), but are blocked by a polypeptide toxin, ω-agatoxin IVA, obtained from a spider venom, suggesting that they are a subtype of the so called P type calcium channels.[29] However, it seems clear that other types of Ca^{2+} channels are also present, and may come into play under certain circumstances. Drugs, such as aminopyridines, which enhance Ca^{2+} influx by blocking the opposing I_K, produce an increase in acetylcholine release and have found occasional clinical use in situations in which facilitated neuromuscular transmission is desirable (see Paskov et al[30] for a review).

Certain antibiotics, notably streptomycin and neomycin, impair acetylcholine release, probably by competing with Ca^{2+} in the terminal Ca^{2+} channels.[31 32]

In recent years, the importance of vesicular membrane proteins has come to be realised. The roles of the vesicular ATPase and the acetylcholine transporter are referred to above. Proteins involved in the anchoring of vesicles and in their fusion with the terminal axon membrane are illustrated in fig 1.2. Their precise roles have not yet been fully elucidated[33] although it is becoming clear that similar mechanisms are responsible for membrane–membrane fusions at most sites in the body.[34]

The small GTP binding protein (G protein) designated Rab3A (fig 1.2a) is specifically associated with neuronal synaptic vesicles. It cycles between a membrane bound (GTP containing) and a free (GDP containing) state.

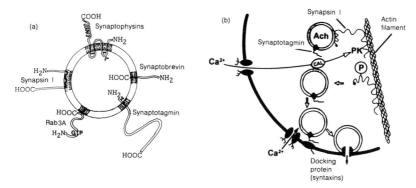

Fig 1.2 (a) Relationship of the major vesicular proteins concerned with acetylcholine release to the synaptic vesicle membrane. Synaptophysins, synaptobrevins, and synaptotagmin are integral membrane proteins. Synapsin I molecules form a cage like structure around the outside of the vesicle and Rab3A is a small G protein bound to the outside surface (see Sudhof and Jahn[33]). (b) The postulated roles of synapsin I and synaptotagmin in Ca^{2+} mediated mobilisation and release of vesicular acetylcholine. The membrane calcium channels are opened by the action potential. The channels closely associated with the docking proteins in the active zones provide for a high local concentration of Ca^{2+} which binds to synaptotagmin. This causes synaptotagmin to fuse with the docking proteins. A fusion pore is formed through the combined membranes, enabling the vesicle contents (acetylcholine, ATP, Ca^{2+}, and probably a binding protein) to escape into the junctional gap. Synapsin I anchors the reserve vesicles to the cytoskeleton. Ca^{2+} entering the axoplasm combines with calmodulin (CAL) and the combination activates protein kinase II (PK) which in turn phosphorylates synapsin I. This frees the vesicles which are then able to migrate to the active zones. Other proteins, represented in (a), are also important in the targeting and release mechanism. Rab3A is concerned in the initial recognition between the vesicle and the docking protein and hence in mobilisation; synaptophysin is probably one of the fusion pore proteins, and synaptobrevin is also essential for release although its precise role has not yet been elucidated

The precise recognition between the vesicle membrane and the active zone of the axonal membrane, that is, the targeting of the vesicle to the release site, seems to be controlled by Rab3A and associated proteins. During the process, GTP is hydrolysed and the GDP bound form of Rab3A is released into the axoplasm. It rebinds to the vesicle only after its GDP has been replaced by GTP. Rab3A appears not to be essential for the exocytosis mechanism but to play an important role in recruitment of vesicles during repetitive stimulation.[35]

Synaptotagmin, synaptophysins, and synaptobrevin (fig 1.2a) are some of the integral vesicular membrane proteins involved in the docking of the vesicles at the release sites, in the formation of the fusion pore that allows the escape of the acetylcholine, and possibly in the reforming of the vesicles. Synaptobrevin is the site of action of botulinum toxin.[36] This toxin is actually an enzyme, a zinc endopeptidase, which cleaves synaptobrevin. Botulinum toxin, which inhibits acetylcholine release, has a number of clinical uses in various types of muscle hypertonia (including blepharospasm and torticollis). It probably inhibits acetylcholine release by inactivating synaptobrevin. Synaptotagmin has the property of binding calcium ions. A simplified view of its function is that, when calcium ions enter the terminal axoplasm on the arrival of a nerve impulse, they bind to synaptotagmin. This induces a conformational change in the synaptotagmin that causes it, in vesicles already in the immediately available store, to fuse with docking proteins (the syntaxins) in the active zones of the terminal axonal membrane. Simultaneously with the fusion of the two proteins, a pore opens through both and rapidly expands so that the vesicular contents are released into the junctional gap. In the absence of Ca^{2+}, synaptotagmin functions as a "vesicle clamp," holding the vesicle in a fusion ready state but blocking release of its contents. Synaptophysin is involved in the formation of the fusion pore. It appears that, under some circumstances, the fusion pore extends, with the result that the vesicular membrane temporarily becomes a part of the axon terminal membrane. Vesicular fusion requires a high concentration of Ca^{2+}, yet release of acetylcholine occurs in response to a single nerve impulse. This is possible because the calcium channels responsible for release are located in the active zones so that the local concentration of Ca^{2+} becomes high even after a single nerve impulse. The Ca^{2+} activated K^+ channels, referred to above and in fig 1.1, are also located close to the calcium channels involved in release.[37] Hence, they are strategically located to hyperpolarise the local membrane and terminate transmitter release.

A toxin, α-latrotoxin, from the venom of the black widow spider, has a specific binding site in the active zones. The toxin causes initial excessive vesicular release of acetylcholine and prevents the vesicles from re-forming, so that the end effect is abolition of acetylcholine release and absence of acetylcholine containing vesicles. The α-latrotoxin binding site is the same site in the active zone to which synaptotagmin binds.[38] It thus appears that α-latrotoxin may behave as a continuously active synaptotagmin, and this observation gives a clear indication that synaptotagmin plays an important role in vesicular fusion. Synaptotagmin may also be a component of the site in the nerve terminals which acts as an antigen giving rise to the circulating autoantibody responsible for the Lambert–Eaton myasthenic syndrome.[39]

Synapsin I (fig 1.2a) is a phosphoprotein that forms a cage like structure around the outside surface of the vesicles. Synapsin I serves to anchor the vesicles in the reserve stores to elements of the cytoskeleton. An additional action of calcium ions on entering the axoplasm is, after combination with calmodulin, to activate the enzyme calcium/calmodulin dependent protein kinase II. This enzyme phosphorylates serine residues in the tail region of synapsin I. As a consequence, the binding affinity of synapsin I for the vesicles is greatly reduced, so that they are freed and able to move towards the active zones (see McGuinness and Greengard[40] for a review). Phosphorylation of synapsin I by calcium activated protein kinases may therefore play an important role, not in immediate release or rapid mobilisation of transmitter, but in the slower mobilisation of transmitter necessary to maintain prolonged high outputs during continuous heavy nerve impulse traffic. As the anchored reserve vesicles are not close to the active zones, opening of additional calcium channels may be necessary to raise the Ca^{2+} concentration of the axoplasm to the level appropriate to activate protein kinase II. This concept is included in the diagram of fig 1.2b, which illustrates the postulated roles of some of the vesicular proteins.

Co-transmitters

Increasingly, nerve fibres, especially those in the brain and those belonging to the autonomic nervous system, are being shown to release more than one transmitter, sometimes several. It now seems that this may also be true for the neuromuscular junction in skeletal muscle.

The vesicles, as well as containing acetylcholine, also contain Ca^{2+}, ATP, and possibly a proteoglycan similar to that present in *Torpedo marmorata* vesicles. All of these are released along with acetylcholine. The Ca^{2+} may simply represent a mechanism for expelling that which enters with the nerve terminal action potential, and the proteoglycan may be an acetylcholine binding molecule. However, the role of the ATP is intriguing. ATP receptors of the P_{2x} subtype, which are coupled to cation channels, are present on both immature and adult muscle cells.[41 42] Those in the motor endplate membrane are similar to nicotinic acetylcholine receptors except that the mean open time of their channels is shorter. Those in the extrajunctional membrane may actually be the acetylcholine receptors. Furthermore, ATP potentiates the action of acetylcholine on nicotinic receptors.[43] ATP receptors of the P_2–G protein coupled type are also present in skeletal muscle. Possibly these are responsible for receptor desensitisation through phosphorylation, and they may play a part in upregulating the receptors.

ATP is rapidly broken down to adenosine, and adenosine (P_1) receptors of both the inhibitory A_1 and excitatory A_2 subtypes have been detected on motor nerve endings.[44 45] Under normal circumstances, activation of the inhibitory A_1 subtype is dominant. Ginsborg and Hirst[46] first showed that adenosine inhibits acetylcholine release in the isolated phrenic nerve–diaphragm preparation of the rat, and this has been confirmed repeatedly in isolated nerve–muscle preparations of rodents and amphibia.[44 47] The inhibitory effect in rodents has been shown to be mediated by an A_1 adenosine receptor[44 47] and to be abolished by pre-treatment with pertussis toxin, indicating the involvement of a G protein. Adenosine acting at an A_1 receptor also inhibits an N type calcium current in the cell bodies of rodent motoneurons, and again a pertussis sensitive G protein is involved.[48 49] It is tempting to relate these results and deduce that the inhibition of a Ca^{2+} current in the terminals is the cause of the reduction in transmitter release. Most evidence indicates, however, that N type channels are not important in neuromuscular transmission in rodents, because the N channel blocker, ω-conotoxin, is without effect on transmission;[50] P type Ca^{2+} channels appear to play the major role as mentioned earlier. It is not yet known whether adenosine inhibits current flow through P type channels, although it seems likely that it does. Adenosine has a ceiling to its effect; it does not abolish acetylcholine release completely. Possibly the component of acetylcholine release that is insensitive to adenosine is triggered by a calcium current that passes through channels that are not affected by adenosine. In the frog, inhibition of calcium currents does not appear to play a part in adenosine's ability to reduce transmitter release.[51] Fig 1.3 illustrates an unpublished experiment carried out by MW Nott and the author about 20 years ago. Adenosine, in a very large dose (75 μg) given close arterially into the tibialis anterior muscle of an anaesthetised cat, although without effect on the twitches (presumably because of the large safety factor in transmitter release), nevertheless produced a pronounced tetanic fade, which was shown to be prejunctional in origin. This effect was blocked by the non-selective adenosine antagonist theophylline. This appears to be the first time that adenosine has been shown to produce an effect on transmission in an intact mammal. At that time, we regarded the

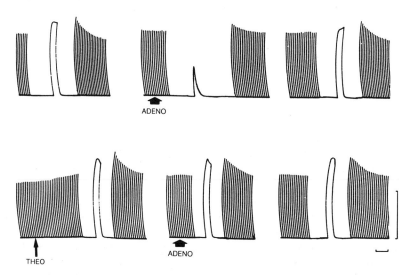

Fig 1.3 Cat, chloralose anaesthesia: maximal twitches of a tibialis anterior muscle were evoked by stimulating the motor nerve at a frequency of 0·1 Hz. Tetani (100 Hz for 25 s) were interposed. At ADENO, 75 μg adenosine were injected close arterially into the muscle. At THEO, 15 mg/kg theophylline were injected intravenously. Time calibration: 1 min; tension calibration: 5 N for the twitches and 20 N for the tetani. Note that the depressed and waning tetanus after adenosine was therefore about twice the amplitude of a twitch. (From an unpublished experiment by WC Bowman and MW Nott in 1973)

effect as unimportant, because of the need for what we considered to be a huge, non-physiological dose, and because the effect occurred only in about 40% of the experiments. More modern experiments have, however, shown that the local endogenous adenosine concentration may be higher than expected, that inactivating mechanisms for adenosine are highly efficient, especially at normal body temperature, and that adenosine, in physiological concentrations in the biophase, does diminish acetylcholine release. It is likely therefore that adenosine does have a role in modulating acetylcholine release at the neuromuscular junction;[52-54] it is probably responsible for the so called neuromuscular depression that follows brief repetitive stimulation. The possible role of adenosine in stimulating acetylcholine synthesis is referred to above. ATP is also released from contracting muscle fibres, providing an additional source of both the nucleotide itself and adenosine.[55]

The adenosine A_2 receptors present on motor nerve endings are generally excitatory in function, serving to enhance acetylcholine output under certain conditions. They belong to the A_{2A} subtype of adenosine receptors[45] and are positively coupled to the adenylate cyclase–cyclic AMP system.[56] Activation of the A_{2A} receptors potentiates other agents (for example, calcitonin gene related peptide and forskolin) which facilitate acetylcholine output through a cyclic AMP mediated mechanism.[57 58] Activation of the same receptors, however, inhibits the facilitatory effect of nicotinic agonists on transmitter release (see below), possibly because cyclic AMP acts to desensitise the prejunctional nicotinic receptors.[59]

In addition to the large numbers of small acetylcholine containing vesicles, a smaller number of large dense core vesicles (LDCVs) containing peptide transmitters have been detected in motor nerve terminals. (The ratio to acetylcholine containing vesicles is about 1:100.) The LDCVs contain the peptide, calcitonin gene related peptide (CGRP).[60] As is the case with other polypeptide transmitters, higher frequencies of stimulation are required to release the contents of the LDCVs at the neuromuscular junction, probably because the LDCVs are not located at the active zones, and an overall high concentration of Ca^{2+} is therefore required to activate the release mechanism. CGRP occurs in sensory nerves and there has been some controversy as to whether, in the mammal, it also occurs in somatic motor nerve terminals.[61] Most evidence indicates that it occurs in both, including the motor nerve terminals of human muscles.[62] CGRP stimulates adenylate cyclase with the production of cyclic AMP. Possibly all its effects are mediated by cyclic AMP. It stimulates a Na^+/K^+ membrane pump which hyperpolarises the membrane,[63] it increases fast contracting muscle contractility[64] and enhances post-tetanic potentiation,[65] it increases receptor desensitisation presumably by giving rise to phosphorylation of the receptor protein,[66] it increases acetylcholine release from the motor nerve,[58] it enhances "non-contractile" Ca^{2+} influx into muscle,[67] and, chronically, it increases the synthesis of acetylcholine receptors,[68] and may therefore play a part in the up and downregulation of receptors.

Prejunctional receptors

Nicotinic acetylcholine receptors

There are two kinds of evidence, biochemical and electrophysiological, that nicotinic receptors exist on the motor nerve endings.[69] The first depends mainly on loading the nerve endings with radiolabelled choline, and measuring its release upon stimulation of the nerve. As the release is blocked by tetrodotoxin (which blocks action potential conduction), it is assumed that the labelled choline has been acetylated in the nerve endings, loaded into the vesicles, and then released as labelled acetylcholine, which is then rapidly hydrolysed back to acetate and tritiated choline so long as acetylcholinesterase remains functional. Many experiments are in fact carried out in the absence of anticholinesterase drugs because these drugs interfere with certain of the effects studied. In this case, a further complication is necessary, because to be able to detect all of the choline released, its uptake back into the nerve endings must be prevented. Hence, the experiments have to be carried out in the presence of hemicholinium which prevents choline uptake. Consequently, acetylcholine synthesis is impaired to an extent because the nerve endings become deficient in choline. The result is that the experiments have to be carried out on a kind of tight-rope in which choline transport is impaired sufficiently to prevent re-uptake of previously released choline, but not sufficiently to abolish neuromuscular transmission.

Under these conditions, small concentrations of many nicotinic agonists, including acetylcholine itself, nicotine, carbachol, dimethylphenyl-piperazinium, suxamethonium (succinylcholine), and decamethonium (the last depending on the species), have been shown to increase the evoked release of acetylcholine measured as tritiated choline.[2 24 70 71] Large concentrations of the same agonists, or even small concentrations left in contact with the preparation, produce a decrease in transmitter release.

Tubocurarine and related nicotinic antagonists prevent the enhanced release evoked by agonists, and in some cases they also prevent the secondary decrease in release. In the absence of an applied nicotinic agonist, tubocurarine, and other reversible nicotinic antagonists, including hexamethonium, reduce the evoked release of labelled choline, which suggests (though it does not prove) that transmitter acetylcholine is itself acting back on the nerve endings to facilitate its own further release. Snake venom neurotoxins (α-bungarotoxin, neuronal bungarotoxin, cobratoxin, erabutoxin-b), providing that they are highly purified, do not inhibit evoked release of labelled choline. According to I Wessler (personal communication) the commercially available α-bungarotoxin contains an impurity that does inhibit release. These observations have been interpreted to mean that nicotinic receptors present on the nerve endings mediate enhanced transmitter release. These receptors differ from postjunctional receptors (for example, they are not blocked by α-bungarotoxin), and from autonomic ganglionic receptors (for example, they are not blocked by neuronal bungarotoxin).

The secondary decrease in evoked transmitter release produced either by large concentrations of agonist, or by prolonged exposure to concentrations that are initially facilitatory, has been interpreted in two ways: excessive agonist activity may lead to depolarisation of the terminal membrane, hence abolishing action potential conduction in the terminals or, assuming that positive feedback by the transmitter itself is continually active, the terminal receptors may become desensitised, and hence abolish the feedback. In fact, both mechanisms may contribute under different conditions, just as is the case with the postjunctional receptors.

In experiments of the type illustrated in fig 1.1, in which nerve terminal waveforms were recorded, it was found that suxamethonium, a nicotinic agonist, enhanced the amplitude of the waveform corresponding to the inward Ca^{2+} current responsible for acetylcholine release.[72] Fig 1.4 illustrates this effect. Recently, the presence of nicotinic receptors containing α_3 subunits has been demonstrated at motor nerve endings by means of specific monoclonal antibodies.[73] Nicotinic receptors containing α_3 subunits[74 75] have a relatively high selectivity for Ca^{2+}, which is compatible with the observation of an enhanced I_{Ca} induced by suxamethonium at the terminals, and is likely to account for the enhanced acetylcholine release induced by nicotinic agonists in general, including suxamethonium.

When acetylcholinesterase is inhibited, high frequency nerve stimulation may cause acetylcholine release to become independent of nerve impulses, to the extent that the transmitter itself generates its own release in what has been described as a regenerative mechanism.[76] This effect, which is blocked by tubocurarine,[77] is explicable in terms of the excess of transmitter producing terminal depolarisation.

Electrophysiological evidence for prejunctional nicotinic receptors depends on the electrical counterparts of the tetanic fade or train-of-four fade (that is, rundown of trains of endplate potentials or endplate currents) that occurs in the presence of tubocurarine and other acetylcholine antagonists. Again (except under special circumstances) the snake toxins are without this effect; they produce a uniform depression of amplitude without evidence of rundown during the train. The voltage clamped motor endplate is an exquisitely sensitive quantitative detector of acetylcholine release from the nerve endings, providing that its sensitivity to acetylcholine does not change during a train. When jets of acetylcholine are applied microiontophoretically to the endplate at the same frequency as the nerve stimulation, the endplate currents remain uniformly partially blocked in the presence of tubocurarine or similarly acting drug; there is no progressive change in sensitivity to acetylcholine. There is a striking rundown of responses, however, during repetitive nerve stimulation (fig 1.5). This result clearly indicates that rundown is a consequence of an action of the acetylcoholine antagonist on the nerve. It should be stated that not all workers have obtained results of this sort,[79] but the large majority have

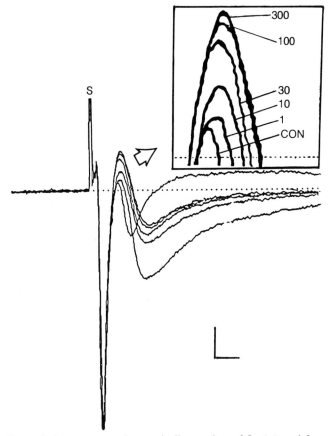

Fig 1.4 Records from an experiment similar to that of fig 1.1 and from the series described in Braga *et al.*[72] I_K has been blocked by 3,4-diaminopyridine to expose the waves corresponding to I_{Ca} and I_{KCa}. Records in the absence (CON) and in the presence of a range of concentrations of suxamethonium (1, 10, 30, 100, and 300 µmol/1) have been superimposed. Each separate waveform is a computer average of 24 recorded waveforms when the response was constant in each concentration. The inset is an enlargement of the waveforms corresponding to I_{Ca}. Suxamethonium produced a concentration dependent increase in Ca^{2+} influx. Calibration: 1 mV, 1 ms. S is the stimulus artefact

concluded that tubocurarine and related drugs act on the nerve endings to impede mobilisation of the transmitter so that release progressively diminishes with repeated nerve shocks.[2] As the drugs that produce this effect are nicotinic antagonists, the conclusion has been drawn that prejunctional nicotinic autoreceptors, stimulated by the released transmitter, mediate mobilisation of the reserve store into the readily releasable store. Hence, availability for release is made to match the requirements of the traffic of nerve impulses. Blockade of the prejunctional autoreceptors by a nicotinic antagonist results in failure of mobilisation to keep pace with the demands of the stimulation frequency, so that fade or rundown of responses

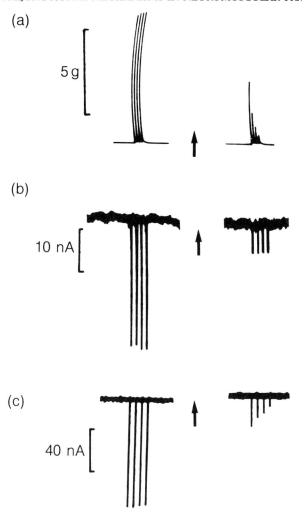

Fig 1.5 Isolated phrenic nerve–hemidiaphragm preparations of rats. All responses are to train-of-four stimulation (2 Hz for 1·9 s) before (left) and in the presence of 5 μmol/l vecuronium (right). (a) Twitches evoked by nerve stimulation; (b) endplate current responses, recorded from a cut muscle fibre clamped at − 80 mV, evoked by jets of acetylcholine applied iontophoretically. (c) Endplate currents (EPCs), recorded from a cut muscle fibre clamped at − 60 mV, evoked by stimulation of the motor nerve. (From an experiment carried out by Dr AJ Gibb and reproduced with permission from Bowmann.[78]) Rundown occurs only when responses are evoked by nerve stimulation. Responses to iontophoretically applied acetylcholine are uniformly depressed; there is no rundown. Similar results are obtained with other tubocurarine like drugs

occurs. A snag with this interpretation is that it is difficult to reverse the electrophysiologically recorded fade with a nicotinic agonist, although partial success has been achieved.[71] The difficulty has been attributed to rapid desensitisation of the prejunctional autoreceptors by externally applied agonist.

It is tempting to merge the results of the biochemical and the electrophysiological experiments completely. The observation[24] that reduced release produced by tubocurarine in the biochemical experiments does not occur as early as the electrophysiological rundown (evident with the second stimulus in a train) has been explained[69] on the grounds that, in the biochemical experiments, release is already impaired by hemicholinium induced synthesis inhibition, and hence the transmitter induced autofacilitation may not immediately be present.

Most workers would accept that neuromuscular blocking drugs exert a prejunctional action to depress transmitter release. Evidence that the biochemical observation of depressed release produced by a neuromuscular blocking drug and the electrophysiological observation of rundown are reflections of the same mechanism lies in the fact that both are independent of the extracellular Ca^{2+} concentration.[32 80] It might be, however, that the converse effect, that is, the ability of stable nicotinic agonists to increase acetylcholine release, occurs through a different mechanism, because this effect does appear to depend on Ca^{2+}. This effect of nicotinic agonists is apparently mediated by prejunctional nicotinic receptors, presumably of the α_3 subunit containing type.

Over 20 years ago, Blaber[81] proposed that the ability of tubocurarine to produce fade and rundown, although prejunctional in origin, was not mediated by nicotinic receptors but rather was a consequence of some other kind of use dependent pharmacological effect. He believed that tubocurarine might exert a type of local anaesthetic action in which it blocked the open Na^+ channels in the nerve endings. Na^+ channel block is clearly not, however, the mechanism involved, because the drug has no effect at all on the waveform representing I_{Na} in the nerve endings. Even so, Blaber's view that some prejunctional action of tubocurarine, unrelated to acetylcholine receptors, is responsible has not yet been disproved. In view of the similarity of their effects, another possibility, suggested by E Rowan (personal communication), is that tubocurarine and related drugs in some way enhance the effect of endogenous adenosine, for example, by impairing its removal from the biophase. Overall it seems most likely, however, that nicotinic acetylcholine receptors are involved because the drugs that produce the various fade phenomena, even though chemically very different to each other in some cases (for example, the short polypeptide, α-conotoxin[82]), are nevertheless all nicotinic receptor antagonists. Hence, it is possible that two different subtypes of nicotinic receptors, both mediating enhanced acetylcholine output, are present on the nerve endings.[24 69] One mediates a Ca^{2+} dependent increase in release, whereas the other mediates mobilisation of transmitter from the reserve to the immediately available store independently of the extracellular Ca^{2+} concentration. The Ca^{2+} dependent increase in release, when activated excessively by the transmitter itself after acetylcholinesterase inhibition, may lead to impairment of evoked release, although at the same time a stimulus independent, so called regenerative release may occur.

It seems that only the mobilisation effect has physiological relevance, being responsible for maintaining transmitter availability during heavy traffic of nerve impulses. Blockade of this effect produces the various fade and rundown phenomena. The evidence that tubocurarine induced rundown is independent of the extracellular Ca^{2+} concentration is compatible with observations such as that illustrated in fig 1.6. The I_{Ca} believed to give rise to acetylcholine release becomes larger with increase in the frequency of stimulation (fig 1.6). Feedback control mediated by nicotinic receptors is not involved in this phenomenon, because tubocurarine in concentrations large enough to produce fade, as well as much larger concentrations, is completely without effect on the I_{Ca}. Hence, if feedback via acetylcholine acting on nicotinic receptors is involved in the maintenance of mobilisation, it must be at a stage that is downstream from Ca^{2+} entry. Effects mediated by nicotinic receptor activation are generally triggered directly by the ion flux through the receptor channels, but this is not invariably the case. For example, stimulation of nicotinic receptors in cultured myotubes leads to phosphatidylinositol breakdown.[83] Possibly some second messenger of this metabolic type mediates the postulated feedback effect of transmitter acetylcholine on mobilisation; it may be that release of intracellular Ca^{2+} is involved.

Figure 1.6 illustrates that, at the same time that the waveform corresponding to I_{Ca} is enhanced by increasing the stimulation frequency, that one corresponding to I_{KCa} is reduced and at 100 Hz it has virtually disappeared. With extracellular recording of this type, the transmembrane potential cannot be detected, but it seems likely that the I_{KCa} may diminish and disappear, simply because the summing positive afterpotentials

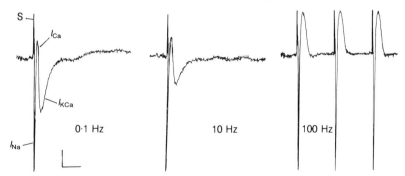

Fig 1.6 Records from an experiment similar to that of fig 1.1. I_K has been blocked by 3,4-diaminopyridine to expose the waves corresponding to I_{Ca} and I_{KCa}. Each panel is a photograph of the oscilloscope screen at a different stimulation frequency (0·1 Hz, 10 Hz, 100 Hz) taken when the responses had become constant after the change in frequency. Increase in frequency of stimulation increased I_{Ca} and reduced I_{KCa}. At 100 Hz, I_{KCa} was absent. Tubocurarine (20 μmol/1) had no effect at all on the waveforms. This concentration of tubocurarine is more than sufficient to block neuromuscular transmission. Calibrations: 2 mV, 2 ms

hyperpolarise the membrane until its potential equals the K^+ equilibrium potential, at which point no further hyperpolarisation can occur.

Nicotinic agonists that are stable to acetylcholinesterase produce repetitive firing in motor nerves, as do anticholinesterase drugs during low frequency nerve stimulation.[84] The effects of anticholinesterase drugs appear to be mediated by preserved transmitter acetylcholine acting on receptors that would otherwise be protected by cholinesterase. The neuronal nicotinic receptors involved in this repetitive firing response appear to be the same ones that mediate the Ca^{2+} dependent increase in acetylcholine release. Their physiological function, if any, is unknown. They may represent a vestigial remnant of receptors that are present at many nerve endings, including some that are non-cholinergic, for example, those at certain locust nerve endings[85] and at synapses in *Aplysia californica*.[86]

Some workers believe that there is also a population of inhibitory nicotinic receptors on the nerve endings. This belief is based on the observation that some neuromuscular blocking drugs, in spite of blocking the amplitude of the endplate potentials (EPPs) or endplate currents (EPCs) in a train, nevertheless increase the quantal content of the first EPP or EPC in that train.[80 87] To explain the fact that the quantal content of the first response in the train is increased by an antagonist, it has been proposed that the quantal content is tonically diminished through nicotinic receptor activation, by the acetylcholine which is spontaneously released from the nerve and possibly from the muscle.[80] Block of this continuous effect by the neuromuscular blocking drug is then said to account for the increased quantal content of the first EPP or EPC in a train. There are, however, difficulties in attempting to explain the effect in this way. First, the enhancement of the quantal content of the first EPP or EPC by the blocking drug is Ca^{2+} dependent,[80] which implies that acetylcholine inhibits release in a Ca^{2+} dependent manner. It is possible to invoke the idea that acetylcholine might do this by leading to the opening of calcium activated K^+ or Cl^- channels which would hyperpolarise the terminal membrane. There is, however, no evidence for such a nicotinic receptor mediated effect at motor nerve terminals. The second problem with this interpretation is that not all neuromuscular blocking drugs produce enhancement of the first response in a train, and there is no subtype of nicotinic receptor yet known that exhibits the same rank order of sensitivity to antagonists.

Blaber[81] was the first to observe that tubocurarine increased the quantal content of the first EPP of a train. He went on to show that what was then erroneously called dimethyltubocurarine (metocurine) did not produce this effect, and he interpreted this observation as evidence that the phenolic –OH groups of tubocurarine were responsible. Phenol itself, and catechol, exert this effect by enhancing the inward Ca^{2+} current, a consequence, as is now known, of blocking K^+ channels.[88] It seems not unlikely that those blocking drugs that produce the effect do so by actions that are unrelated to nicotinic receptors. Gallamine is another example, and its molecule contains three tetraethylammonium like moieties, another structure known to block K^+ channels. Recently, a number of aminosteroidal blocking drugs have been shown to block certain Ca^{2+} channels in smooth muscle.[89] It is a common observation in pharmacology that close relatives of molecules which exert one type of effect may exert the opposite type of effect at a different site.

Muscarinic receptors

Some workers have denied the presence of muscarinic receptors on motor nerve endings, but most are of the opinion that such receptors do exist,[2 24] although the physiological circumstances under which they might be activated are not known. It seems that both inhibitory and excitatory muscarinic autoreceptors are present,[90] acting to reduce and facilitate respectively nerve impulse evoked acetylcholine release. The particular subtypes of muscarinic receptors involved are not clear, and there is some contradiction in the literature. Wessler and his coworkers[91 92] found that the facilitatory muscarinic receptor was blocked by pirenzepine (a relatively selective M_1 receptor antagonist), but others[48] found that pirenzepine blocked the ability of acetylcholine to depress the terminal Ca^{2+} current, which is presumably mediated by the inhibitory muscarinic receptor. The second messengers formed after activation of the muscarinic receptors are not yet definitely known, although a pertussis sensitive G protein appears to be involved in the activation of the inhibitory receptor; adenylate cyclase and diacylglycerol are apparently not involved.[48] The inhibitory effect of adenosine, and the inhibitory effect of acetylcholine acting on muscarinic receptors, are additive in their effects.[48] The nicotinic, Ca^{2+} dependent facilitatory mechanism takes precedence over the muscarinic inhibitory mechanism. When the nicotinic mechanism was fully activated, muscarinic receptor mediated inhibition could not be brought into play.[93]

Enhanced acetylcholine release in myasthenia gravis has been attributed to antibody mediated blocking of inhibitory prejunctional muscarinic receptors.[94] In mice with passively transferred Lambert–Eaton myasthenic syndrome, atropine produced a greater than normal increase in acetylcholine release from motor nerve endings.[95] The explanation put forward was that such mice are in an especially sensitive condition in relation to Ca^{2+} influx because the Lambert–Eaton myasthenic syndrome is characterised by impaired Ca^{2+} influx into motor nerve endings.

It is well known that the motor nerve exerts a number of trophic influences on the innervated muscle. It appears that an influence in the reverse direction also occurs. Thus, when rats were treated with α-bungarotoxin, the amplitude of miniature EPPs was rapidly reduced to about 60% of the control amplitude. During the next few days of treatment, the quantal content of the EPP gradually increased to reach a plateau after 30 days or so. It thus appeared that some kind of retrograde signal from muscle to motor nerve terminals (could it be muscle acetylcholine?) caused an increase in the release of acetylcholine to compensate for the postjunctional decrease in sensitivity.[96] Perhaps a similar mechanism operates in myasthenia gravis.

Adrenoceptors

It has been known for many years that, in spite of there being no noradrenergic nerve endings in the vicinity, motor nerve terminals nevertheless possess adrenoceptors which, when activated, facilitate the release of acetylcholine evoked by nerve impulses. The effect is especially obvious during partial curarisation when adrenaline (epinephrine) produces a clear, though short lasting, anti-curare effect.[97 98] Early experiments indicated that the effect in anaesthetised animals and in isolated nerve–muscle preparations was mediated by α-adrenoceptors; β-adrenoceptors did not appear to be involved.[99 100]

Kuba[100] showed that the action of adrenaline, and noradrenaline (norepinephrine), was to increase the quantal content of the EPP by increasing the probability of release, and he and his coworker[101 102] suggested that the mechanism of action involved potentiation of the ability of Ca^{2+} to cause release of acetylcholine. The receptors mediating the facilitatory effect on acetylcholine release have characteristics that are closest to the α_1 subtype of adrenoceptors,[103 104] although it is not yet known to which subgroup (α_{1A}, α_{1B}, or α_{1D}) they belong, or if they form a fourth subgroup.

In contrast to the earlier workers, Wessler and his coworkers,[105 106] while agreeing that α_1-adrenoceptors play an important part, also found evidence of facilitatory prejunctional β_1-adrenoceptors. This is a rather surprising result, because most β_1-adrenoceptors are innervated by sympathetic nerve fibres. Generally speaking, it is β_2-adrenoceptors that are not innervated and which respond, physiologically, to adrenal medullary adrenaline. It is also surprising in that in both in vivo and intact in vitro preparations, the non-specific β-adrenoceptor agonist[99] isoprenaline was without anti-curare effect and did not augment EPPs.[100]

In the experiments in which isoprenaline has been shown to increase transmitter output,[105 106] the release of radiolabelled choline was measured. As explained above, this type of experiment demands the presence of hemicholinium which to an extent must impair acetylcholine synthesis. Agents that enhance the formation of cyclic AMP are known to stimulate acetylcholine synthesis,[107] and it is therefore pertinent to wonder to what extent enhanced synthesis, under the vulnerable conditions of the experiment, as distinct from an action on the release mechanism, contributed to the increased β-receptor mediated transmitter output. Other agents reported to increase acetylcholine output by a cyclic AMP mechanism (for example, CGRP and adenosine on A_2 receptors) have been studied in a similar way. However, Wessler[106] obtained evidence that the β_1 adrenoceptors were coupled, directly or indirectly, to ω-conotoxin (GVIA) sensitive N type calcium channels, indicating that enhanced synthesis cannot be the only mechanism involved, even though the role of N type calcium channels in acetylcholine release has not been clarified.

The question arises as to whether the effects of adrenal medullary adrenaline and noradrenaline on transmitter release have any relevance to events in human patients. Vizi[104] gives reasons for concluding that they have. He suggests that, at the end of a surgical operation with partial curarisation still present, an elevated plasma catecholamine concentration arising from operative stress is within the levels that affect neuromuscular transmission.

1 Bowden REM, Duchen LW. The anatomy and pathology of the neuromuscular junction. In Zaimis E, ed, *Neuromuscular junction. Handbook of experimental pharmacology,* vol 42. Berlin: Springer-Verlag, 1976:23–97.

2 Bowman WC. *Pharmacology of neuromuscular function.* London: Wright, 1990.

3 Brismar T. Distribution of K-channels in the axolemma of myelinated fibres. *Trends Neurosci* 1982;5:179–81.

4 Brigant JL, Mallart A. Presynaptic currents in mammalian motor endings. *J Physiol* 1982;333:619–36.

5 Penner T, Dreyer F. Two different presynaptic calcium currents in mouse motor nerve terminals. *Pflügers Arch Eur J Physiol* 1986;406:190–7.

6 Anderson AJ, Harvey AL, Rowan EG, Strong PN. Effects of charybdotoxin, a blocker of Ca^{2+}-activated K^+ channels, on motor nerve terminals. *Br J Pharmacol* 1988; 95:1329–35.

7 Jope RS. High affinity choline transport and acetyl-CoA production in brain and their roles in the regulation of acetylcholine synthesis. *Brain Res Rev* 1979;1:313–44.

8 Tucek S. *Acetylcholine synthesis in neurons.* London: Chapman & Hall, 1978.

9 Wessler I, Kilbinger H. Release of [³H] acetylcholine from a modified rat phrenic nerve-hemidiaphragm preparation. *Naunyn Schmiedebergs Arch Pharmacol* 1986;334:357–64.

10 Tucek S. Regulation of acetylcholine synthesis in the brain. *J Neurochem* 1985; 44:11–24.

11 Collier B. The synthesis and storage of acetylcholine in mammalian cholinergic nerve terminals. In: Avioli M, Reader TA, Dykes RW, Gloor P, eds, *Neurotransmitters and cortical function: from molecules to mind.* New York: Plenum, 1988:261–76.

12 Birks RI. The role of sodium ions in the metabolism of acetylcholine. *Can J Biochem Physiol* 1963;41:2573–9.

13 Tandon A, Collier B. Increased acetylcholine content induced by adenosine in a sympathetic ganglion and its subsequent mobilization by electrical stimulation. *J. Neurochem* 1993;60:2124–33.

14 Tandon A, Collier B. The role of endogenous adenosine in a postsimulation increase in the acetylcholine content of a sympathetic ganglion. *J Neurosci* 1994;14:4927–36.

15 Stone TW. Physiological roles for adenosine and adenosine 5'-triphosphate in the nervous system. *Neuroscience* 1981;6:523–55.

16 Bowman WC, Marshall IG. Inhibition of acetylcholine synthesis. In: Cheymol J, ed, *Neuromuscular blocking and stimulating agents,* vol. 1. *International encyclopedia of pharmacology and therapeutics,* Section 14. Oxford: Pergamon, 1972:357–90.

17 MacIntosh FC, Collier B. Neurochemistry of cholinergic terminals. In: Zaimis E, ed, *Neuromuscular junction. Handbook of experimental pharmacology,* vol 42. Berlin: Springer-Verlag, 1976:99–228.

18 Collier B, Boska P, Lovat S. Cholinergic false transmitters. *Prog Brain Res* 1979; 49:107–21.

19 Miledi R, Molenaar PC, Polak RL. An analysis of acetylcholine in frog muscle by mass fragmentography. *Proc R Soc Lond [Biol]* 1977;197:285–97.

20 Miledi R, Molenaar PC, Polak RL, Tas JWM, van der Laaken T. Neuronal and nonneuronal acetylcholine in the rat diaphragm. *Proc R Soc Lond [Biol]* 1982;214:153–68.

21 Molenaar P. Synthesis, storage and release of acetylcholine. In: Vincent A, Wray D, eds, *Neuromuscular transmission.* Manchester: Manchester University Press, 1990:62–81.

22 Dennis MJ, Miledi R. Electrically induced release of acetylcholine from denervated

Schwann cells. *J Physiol* 1974;237:431–52

23 Wessler I, Sandmann J. Uptake and metabolism of [^{3}H]choline by the rat phrenic nerve-hemidiaphragm preparation. *Naunyn Schmiedebergs Arch Pharmacol* 1987;335:231–7.

24 Wessler I. Acetylcholine at motor nerves: storage, release and presynaptic modulation by autoreceptors and adrenoceptors. *Int Rev Neurobiol* 1992;34:283–384.

25 Parsons SM, Prior C, Marshall IG. Acetylcholine transport, storage and release. *Int Rev Neurobiol* 1993;35:279–90.

26 Marshall IG, Prior C. Update on the acetylcholine receptor and the neuromuscular junction. *Ballières Clinical Anaesthesiology* 1994;8(2):1–17.

27 Vizi ES. In favour of the vesicular hypothesis: neurochemical evidence that vesamicol (AH 5183) inhibits stimulation-evoked release of acetylcholine from neuromuscular junction. *Br J Pharmacol* 1989;98:898–902.

28 Smith DO. Routes of acetylcholine leakage from cytosolic and vesicular compartments of rat motor nerve terminals. *Neurosci Lett* 1992; 135:5–9.

29 Hong SJ, Chang CC. Inhibition of acetylcholine release from mouse motor nerve by a P-type calcium channel blocker. *J Physiol* 1995;482(2):283–90.

30 Paskov DS, Agoston S, Bowman WC. 4-Aminopyridine hydrochloride (Pymadin). In: Kharkevich DA, ed, *New neuromuscular blocking agents. Handbook of experimental phartmacology.* Berlin: Springer-Verlag, 1986:679–717.

31 Singh YN, Marshall IG, Harvey AL. Depression of transmitter release and postjunctional sensitivity during neuromuscular block produced by antibiotics. *Br J Anaesth* 1979; 51:1027–33.

32 Vizi ES, Chaudrey IA, Goldiner PL, Ohta Y, Nagashima H, Foldes FF. The pre- and postjunctional components of the neuromuscular effect of antibiotics. *J Anesth* 1991;5:1–9.

33 Sudhof TC, Jahn R. Proteins of synaptic vesicles involved in exocytosis and membrane recycling. *Neuron* 1991;6:665–77.

34 Monck JR, Fernandez JM. The exocytotic fusion pore and neurotransmitter release. *Neuron* 1994;12:707–16.

35 Geppert M, Bolshakov VY, Siegelbaum SA, Takei K, De Camilli P, Hammer RE, Sudhof TC. The role of Rab3A in neurotransmitter release. *Nature* 1994;369:493–7.

36 Montecucco D, Shiavo G. Tetanus and botulinum neurotoxins: a new group of zinc proteases. *Trends Biochem Sci* 1993;18:324–7.

37 Robitaille R, Garcia ML, Kaczorowski GJ, Charlton MP. Functional colocalization of calcium and calcium-gated potassium channels in control of transmitter release. *Neuron* 1993;11:645–55.

38 Petrenko AG, Perin MS, Davletov BA, Ushkaryov YA, Getterp M, Suchof TC. Binding of synaptotagmin to the α-latrotoxin receptor implicates both in synaptic vesicle exocytosis. *Nature* 1991;353:65–8.

39 Leveque C, Hoshino T, David P, *et al.* The synaptic vesicle protein synaptotagmin associates with calcium channels and is a putative Lambert-Eaton myasthenic syndrome antigen. *Proc Natl Acad Sci USA* 1992;89:3625–9.

40 McGuiness TL, Greengard P. Protein phosphorylation and synaptic transmission. In: Sellin LC, Libelius R, Thesleff S, eds, *Neuromuscular junction.* Amsterdam: Elsevier, 1988:111–24.

41 Lu Z, Smith DO. Adenosine 5'-triphosphate increases acetylcholine channel opening frequency in rat skeletal muscle. *J Physiol* 1991;436:45–56.

42 Mozrzymas JW, Ruzzier F. ATP activates junctional and extrajunctional acetylcholine receptor channels in isolated adult rat muscle fibres. *Neurosci Lett* 1992;139:217–20.

43 Fu W-M. Potentiation by ATP of the postsynaptic acetylcholine response at developing neuromuscular synapses in *Xenopus* cell culture. *J Physiol* 1994;477:449–58.

44 Sebastião AM, Stone TW, Ribeiro JA. The inhibitory adenosine receptor at the neuromuscular junction and hippocampus of the rat: antagonism by 1,3,8-substituted xanthines. *Br J Pharmacol* 1990;101:453–9.

45 Correia-de Sá P, Sebastião AM, Ribeiro JA. Inhibitory and excitatory effects of adenosine receptor agonists on evoked transmitter release from phrenic nerve endings of the rat. *Br J Pharmacol* 1991;103:1614–20.

46 Ginsborg BL, Hirst GDS. The effect of adenosine on the release of the transmitter from the phrenic nerve of the rat. *J Physiol* 1972;224:629–45.

47 Nagano O, Foldes FF, Nakatsuka H, Reich D, Ohta Y, Sperlagh B, Vizi ES. Presynaptic A_1-purinoceptor-mediated inhibitory effects of adenosine and its stable analogues on the

mouse hemidiaphragm preparation. *Naunyn Schmiedebergs Arch Pharmacol* 1992; **346**:197–202.

48 Hamilton BR, Smith DO. Autoreceptor-mediated purinergic and cholinergic inhibition of motor nerve terminal calcium currents in the rat. *J Physiol* 1991;**432**:327–41.

49 Mynlieff M, Beam KG. Adenosine acting at an A_1 receptor decreases N-type calcium current in mouse motoneurons. *J Neurosci* 1994;**14**:3628–34.

50 Sano K, Enomoto K, Maeno T. Effects of synthetic ω-conotoxin, a new type of Ca^{2+}-antagonist on frog and mouse neuromuscular transmission. *Eur J Pharmacol* 1987; **141**:235–41.

51 Silinsky EM, Solsona CS. Calcium currents at motor nerve endings: absence of effects of adenosine receptor agonists in the frog. *J Physiol* 1992;**457**:315–28.

52 Meriney SD, Grinnell AD. Endogenous adenosine modulates stimulation-induced depression at the frog neuromuscular junction. *J Physiol* 1991;**443**:441–55.

53 Redman RS, Silinsky EM. A selective adenosine antagonist (8-cyclopentyl-1,3-dipropylxanthine) eliminates both neuromuscular depression and the action of exogenous adenosine by an effect on A_1 receptors. *Mol Pharmacol* 1993;**44**:835–40.

54 Redman RS, Silinsky EM. ATP released together with acetylcholine as the mediator of neuromuscular depression at frog motor nerve endings. *J Physiol* 1994;**477**:117–27.

55 Smith DO. Sources of adenosine released during neuromuscular transmission in the rat. *J Physiol* 1991;**432**:343–54.

56 Correia-de-Sá P, Ribeiro JA. Evidence that the presynaptic A_{2A}-adenosine receptor is positively coupled to adenylate cyclase. *Naunyn Schmiedebergs Arch Pharmacol* 1994; **349**:514–22.

57 Correia-de-Sá P, Ribeiro JA. Facilitation of [^{3}H]Ach release by forskolin depends on A_{2A}-adenosine receptor activation. *Neurosci Lett* 1993;**151**:21–6.

58 Correia-de-Sá P, Ribeiro JA. Potentiation by tonic A_{2A}-adenosine receptor activation of CGRP-facilitated [^{3}H]-Ach release from rat motor nerve endings. *Br J Pharmacol* 1994;**111**:582–8.

59 Correia-de-Sá P, Ribeiro JA. Tonic adenosine A_{2A} receptor activation modulates nicotinic autoreceptor function at the rat neuromuscular junction. *Eur J Pharmacol* 1994; **271**:349–55.

60 Popper P, Micevych PE. Localization of calcitonin gene-related peptide and its receptors in a striated muscle. *Brain Res* 1989;**496**:180–6.

61 Sakaguchi J, Inuishi Y, Kashihara Y, Kuno M. Release of calcitonin gene-related peptide from nerve terminals in rat skeletal muscle. *J Physiol* 1991;**434**:257–70.

62 Mora M, Marchi M, Polak JM, Gibson SJ, Cornelio F. Calcitonin gene-related peptide immunoreactivity of the human neuromuscular junction. *Brain Res* 1989; **492**:404–7.

63 Andersen SLV, Clausen T. Calcitonon gene-related peptide stimulates active Na^+–K^+ transport in rat soleus muscle. *Am J Physiol* 1993;**264** (*Cell Physiol* **33**): C419–29.

64 Takami K, Kawai Y, Uchida S. Effects of CGRP on contraction of striated muscle in the mouse. *Neurosci Lett* 1985;**60**:227–30.

65 Fleming NW, Lewis BK. CGRP and skeletal muscle. Abstract 4f in *Proceedings of the 4th International Neuromuscular Meeting: 50 years of curare*, Montréal, 1992.

66 Mulle C, Benoite P, Pinse C, Roa M, Changeux JP. Calcitonon gene-related peptide enhances the rate of desensitization of the nicotinic acetylcholine receptor in cultured mouse muscle cells. *Proc Natl Acad Sci USA* 1988;**85**:5728–32.

67 Kimura I, Tsuneki H, Dezaki K, Kimura M. Enhancement by calcitonin gene-related peptide of nicotinic receptor operated noncontractile Ca^{2+} mobilization at the mouse neuromuscular junction. *Br J Pharmacol* 1993;**110**:639–44.

68 Fontaine B, Klarsfeld A, Changeux J-P. Calcitonin gene-related peptide and muscle activity regulate acetylcholine receptor α-subunit mRNA levels by distinct intracellular pathways. *J Cell Biol* 1987;**105**:1337–42.

69 Bowman WC, Gibb AJ, Harvey AL, Marshall IG. Prejunctional actions of cholinoceptor agonists and antagonists and of anticholinesterase drugs. In: Kharkevich DA, ed, *New neuromuscular blocking agents. Handbook of experimental pathology*, vol 79. Berlin: Springer Verlag, 1986:141–70.

70 Kimura I, Okazaki M, Uwano T, Shinjiro K, Kimura M. Succinylcholine-induced acceleration and suppression of electrically evoked acetylcholine release from mouse phrenic nerve-hemidiaphragm muscle preparation. *Jpn J Pharmacol* 1991;**57**:397–409.

71 Bowman WC, Prior C, Marshall IG. Presynaptic receptors in the neuromuscular junction. *Ann NY Acad Sci* 1990;**604**:69–81.

72 Braga MFM, Rowan EG, Harvey AL, Bowman WC. Interactions between suxamethonium and non depolarizing neuromuscular blocking drugs. *Br J Anaesth* 1994; **72**:198–204.

73 Tsunkei H, Kimura I, Dezaki K, Kimura M, Sala C, Fumagalli G. Immunohistochemical localization of neuronal nicotinic receptor subtypes at the pre- and postjunctional sites in mouse diaphragm muscle. *Neurosci Lett* 1995;**406**:13–16.

74 Vernino S, Amador M, Luetje CW, Patrick J, Dani JA. Calcium modulation and high calcium permeability of neuronal nicotinic acetylcholine receptors. *Neuron* 1992; **8**:127–34.

75 Sargent PB. The diversity of neuronal nicotinic acetylcholine receptors. *Ann Rev Neurosci* 1993;**16**:403–43.

76 Chang CC, Hong SJ. A regenerating release of acetylcholine from mouse motor nerve terminals treated with anticholinesterase agents. *Neurosci Lett* 1986;**69**:203–7.

77 Hong SJ, Chang CC. Antagonism by tubocurarine and verapamil of the regenerative acetylcholine release from mouse motor nerve. *Eur J Pharmacol* 1989;**162**:11–17.

78 Bowman WC. Presynaptic nicotinic autoreceptors. *Trends Pharmacol Sci* 1989;**101**:136.

79 Bradley RJ, Sterz R, Peper K, Chan W-C, Zhang G. Evidence that postsynaptic effects of d-tubocurarine or α-toxin cause fade at the neuromuscular junction. *Ann NY Acad Sci* 1990;**604**:548–51.

80 Tian L, Prior C, Dempster J, Marshall IG. Nicotinic antagonist-produced frequency-dependent changes in acetylcholine release from rat motor nerve terminals. *J Physiol* 1994;**476**:517–29.

81 Blaber LC. The prejunctional actions of some nondepolarizing blocking drugs. *Br J Pharmacol* 1973;**47**:109–16.

82 Blount K, Johnson A, Prior C, Marshall JG. α-Conotoxin GI produces tetanic fade at the rat neuromuscular junction. *Toxicon* 1992;**30**:835–42.

83 Adamo S, Zani BM, Nervi C, Senni MI, Molinaro M, Eusebi F. Acetylcholine stimulates phosphatidylinositol turnover at nicotinic receptors of cultured myotubes. *FEBS Lett* 1981;**190**:161–4.

84 Riker WF. Prejunctional effects of neuromuscular blocking and facilitatory drugs. In Katz RL, ed, *Muscle relaxants,* vol 3. Amsterdam: North Holland, 1975:59–102.

85 Fulton BP, Usherwood PNR. Presynaptic acetylcholine action at the locust neuromuscular junction. *Neuropharmacology* 1977;**16**:877–80.

86 Baux G, Tauc L. Presynaptic actions of curare and atropine on quantal acetylcholine release at a central synapse of *Aplysia. J Physiol* 1987;**388**:665–80.

87 Wilson DF. Influence of presynaptic receptors on neuromuscular transmission in rat. *Am J Physiol* 1982;**242**:366–72.

88 Ito I, Maeno T. Catechol: a potent and specific inhibitor of the fast potassium channel in frog primary afferent neurones. *J Physiol* 1986;**373**:115–27.

89 Fiddes S, Prior C. In vitro smooth muscle relaxant activity of a series of vecuronium analogues in the rat aorta. *J Pharm Pharmacol* 1994;**46**:911–16.

90 Wessler I, Karl M, Mai M, Diener A. Muscarinic receptors on the rat phrenic nerve, evidence for positive and negative muscarinic feedback mechanisms. *Naunyn Schmiedebergs Arch Pharmacol* 1987;**335**:605–12.

91 Wessler I, Diener A, Offermann M. Facilitatory and inhibitory muscarine receptors on the rat phrenic nerve; effects of pirenzepine and dicyclomine. *Naunyn Schmiedebergs Arch Pharmacol* 1988;**338**:138–42.

92 Wessler I. Control of transmitter release from the motor nerve by presynaptic nicotinic and muscarinic autoreceptors. *Trends Pharmacol Sci* 1989;**10**:110–14.

93 Vizi ES, Somogyi GT. Prejunctional modulation of acetylcholine release from the skeletal neuromuscular junction: link between positive (nicotinic) and negative (muscarinic) feedback modulation. *Br J Pharmacol* 1989;**97**:65–70.

94 Michaelson DM, Korczyn AD, Sokolovsky M. Antibodies to muscarinic acetylcholine receptors in myasthenia gravis. *Biochem Biophys Res Commun* 1982;**104**:52–7.

95 Takamori M, Sakajiri K, Hamada T. Atropine modulates presynaptic functions in mice with passively transferred Lambert–Eaton myasthenic syndrome. *Muscle Nerve* 1993; Jan:115–16.

96 Plomp JJ, van Kempton GThH, Molenaar PC. Adaptation of quantal content to decreased postsynaptic sensitivity at single endplates in α-bungarotoxin-treated rats. *J Physiol* 1992;**458**:487–99.

97 Bowman WC, Nott MW. Actions of sympathomimetic amines and their antagonists on skeletal muscle. *Pharmacol Rev* 1969;**21**:27–72.

98 Bowman WC. Effects of adrenergic activators and inhibitors on skeletal muscles. In: Szekeres L, ed, *Adrenergic activators and inhibitors. Handbook of experimental pharmacology* vol 54. Berlin: Springer-Verlag, 1980:47–128.

99 Bowman WC, Raper C. Effects of sympathomimetic amines on neuromuscular transmission. *Br J Pharmacol* 1966;**27**:313–31.

100 Kuba K. Effects of catecholamines on the neuromuscular junction in the rat diaphragm. *J Physiol* 1970;**211**:551–70.

101 Kuba K, Tomita T. Noradrenaline action on nerve terminal in rat diaphragm. *J Physiol* 1971;**217**:19–31.

102 Kuba K, Tomita T. Effects of noradrenaline on miniature endplate potentials and on endplate potentials. *J Theor Biol* 1972;**36**:81–8.

103 Malta E, McPherson GA, Raper C. Comparison of prejunctional α-adrenoceptors at the neuromuscular junction with vascular postjunctional α-adrenoceptors in cat skeletal muscle. *Br J Pharmacol* 1979;**65**:249–56.

104 Vizi ES. Evidence that catecholamines increase acetylcholine release from neuromuscular junction through stimulation of alpha-1 adrenoceptors. *Naunyn Schmiedebergs Arch Pharmacol* 1991;**343**:435–8.

105 Wessler I, Ladwein E, Szrama E. Stimulation of α_1-adrenoceptors increases electrically evoked [^{3}H] acetylcholine release from the rat phrenic nerve. *Eur J Pharmacol* 1989;**174**:77–83.

106 Wessler I, Holzer G, Künster A. Stimulation of β_1-adrenoceptors enhances electrically evoked [^{3}H]-acetylcholine release from rat phrenic nerve. *Clin Expl Pharmacol Physiol* 1990;**17**:23–32.

107 Blusztajn JK, Venturini A, Jackson DA, Lee HJ, Wainer BH. Acetylcholine synthesis and release is enhanced by dibutyryl cyclic AMP in a neuronal cell line derived from mouse septum. *J Neurosci* 1992;**12**:793–9.

2: Postjunctional mechanisms involved in neuromuscular transmission

FRANÇOIS DONATI, DAVID R BEVAN

Muscle cells are designed to contract in response to stimuli originating in nerve cells, to produce force and movement. Both nerve and muscle cells can generate and propagate action potentials, that is, they are excitable. In peripheral nerve, the role of action potentials is to carry information from the central nervous system to a group of muscle cells, or fibres, located at a certain distance in the body. In muscle, the action potential precedes and leads to the contraction process. Thus, its role is to ensure a uniform and synchronous contraction along the whole length of the muscle fibre. Action potentials do not propagate across the neuromuscular junction. Transmission takes place because the nerve ending releases acetylcholine, which in turn binds to specialised receptors located at the endplate. This chapter deals with the physiological processes taking place postjunctionally, that is, between the binding of acetylcholine and the contraction process.

The endplate

The nerve terminal is in close approximation with a specialised area of muscle cell membrane, called the endplate. The muscle and nerve cells are separated by a narrow gap, about 50 nm (50×10^{-9} m) wide, called the junctional cleft. This space contains a basement membrane, fibrous strands for mechanical stability, and acetylcholinesterase molecules.[1 2] If one peeled off the nerve terminal from the muscle cell, the endplate would appear, in mammals, as an oval shaped depression, where the muscle membrane forms a network of primary and secondary folds[3] (fig 2.1). The crests of these folds have a high density of acetylcholine sensitive receptors. The troughs of the folds have a high density of sodium channels, which play an important role in action potential propagation.[4] The space between the folds contains a large quantity of acetylcholinesterase.

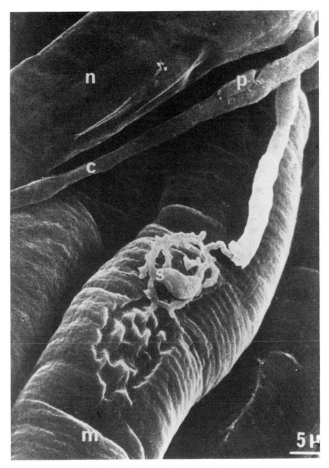

Fig 2.1 The neuromuscular junction and surrounding area. The nerve terminal(s) can be seen as branching from the nerve (n) and is peeled off from the endplate, showing the postjunctional folds. The muscle cell is shown by m and the letter c denotes a capillary[3]

Most mammalian muscle cells have only one endplate, normally located near the midpoint between origin and insertion. In humans, only extraocular muscles, and a proportion of muscles of the larynx, upper oesophagus, middle ear, and face, may have multiple endplates for each fibre.[1] Muscle is made up of many cells which run parallel to each other, and the neuromuscular junctions of focally innervated muscle (one junction per fibre) are located in a relatively narrow band. Thus, the length of muscle cell depends on the length of the muscle itself (up to 50 cm). The long diameter of an oval shaped neuromuscular junction is 20–50 μm (0·002–0·0005 cm). Therefore, the neuromuscular junction occupies just a tiny part, typically from 0·5 to 0·01%, of the length of a muscle cell, and muscle action potentials are required to carry the information from the

29

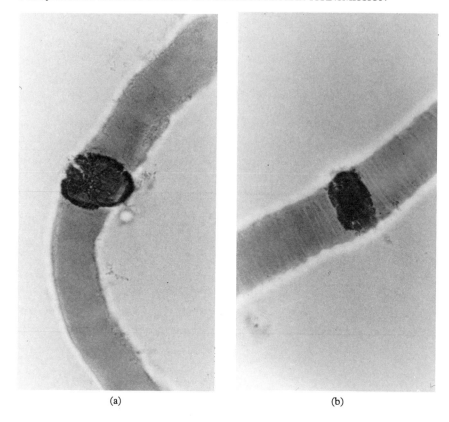

(a)   (b)

Fig 2.2 Goat muscle fibres shown with an optical microscope. The fibres were cut near the neuromuscular junction, which appears darker because of acetyl-cholinesterase staining. Muscle fibres vary in size, but the size of the neuromuscular junction tends to remain relatively constant. Thus, small fibres tend to have junctions which occupy a large portion of their diameter, and large fibres have junctions which are smaller than their respective diameters. (a) Thyroarytenoid muscle; (b) cricoarytenoid muscle; (c) soleus; (d) rectus abdominis; (e) masseter. Diameter of muscle fibre is about 25–30 μm in (a) and (b) and (e) and 40–45 μm in (c) and (d). (Courtesy of C Ibebunjo)

junction to all parts of the muscle cell. For comparison purposes, if the neuromuscular junction had the size of the period at the end of this sentence, the corresponding muscle cell could be as long as an average size room.

It is also important to consider size relationships within the neuro-muscular junction itself. The endplate is 20–50 μm lengthwise and 15–30 μm across. It covers as little as one half the diameter of the muscle cell and sometimes extends over the edges (fig 2.2). The nerve terminal is very close to all this surface, the thickness of the junctional cleft being only one thousandth the diameter of the endplate. It follows that access to the postjunctional receptor is relatively easier for acetylcholine, which is released from the nerve terminal, only 50 nm away from the receptor, than

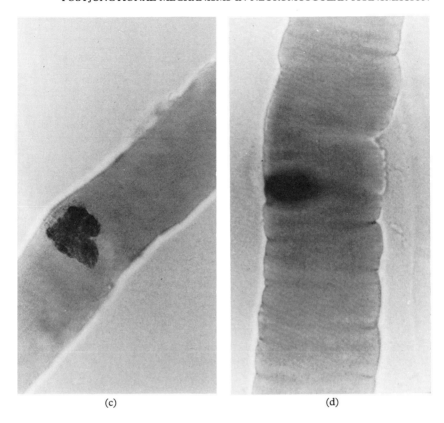

(c)   (d)

Fig 2.2 *continued*

for muscle relaxants, which can gain access to the receptor only by sneaking in through the edges of the junctional cleft. This anatomical feature lends credence to the concept of buffered diffusion, or restricted diffusion, which is discussed below.

Structure of the acetylcholine receptor

Recent advances in molecular biology have led to the characterisation of the structure of the acetylcholine receptor, which belongs to the class of agonist activated channels. Functionally, these receptors require binding with a chemical compound, either an endogenous neurotransmitter or an exogenous pharmacological agent, to activate. Structurally, agonist (acetylcholine, glycine, γ-aminobutyrate or GABA, or serotonin) activated channels all have protein subunits arranged like a rosette or doughnut.[56] The nicotinic acetylcholine receptor at the endplate has five subunits, two of which, called α, are similar. The other subunits are called β, δ, and ε, respectively. Another type of nicotinic receptor has a γ subunit instead of an ε. The receptor with the γ subunit is called the "extrajunctional" or the "fetal" receptor because it is found, in relatively low numbers, in skeletal

31

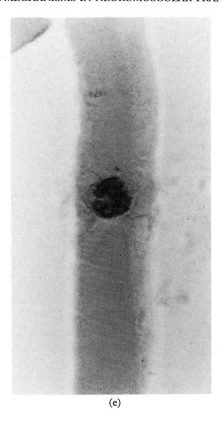

(e)

Fig 2.2 *continued*

muscle outside the neuromuscular junction, and in immature junctions. The receptor containing the ε subunit is the "junctional" or the "adult" receptor.

Junctional and extrajunctional receptors have many characteristics in common. Their molecular weight is about 250 000 daltons. They lie across the whole thickness of the muscle cell membrane. The part that projects extracellularly is relatively bulky, compared with the intracellular portion. The thickness of the doughnut, or the distance from the intracellular to the extracellular extremes, is 11 nm, greater than the thickness of the bilayer membrane (4 nm)[7] (fig 2.3). The extracellular "mouth" of the channel is somewhat wider (8·5 nm) than the rest of the receptor. Each of the subunits is a protein. It appears that each of them has four membrane domains, that is, it crosses the membrane four times.[5-7] Both carboxy and amino ends lie on the extracellular side of the membrane. The channel, or hole of the doughnut, is lined with the second membrane domain of each of the subunits.[6 7]

The α subunit has 437 amino acids, or residues, and its molecular weight is 40 000 daltons. It is the smallest of the subunits, the others ranging in

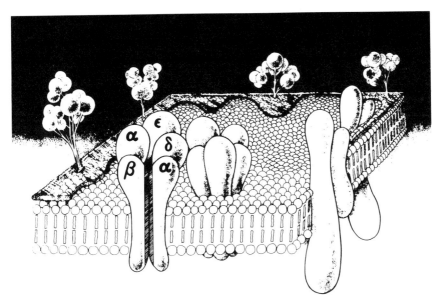

Fig 2.3 View of the junctional, or adult, acetylcholine receptor, and the surrounding membrane. It is made up of five subunits, all of which cross the membrane completely. Each of the two α subunits contain the acetylcholine recognition site. The membrane also contains other proteins (shown here as potato shaped structures). The acetylcholinesterase enzyme is represented here as a stalk to which multiple balloons are attached[2]

molecular weight between 49 000 and 67 000 daltons.[6] Acetylcholine binds to the α subunit, probably at a site located between amino acid 172 and 201 from the N terminal end.[6] This segment is located extracellularly, before the first membrane domain. Channel activation takes place if two molecules of acetylcholine, or another agonist, bind simultaneously both α subunits.[2] This binding produces a conformational change in the protein structure of the receptor, which causes an opening of the channel or the hole of the receptor. The affinity of each α binding site is probably different from the other because, although identical, the subunits have a different environment.[6] One of these is surrounded by a β and a δ subunit, and the other has a β and an ε subunit as neighbours. Substituting the ε for a γ subunit changes the affinity for both agonists and antagonists.[2]

The density of acetylcholine receptors has been evaluated as 10 000–20 000/μm^2 of endplate area.[12] This indicates that the receptors are tightly packed. If the endplate was a smooth structure, a membrane containing 10 000 receptors/μm^2 would be 62% occupied by these receptors, assuming a diameter of 8·5 nm for each receptor.[7] The presence of junctional folds allows more "standing room" for receptors, and for the other proteins such as sodium channels, which are necessary for proper cell function. Considering neuromuscular junction areas of 500–1500 μm^2, the number of receptors per endplate is of the order of 10^7.

Extrajunctional receptors

The density of extrajunctional receptors, characterised by a γ instead of an ε subunit, is many orders of magnitude less than junctional receptors. During development, only the extrajunctional, or fetal, type is formed. Innervation inhibits the incorporation of extrajunctional receptors into the muscle cell membrane, and promotes the formation and insertion of junctional receptors at the endplate. Disuse without denervation, resulting from stroke or prolonged immobilisation, may increase the number of extrajunctional receptors at the endplate. Denervation causes proliferation of extrajunctional receptors throughout the muscle cell membrane, that is, both junctionally and extrajunctionally. Extrajunctional receptors are more sensitive to agonists, such as acetylcholine and suxamethonium (succinyl-choline), and less sensitive to agonists (non-depolarising relaxants) than junctional receptors.[28] This might explain the relative resistance to non-depolarising agents observed with immobilisation and disuse.

Function of the acetycholine receptor

The size of the open channel (0·65 nm) is large enough to let cations pass through indiscriminately. Concentration gradients favour outward move-ment of potassium ions and inward movement of sodium ions, because of the ionic composition of intracellular and extracellular fluid. In addition, entry of sodium ion is enhanced by a favourable electrical gradient, because the potential inside the cell is negative and attracts positive ions. Similarly, this electrical gradient puts a brake on the outward movement of potassium ions. The net effect is a transfer of positive charges from the outside to the inside of the cell, making the inside less negative. A depolarisation occurs.

The open time of the channel is agonist dependent, but does not depend on how long the agonist stays bound to the α subunits. For instance, junctional receptors activated by acetylcholine have a mean open time of 1 ms, in spite of the fact that acetylcholine may come off the receptor and be broken down in a much shorter time. Extrajunctional (or fetal) receptors have a longer (6 ms) open time. Conductance of these receptors has been evaluated at 50 and 35 picosiemens (pS) respectively. During one opening of junctional receptors, as many as 100 000 sodium ions might be allowed to go through.[7]

Opening of only one channel is insufficient to change the resting potential to any significant extent. Spontaneous release of one vesicle, or quantum, which may be made up of 10 000 or so acetylcholine vesicles, produces simultaneous activation of several receptors, and this can be recorded in vitro as a small change (0·5–1 mV) in endplate potential. This miniature endplate potential, or MEPP, is insufficient, however, to lead to the generation of an action potential. When the nerve terminal is invaded by a nerve action potential, simultaneous release of the contents of a large number of vesicles takes place, discharging as many as 1–1·5 million acetylcholine molecules. It is difficult to determine how many receptors are actually activated by this massive bombardment with acetylcholine. An unknown proportion of the released acetylcholine is broken down en route to the endplate by acetylcholinesterase. Furthermore, only receptors which simultaneously bind two acetylcholine molecules will be activated. On the other hand, the efficiency of the system is enhanced by the close proximity of the areas of release, called active zones, to the crests of the folds, where receptors are densely packed. Considering that the numbers mentioned above are rough estimates coming from various sources, one could estimate, as a very crude approximation, that several hundred thousand receptors open simultaneously. This is considerably less than the 10 million receptors at the endplate, but is sufficient to produce a potential change or EPP, which is large enough to trigger an action potential in muscle.

Excitation of muscle

The simultaneous opening of several hundred thousand channels at the endplate produces an inward current of positively charged sodium ions, making the endplate and the neighbouring area electrically more positive than the rest of the muscle cell. When the membrane potential is depolarised to a potential of about -50 to -40 mV, sodium channels are activated. Sodium channels are, similar to acetylcholine receptors, protein structures shaped like a doughnut which lie across the full thickness of the cell membrane (fig 2.4). Unlike acetylcholine receptors, sodium channels do not respond to agonists, but are activated in response to changes in electrical potential across the cell membrane. The sodium channel is activated if the transmembrane potential is depolarised above a certain threshold. Structurally, sodium channels differ from agonist activated channels in two respects. First, the doughnut is made up of a single protein subunit instead of several, and second, contrary to acetylcholine channels, sodium channels project intracellularly more than extracellularly.[4]

The endplate and the surrounding area, also called the perijunctional area, are rich in sodium channels.[23] Unlike acetylcholine receptors, which let most cations pass through, sodium channels discriminate between ions and allow inward movement of sodium ions almost exclusively. As the sodium concentration is lower inside the cell than outside, opening of sodium channels produces an influx of sodium ions, and this movement leads to an excess of positive ions on the inside of the cell. Thus, the electrical potential inside the cell becomes more positive. This increase in membrane potential produces a positive feedback mechanism. Sodium channels open in response to depolarisation, which produces more depolarisation, which in turn causes more sodium channels to open. An action potential is generated and is propagated because of the presence of sodium channels along the whole length of muscle. The process is terminated by inactivation of sodium channels, which occurs when the membrane potential is held above threshold during a certain time (a few

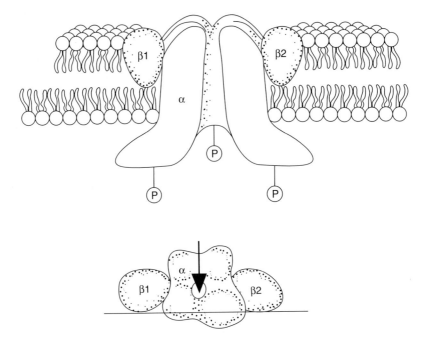

Fig 2.4 View of a sodium channel within the membrane. The α subunit is doughnut shaped and crosses the membrane completely (top). Two smaller units (β_1 and β_2), which lie in the external half of the membrane, are also present. The bottom drawing represents the sodium channel viewed from the outside of the membrane[3]

milliseconds), and activation of potassium channels, which tend to restore the membrane potential towards its resting value.

Excitation–contraction coupling

During normal transmission, an action potential is generated at the endplate and spreads simultaneously to both ends of the muscle cell. Conduction velocity of this electrical impulse is less in muscle (5–10 m/s) than in nerve (50–100 m/s). Nevertheless, a long, 50 cm muscle will depolarise in a relatively short time—50 ms or less—and a short muscle, such as the adductor pollicis, will take less than 5 ms to do so. If all muscle cells, or fibres, of a muscle are activated simultaneously, as occurs when the nerve is stimulated electrically with a stimulator, action potentials will propagate in all muscle fibres simultaneously. The sum of these electrical events can be measured as an electromyographic (EMG) signal. The EMG signal is normally obtained with one electrode overlying the neuromuscular junction, usually the midpoint of the muscle, and the other electrode positioned near the origin or the insertion of the muscle. The shape and magnitude of EMG signals obtained extracellularly with surface electrodes, for example, are different from those of intracellular EMGs, but they have the advantage of reflecting the activity of the whole muscle instead of single

36

fibres. The size, shape, and duration of the EMG signal depend on the geometry of the muscle and the position of the electrodes. For the muscles of the hand (adductor pollicis, first dorsal interosseous, abductor digiti minimi), which are commonly used for monitoring purposes, the EMG signal, in the absence of neuromuscular blockers, is typically 5–20 mV and its duration 5–10 ms (fig 2.5).[9]

A muscle action potential produces opening of calcium channels, which are morphologically similar to sodium channels. Functionally, calcium channels are voltage dependent and ion specific. They open when the membrane is depolarised, as occurs normally with an action potential, and calcium ions move along their concentration gradient. The sarcoplasm, or protoplasm of the muscle cell, is a calcium poor environment, and opening of calcium channels produces a sudden increase in intercellular calcium ion concentration. Calcium binds with the intracellular protein troponin, and

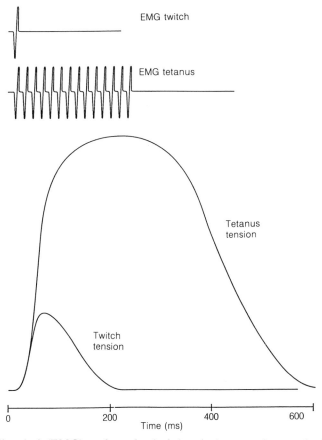

Fig 2.5 Electrical (EMG) and mechanical (tension) events in muscle following single twitch and tetanic stimulations. The EMG signal occurs earlier and is shorter than the contraction. During tetanic stimulation, the EMG signals remain separate, but there is fusion of the individual twitches, which form a tetanus

37

this interaction removes the inhibitory effect of troponin on actin and myosin, two interdigitating proteins which form the skeleton of the muscle fibre. Interaction between actin and myosin produces binding of these interdigitating structures, and the net effect is a contraction. When all muscle fibres contract, as occurs in response to evoked nerve stimulation, an increase in tension is observed shortly after the EMG signal. Relaxation occurs when intracellular calcium concentration decreases to normal levels. This occurs because of binding of the ion to intracellular proteins and active pumping of the ion outside of the cell and especially into specialised reservoirs, the sarcoplasmic reticulum, which are characteristic of muscle cells. The time course of a muscle contraction (100–200 ms) is slower than that of the electrical event (5–10 ms) which precedes it. If a nerve is stimulated at a relatively high frequency (> 10 Hz), the muscle does not have time to relax between stimulations. This causes fusion, or adding up, of contractions, and a tetanus is observed. The net result is a force of contraction greater than that associated with a single twitch. Malignant hyperthermia is thought to be a disorder of calcium homoeostasis in muscle, resulting in an excess of intracellular calcium, which in turn causes uncontrolled rigidity.

Excitation–contraction coupling refers to the relationship between the EMG signal and the force of contraction. Neuromuscular blocking drugs do not affect excitation–contraction coupling because they decrease both the electrical and mechanical events proportionally. Dantrolene, on the other hand, is an example of an agent that does not affect the electrical event (EMG), but leads to a decrease in the force of contraction. Thus, dantrolene affects excitation–contraction coupling.

Interaction of non-depolarising agents with the receptor

The main action of non-depolarising neuromuscular blocking agents is to antagonise the action of acetylcholine in a competitive manner. These drugs compete for the same site as acetylcholine on the α subunit of the acetylcholine receptor. As acetylcholine must bind to both α subunits of the receptor to produce activation, it is sufficient for blocking agents to bind to only one site to produce their effect. It is not necessary, however, for all receptors to be activated to generate an EPP of sufficient magnitude to reach threshold. In fact, only a small proportion of the receptors need to be activated (margin of safety of neuromuscular transmission). As a consequence, a large proportion of receptors must be blocked before neuromuscular blockade is manifest.

Evaluation of the degree of this margin of safety for neuromuscular blocking drugs was attempted many years ago by measuring the degree of depolarisation produced by an agonist (carbachol or suxamethonium) in the presence of various contractions of d-tubocurarine. Twitch depression was also measured in the presence of d-tubocurarine but in the absence of an agonist. The preparation used was the anterior tibial muscle of the cat. The main assumption here was that the degree of depolarisation produced by the agonist was proportional to the percentage of free receptors. Neuromuscular blockade, defined as depression of single twitch height, was found to be detectable when 75% of receptors were occupied, and was complete when this proportion reached 92%.[10] This does not imply that, when 75–92% of receptors are occupied, all endplates in a given muscle conduct partially. It means that, in the 75–92% range, threshold is not reached at some endplates, but fibres in which threshold is reached contract normally. For example, 60% twitch depression implies that threshold was not reached at 60% of the endplates in the muscle involved and these fibres did not contract, but a normal action potential and contraction took place in the remaining 40% of fibres.

This range of receptor occupancy varies slightly with species, and between muscles within the same species. For example, the diaphragm of the cat has a greater margin of safety than peripheral muscle.[11] Obviously, these elaborate experiments have not been attempted in humans. Considering the limitations of the technique used, the interspecies variability, and the differences between muscles within the same organism, it is inappropriate to claim that neuromuscular blockade occurs over the same receptor occupancy range as in the cat tibialis anterior. Nevertheless, the concept of margin of safety is certainly just as valid in humans as in animals, although the magnitude of this effect might be quantitatively different.

Another possible mode of action of neuromuscular blocking drugs is channel blockade. When receptors are activated by acetylcholine, all positively charged ions are attracted to the mouth of the channel, including muscle relaxants. Contrary to sodium ions which are small enough to squeeze through the open channels, non-depolarising agents are, however, large molecules which are likely to plug the open channel. This non-competitive effect is likely to be quantitatively minor, for two reasons. First, the concentration of non-depolarising agents that produce blockade is normally too small to produce a significant effect. For d-tubocurarine, it has been estimated that, at equilibrium, one molecule was free for every 300 bound.[12] This implies that the proportion of molecules available for open channel blockade is only one in 300, and this effect could represent only 0·3% of total receptor occupancy. For a more potent relaxant, such as vecuronium, the importance of such a mechanism is probably even less. At 90% blockade, the free concentration of the drug is about 0·17 μmol/l, or 10^{17} molecules per litre. Assuming a junction 1000 μm^2 in area and a synaptic cleft 50 nm wide, the junctional area has a volume of 50×10^{-15} l. This means only 5000 free vecuronium molecules for more than 10 000 000 receptors, or one free for every 2000 bound. The second reason for discarding the importance of channel blockade is the demonstrated effectiveness of anticholinesterase agents as anti-curare drugs.[2] Inhibition of acetylcholinesterase increases the half life of acetylcholine at the neuromuscular junction, so that one molecule of the neurotransmitter can bind several times to receptors, instead of only once. This has the same effect as increasing the concentration of a competitive agonist, and reduces the effectiveness of the competitive antagonist, the relaxant. Repeated activation of receptors would, however, increase the probability of channel blockade by relaxant molecules. The effectiveness of anticholinesterase agents in reversing neuromuscular blockade suggests that the competitive action (acetylcholine and relaxants binding to the same site) is quantitatively more important than channel blockade.

Access to the junction

It appears that neuromuscular blocking drugs act at the receptor as soon as binding occurs and the effect stops as soon as the drug molecule comes off the receptor. Most of the delay in action seems to originate from the restricted space which the neuromuscular junction constitutes. When d-tubocurarine is applied iontophoretically, that is, by means of an electrode located in the vicinity of the junction, the full effect takes a few seconds. The same phenomenon is observed for offset of action. If the nerve terminal is removed, both onset and offset are much more rapid.[12] This phenomenon has been called "buffered diffusion," and is explained as follows. When a high concentration of relaxant arrives in the vicinity of the neuromuscular junction, as may happen during iontophoretic application or after intravenous injection, drug molecules are driven towards the junctional cleft, because of the existence of a concentration gradient. As pointed out previously, the existence of a high density of receptors implies that most molecules gaining access to the junctional cleft bind to receptors, which tends to lower the concentration of free drug molecules in the area. Thus, more molecules are driven in, and these new molecules are also likely to be bound. This process continues until the concentrations of free drug within and outside the junctional cleft are equal. To use the vecuronium example mentioned above, if a concentration sufficient to establish 90% blockade is provided ($0 \cdot 17 \ \mu\text{mol/l}$) outside a neuromuscular junction containing 10 000 000 receptors, 9000 000 molecules need to be transferred to bind 90% of the receptors (actually this value is greater, because there are two binding sites per receptor, but for the purpose of the demonstration, it is sufficient to assume only one binding site per receptor), plus 4500 free molecules (one per 2000 bound). At equilibrium, the junction contains 2000 times as many vecuronium molecules as a neighbouring area of similar volume. Before this equilibrium is reached, 2000 times as many molecules need to be transferred to the neuromuscular junction than to any area of comparable size. Thus, the process is likely to be 2000 times as long!

The same process occurs with recovery, but in reverse. If the concentration outside the junctional cleft decreases rapidly to zero, as is the case if iontophoretic application of muscle relaxants is stopped, a concentration gradient favouring exit of the relaxant drug is established. The presence of many free binding sites means, however, that the relaxant molecule is more likely to bind to a receptor than to exit the junction. On average, a relaxant molecule binds and unbinds repeatedly before it has a chance to leave the junctional cleft. This process is, however, unlikely to be important for most drugs, because the drug concentration outside the junction, which is mirrored by plasma concentration, does not decrease rapidly. The only possible exception is mivacurium, which is the only drug that has a recovery index (6–8 min) exceeding by far its terminal elimination half life (2 min).[13]

The extent of buffered diffusion is predicted to be directly related to potency. If one applies a potent drug, for example, doxacurium, by means of an electrode located near the junction, and a certain degree of blockade is attained, for instance 90%, the concentration at equilibrium will be 100 times less than the concentration of gallamine, which has one hundredth of the potency, for the same degree of blockade. In other words, the concentration gradient will be 100 times greater in the case of gallamine, indicating that the initial transfer of drug from the outside to the inside of the junctional cleft will be 100 times faster in the case of gallamine. At equilibrium, 9000 000 molecules of doxacurium will be bound versus 1000 free. In the case of gallamine, 9000 000 will be bound versus 100 000 free, reflecting the fact that gallamine has one hundredth the potency of doxacurium. Thus, the total number of molecules is almost identical (9001 000 versus 9100 000), but the rate of transfer is much faster in the case of gallamine, because its concentration outside the junction is 100 times greater. This relationship between speed of onset and potency has been demonstrated in vitro[14] (fig 2.6), and this phenomenon has also been reported in vivo in the cat,[15] and in anaesthetised patients.[16] Gallamine has a faster onset of action than equipotent doses of the more potent pancuronium, rocuronium is faster acting than the more potent vecuronium, and doxacurium, the most potent non-depolarising agent in clinical use, has the slowest onset time.

Effect of depolarising drugs

There is no consensus regarding the exact mechanism by which suxamethonium and other depolarising agents cause muscle paralysis, but two separate phenomena, which may not be mutually exclusive, may explain the paralysing effect of these drugs. Suxamethonium is an agonist like acetylcholine. Simultaneous binding of the drug to the α subunits normally opens the channel and depolarisation is produced. This initial depolarisation was thought to be the source of the fasciculations which suxamethonium produces, but this is now considered to be a prejunctional phenomenon.[17] Depolarisation, whether produced by suxamethonium, acetylcholine, or any other depolarising agent, causes desensitisation, which implies a lack of responsiveness to further agonist. Normally, acetylcholine is hydrolysed so rapidly that it has no potential for causing desensitisation.

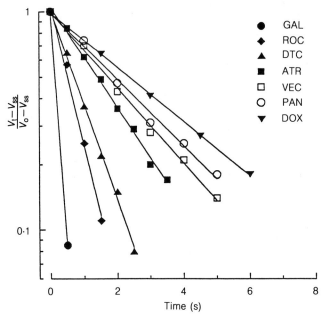

Fig 2.6 Time course of onset of effect of muscle relaxants applied iontophoretically, that is, by means of a microelectrode to the endplate. The time constant of the effect varies directly with the potency of the drug, being fastest for the least potent (gallamine—GAL), and slowest for the most potent (doxacurium—DOX). Intermediate values are found for the other agents (ROC, rocuronium; DTC, d-tubocurarine; ATR, atracurium; VEC, vecuronium; PAN, pancuronium)[14]

Suxamethonium remains, however, at the neuromuscular junction for many minutes, instead of a fraction of a millisecond, and it has the potential to produce desensitisation. The other mechanism which might be implicated is the inactivation of sodium channels. If the endplate is maintained in a depolarised state because of the continued presence of suxamethonium, the sodium channels present at the endplate and the perijunctional area will be inactivated, because prolonged depolarisation from any cause produces this effect. This means that further depolarisation of the endplate will not generate an action potential, because of the inactivation of the junctional and perijunctional area.[2]

Fate of acetylcholine and anticholinesterase drugs

The action of acetylcholine is terminated by the rapid action of acetylcholinesterase. If such a rapid hydrolysis did not take place, the neurotransmitter would have to leave the synaptic cleft, and would most probably bind again to other receptors because of buffered diffusion. Drugs such as neostigmine and edrophonium have a profound inhibiting action on acetylcholinesterase. As expected, the endplate potential has a larger amplitude and a longer duration in the presence of neostigmine. Inhibition of acetylcholinesterase is not, however, the only action of these drugs because an additional effect can be measured in spite of previous treatment with an irreversible acetylcholinesterase inhibitor.[19]

The anticholinesterase agents are not true antagonists of non-depolarising neuromuscular blockers. Their action is mainly by increasing the amount of the endogenous agonist, acetylcholine, at the endplate, shifting the competitive interaction between relaxant and acetycholine in favour of acetylcholine. Increased acetylcholine has been thought of as displacing relaxant molecules or knocking them off the receptor. In fact, relaxant molecules bind and unbind repeatedly, in a dynamic equilibrium, and the probability of binding again decreases if a competitor (acetylcholine) is present. Similarly, if the probability of rebinding to a receptor decreases for the relaxant, it has more chance of leaving the junctional cleft, provided that the concentration outside the junction is low enough. This might explain why anticholinesterase drugs are more effective with short acting drugs, which are characterised by a rapid decline in plasma concentrations.

The mechanism of action of anticholinesterase drugs has another consequence: a ceiling effect. Even if the enzyme is 100% inhibited, the amount of acetylcholine at the endplate is limited, because only a limited amount is released. Thus, increasing the amount of pyridostigmine, edrophonium, or neostigmine beyond a certain point does not increase their ability to antagonise the blocking effect of muscle relaxants.[20]

Future trends

The tendency in modern anaesthetic practice is to rely on drugs with a specific mechanism of action with as few side effects as possible. This militates against the use of depolarising agents and anticholinesterase drugs, which have multiple, complicated effects. Non-depolarising neuromuscular blocking agents are much more specific in their action, but future representatives of their class will need to fill the niche that is occupied by agents such as suxamethonium, neostigmine, and edrophonium. In other words, the relaxant drugs of the future will need to have a non-depolarising, competitive mode of action, but their onset and recovery will need to be rapid. Current knowledge of neuromuscular physiology indicates that the ideal agent would have to have low potency and be cleared rapidly from the plasma.

1 Bowman WC. *Pharmacology of neuromuscular function,* 2nd ed. London: Wright, 1990.
2 Standaert FG. Neuromuscular physiology and pharmacology. In: Miller RD, ed, *Anaesthesia,* 4th edn. New York: Churchill Livingstone, 1994:731–54.
3 Matsuda Y, Oki S, Kimota K, Nagano Y, Nojima M, Desaki J. Scanning electron microscopic study of denervated and reinervated neuromuscular junction. *Muscle Nerve* 1988;11:1266–71.
4 Catterall WA. Cellular and molecular biology of voltage-gated sodium channels. *Physiol Rev* 1972;72:S15–48.
5 Andersen OS, Koppe RE II. Molecular determinants of channel function. *Physiol Rev* 1992;72:S89–158.

6 Marshall IG, Prior C. Update on the acetylcholine receptor and the neuromuscular junction. *Ballières Clin Anaesthesiol* 1994;**8**:299–313.
7 Sastry BVR. Nicotinic receptor. *Anaesth Pharmacol Rev* 1993;**1**:6–19.
8 Martyn JAJ, White DA, Gronert GA, Jaffe RS, Ward JM. Up- and down-regulation of skeletal muscle acetylcholine receptors. Effects of neuromuscular blockers. *Anesthesiology* 1992;**76**:822–43.
9 Kalli I. Effect of surface electrode position on the compound action potential evoked by ulnar nerve stimulation during isoflurane anaesthesia. *Br J Anaesth* 1990;**65**:494–9.
10 Paton WDM, Waud DR. The margin of safety of neuromuscular transmission. *J Physiol* 1967;**191**:59–90.
11 Waud BE, Waud DR. The margin of safety of neuromuscular transmission in the muscle of the diaphragm. *Anesthesiology* 1972;**37**:417–22.
12 Armstrong DL, Lester HA. The kinetics of tubocurarine action and restricted diffusion within the synaptic cleft. *J Physiol* 1979;**294**:365–86.
13 Head-Rapson AG, Devlin JC, Parker CJR, Hunter JM. Pharmacokinetics of the three isomers of mivacurium and pharmacodynamics of the chiral mixture in hepatic cirrhosis. *Br J Anaesth* 1994;**73**:613–18.
14 Law-Min JC, Bekevac I, Glavinovic MI, Donati F, Bevan DR. Iontophoretic study of speed of action of various muscle relaxants. *Anesthesiology* 1992;**77**:351–6.
15 Bowman WC, Rodger IW, Houston J, Marshall RJ, McIndewar LI. Structure–action relationships among some deacetoxy analogues of pancuronium and vecuronium in the anesthetized cat. *Anesthesiology* 1988;**69**:57–62.
16 Kopman AF. Pancuronium, gallamine, and *d*-tubocurarine compared: Is speed of onset inversely related to drug potency. *Anesthesiology* 1989;**70**:915–20.
17 Hartmann GS, Fiamengo SA, Riker WF Jr. Succinylcholine: mechanism of fasciculations and their prevention by *d*-tubocurarine and diphenylhydantoin. *Anesthesiology* 1986; **65**:405–13.
18 Braga MFM, Rowan EG, Harvey AL, Bowman WC. Prejunctional action of neostigmine on mouse neuromuscular preparations. *Br J Anaesth* 1993;**70**:405–10.
19 Fiekers JF. Interactions of edrophonium, physostigmine and methanesulfonyl fluoride with the snake end-plate acetylcholine receptor complex. *J Pharmacol Expl Ther* 1985; **234**:539–49.
20 Bartkowski RR. Incomplete reversal of pancuronium neuromuscular blockade by neostigmine, pyridostigmine, and edrophonium. *Anesth Analg* 1987;**66**:594–8.

3: Central control of neuromuscular transmission

EDWARD S WEGRZYNOWICZ, KENT S PEARSON, MARTIN D SOKOLL

Anaesthetists frequently use relatively specific neuromuscular blocking agents that act at the postjunctional membrane (endplate) to block neuromuscular transmission. We often, however, ignore the contribution of the central nervous system in the control of neuromuscular transmission, forgetting that the action potential that causes the final release of acetylcholine at the motor unit is the result of spatial and temporal summation of excitatory and inhibitory input occurring in the anterior (ventral) horn of the spinal cord. The rich input to the α motoneuron comes from a variety of sources, including the cerebral cortex, cerebellum, midbrain and brain stem nuclei, red nucleus, vestibular nucleus, and reticular formation. In addition to central input the α motoneuron receives modulating impulses from control sensors within muscles and tendons through monosynaptic and polysynaptic spinal reflex arcs.

Review of neuromuscular transmission

A recent paper by King and Rampil indicates that at least some of what we think of as volatile anaesthetic MAC (minimum alveolar concentration) may be the result of spinal α motoneuron depression. Using electromyographic techniques they demonstrated that isoflurane decreases impulses arising in the spinal portion of motoneurons. This indicates that nocifensor behaviour can be affected at the spinal cord level by alterations in motor function.[1] Any anaesthetic or disease process that alters either the function or the input to the motoneuron will affect neuromuscular transmission.

Neuromuscular transmission is modulated in the central nervous system through mechanisms that determine whether or not an action potential is generated in the motoneuron, causing release of acetylcholine at the neuromuscular junction. The final common pathway is the α motoneuron—a large, efferent, myelinated, fast conducting neuron, whose cell

45

body (soma) lies in the anterior horn grey matter of the spinal cord. The integration of excitatory and inhibitory information at the soma of the α motoneuron determines whether or not a depolarisation propagates towards the neuromuscular junction in the form of an action potential.

In ascending order neuromuscular transmission is regulated by the following:

1 Postjunctional nicotinic cholinergic cation channels
2 Prejunctional acetylcholine receptors
3 Voltage activated calcium channels
4 Acetylcholine synthesis, storage, release, metabolism, and recycling.

Postjunctional nicotinic cholinergic cation channels

A channel is composed of five linear transmembrane proteins, two α, and one each of β, δ, and ε subunits.[2] An acetylcholine molecule must interact with the active site on each of the α subunits to cause a conformational change in the receptor. Thus two molecules of acetylcholine are required to activate the endplate channel allowing small cations such as Na^+ and K^+ to flow down their concentration gradients. Once acetylcholine has opened 5–20% of the channels at the endplate, the summated endplate potential reaches threshold activating, voltage dependent Na^+ channels. A muscle action potential (MAP) then occurs allowing calcium entry and subsequent muscle contraction. The muscle tension developed is dependent on repetitive, additive, and fused contractions, not on the magnitude of the action potential.

Prejunctional acetylcholine receptors

These receptors are similar to the postjunctional receptors, but are thought to be specific for sodium because sodium is necessary for the synthesis and mobilisation of acetylcholine, although not needed for release. Evidence for this is that d-tubocurarine interaction with these receptors decreases mobilisation of acetylcholine causing fade when the motoneurons are stimulated at high rate.

Voltage activated calcium channels

The release of acetylcholine at the prejunctional terminal of the neuromuscular junction is highly dependent on calcium. When the nerve action potential reaches the nerve terminal it causes a conformational change in both fast ("P") and slow ("L") calcium channels. The fast channels are not affected by conventional calcium channel antagonists. The P channels play a prominent role during depolarisation. The L channels are important in allowing additional calcium ions to enter the nerve terminal, where they bind to the glycoprotein synaptophysin allowing acetylcholine vesicles to fuse with the prejunctional membrane and discharge their contents into the neuromuscular junctional cleft. Calcium channel blockers affect the slow L channels, slightly augmenting the effects of neuromuscular block.[3] Calcium and magnesium have antagonistic roles at the prejunctional terminal. Although magnesium will pass through the calcium channel it does not promote the release of acetylcholine into the junctional cleft.

Acetylcholine synthesis, storage, release, metabolism, and recycling

Acetylcholine is synthesised, stored, released, metabolised, and recycled at the nerve terminal and neuromuscular junction. Acetylcholine processing is graphically represented in fig 3.1. Black widow spider venom causes massive release of acetylcholine vesicles depleting prejunctional stores. Hemicholinium-3 blocks the reuptake of choline (produced by the hydrolysis of acetylcholine by acetylcholinesterase) into the nerve terminal; this also depletes prejunctional stores of acetylcholine.

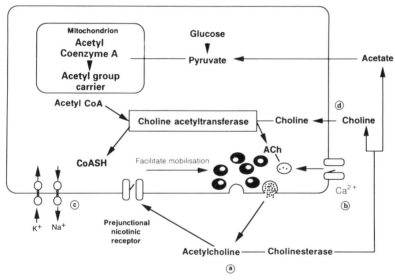

Fig 3.1 A diagrammatic representation of the prejunctional nerve terminal of the α motoneuron which is specialised for the manufacture, mobilisation, release, and resynthesis of acetylcholine. (a) Acetylcholine is metabolised by cholinesterase to choline and acetate which undergo re-uptake into the motoneuron. In addition to interaction with postjunctional receptor acetylcholine interacts with prejunctional nicotinic receptor facilitating additional release. (b) Prejunctional calcium receptor allows calcium influx facilitating release of acetylcholine vesicles. Botulinum binds to these channels irreversibly. (c) Catecholamines indirectly activate Na^+/K^+ pump facilitating acetylcholine release. (d) Choline re-uptake can be blocked by hemicholinium-3 causing a depletion of transmitter available for release

The motoneuron soma receives projections from the peripheral nervous system as well as higher centres. Peripheral nervous system input into action potential propagation in the α motoneuron occurs at the spinal cord level. The simplest of these reflexes is the monosynaptic stretch (myotactic) reflex. When a muscle spindle is stretched, Ia afferent nerve fibres from the spindles make monosynaptic excitatory connections with α motoneurons in the anterior horn of the spinal cord that innervate the same (homonymous) muscles as well as synergistic muscles. The same Ia fibre whose cell body resides in the dorsal root ganglion also synapses with Ia inhibitory interneurons. The inhibitory interneurons synapse with α motoneurons that innervate antagonist muscles. Both the Ia inhibitory interneuron and the motoneuron receive descending input from corticospinal and other pathways. This action coordinates opposing muscles and counteracts the passive stretch of muscles, thereby contributing to muscle tone.

A complementary peripheral control mechanism is the Ib afferent neurons, mediating an inverse myotactic reflex. These cell bodies also lie in the dorsal root ganglion. Ib afferent fibres form excitatory connections with interneurons which, in turn, form inhibitory synapses with the $A\alpha$ motoneurons innervating the homonymous muscle. The same Ib fibre also forms polysynaptic excitatory connections with excitatory interneurons innervating antagonist muscles. When a Golgi tendon organ, which lies in series with a muscle, is stretched, the homonymous muscle is inhibited, whereas the antagonistic muscle is excited. Ib afferent fibres have numerous sensors, and also receive input from joint and cutaneous receptors. Descending pathways also provide both excitatory and inhibitory inputs to Ib interneurons, further modulating muscle coordination.

An additional spinal modulating pathway includes the Renshaw (named for Birdsley Renshaw who described it in 1941) interneuron. Generally inhibitory in nature, the Renshaw cells project to both homonymous $A\alpha$ motoneurons and inhibitory Ia interneurons innervating antagonistic motoneurons. A Renshaw cell receives both excitatory and inhibitory synaptic inputs from descending pathways, and excitatory input from homonymous α motoneurons which it inhibits itself. The Renshaw cells inhibit homonymous $A\alpha$ motoneurons while simultaneously disinhibiting $A\alpha$ motoneurons to antagonist muscles. By changing the excitability of the Renshaw cell, higher motor centres adjust the sensitivity of the motoneuron to both descending and afferent input. The divergent connections of the Renshaw interneurons to motoneurons affecting the whole joint controls the excitability of the entire myotactic unit.

A final peripheral modulating mechanism acting in the spinal cord is the flexion withdrawal reflex. Cutaneous afferent $A\delta$ fibres from nociceptors (whose cell bodies reside in the dorsal root ganglion) project to excitatory interneurons in the dorsal grey matter of the spinal cord. These interneurons in turn project to inhibitory neurons that act on the α motoneurons innervating the extensor muscles of the ipsilateral limb. They also supply excitatory input to interneurons that have excitatory synapses with the α motoneuron supplying the ipsilateral flexors. The same $A\delta$ fibres inhibit the flexors of the contralateral limb via polysynaptic pathways while exciting the Aα motoneurons to the extensor muscles. This produces a withdrawal from a cutaneous noxious stimulus while facilitating weight transfer to the contralateral limb. These spinal reflex pathways are illustrated in fig 3.2.

Anaesthetics can also alter neuromuscular function at higher levels by interfering with action potential propagation or synaptic transmission anywhere along the cortical spinal axis. Volitional or planned movement involves the integration of complex descending pathways. Information concerning volitional movement is relayed from the cerebral cortex to the lateral lobe of the cerebellum, where it is processed and sent back to the motor cortex through the dentate nucleus. Then signals are relayed, from the motor cortex, through descending pathways to the appropriate α motoneuron as well as back to the cerebellum. Sensory and positional information is then relayed to the cerebellum and cerebral cortex. Purkinje cells of the cerebellum project to nuclei interposed between the motor cortex and descending pathways which receive input from lower spinal levels via the spinocerebellar pathways. They receive proprioceptive information from muscles participating in volitional movement and modulate the interposed cerebellar nuclei. When the cerebral cortex decides on movement, a duplicate message goes to both the cerebellum and the spinal cord. In the cerebellum, interaction of this message with other sensory input (that is, information from the muscle spindles, pressure sensors, and proprioceptors) results in secondary information being passed to the spinal cord to permit the correct muscle groups to come into play at

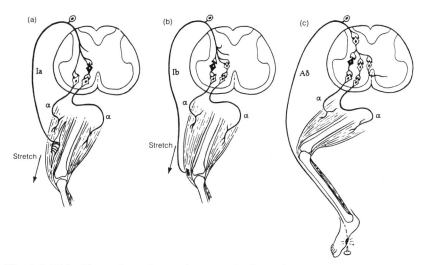

Fig 3.2 This illustration shows the organisation of synaptic connection for maintenance of myotactic reflexes and muscle tone and their organisation at the spinal cord level. (a) The muscle spindle myotactic reflex arc; (b) Golgi tendon organ inverse myotactic response arc; and (c) the flexor reflex. (From Nicholls, Martin, and Wallace. *From neuron to brain*, 3rd edn, 1992, with permission of Sinauer Associates Inc., Publishers, Sunderland, Massachusetts, USA)

the moments they are needed. Normal tone of muscles is maintained not only by reflex arcs, but also by the summation of nervous impulses to the anterior grey matter of the cord and α motoneurons from the central nervous system (CNS). Part of this system is the γ motor system which receives inputs from the vestibulospinal, olivospinal, and tectospinal tracts. Gamma efferent activity alters muscle tension within the muscle spindles, thus altering Ia afferent impulses involved in monosynaptic and poly-synaptic reflex arcs affecting α motoneuron activity. This cerebral and cerebellar control of the α and γ motoneuron system is demonstrated in fig 3.3.

The CNS also controls neuromuscular transmission via humoral and indirect transmitter mechanisms. At first glance the inputs to skeletal muscle are much simpler than to neurons in the CNS. The input is only excitatory. The completion of transmission, resulting in the production of an MAP, is determined by the magnitude of the temporal summation of the postjunctional endplate. If sufficient acetylcholine quanta are released the muscle fibre will depolarise. In spite of this apparent simplicity, direct

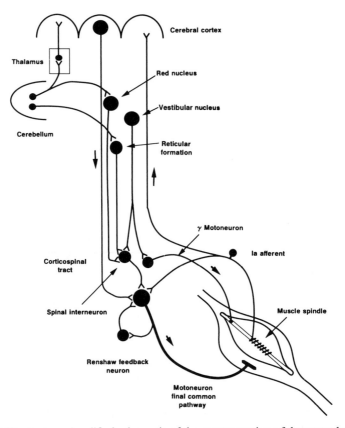

Fig 3.3 Illustrates a simplified schematic of the motor portion of the central nervous system and the relation to the α motoneuron final common pathway

cholinergic transmission is modulated by a number of substances. Noradrenaline (norepinephrine) released from varicosities along sympathetic axons and adrenaline (epinephrine) released by the adrenal medulla both facilitate neuromuscular transmission. Adrenaline and noradrenaline act on a variety of receptors that are indirectly coupled to effector proteins. The β_2 and α-adrenergic receptors are found in skeletal muscle and α_1 receptors are found in prejunctional nerve terminals. Activation of the α_1-adrenergic receptor on the prejunctional nerve terminal increases the number of acetylcholine quanta released in response to an action potential. Postjunctional β_2 receptor stimulation activates the Na^+/K^+ pump in muscle fibres, causing hyperpolarisation.[4 5] Postjunctional hyperpolarisation leads to muscle action potentials of greater amplitude and duration.

α Motoneurons express a variety of molecules involved in intercellular communication. In addition to acetylcholine, mammalian motoneurons make connections and the neuroactive peptides calcitonin gene related peptide (CGRP) and cholecystokinin. These compounds, although not active in transmission itself, may be responsible for the maintenance of the neuromuscular junction.[6] Although impulse transmission at the neuromuscular junction is mediated by acetylcholine, a number of other chemical factors such as steroid hormones, catecholamines, and peptides may also affect the structure and function of the α motoneuron/neuromuscular junction axis.[7] Receptors for a variety of transmitters and hormones are present on the soma of the α motoneuron as well as at the neuromuscular junction. These phenomena have been investigated mainly in the spinal nucleus of the bulbocavernosus (SNB). This nucleus is mainly involved in stereotypical reproductive behaviour. Although these concerns are not of major physiological interests to the anaesthetist, this evidence nevertheless demonstrates the presence of modulation of neuromuscular activity by mechanisms other than corticospinal mechanisms. The α motoneuron as well as the neuromuscular junction may be modulated by a variety of hormones, neurotransmitters, and peptides.

Given the amazing complexity of the CNS's link to the periphery, it is not surprising that a number of diseases cause abnormalities of the function of the nervous system. The damage can occur at any level from the muscle itself to the central processing of data controlling muscle movement. This section will review several disease states that have potential impact on the anaesthetic management of patients with these diseases.

Diseases of the motor nerves

Diseases of the motor unit have great potential for disability and early death. As discussed above, the motor unit consists of the cell body of the motoneuron, the axon of the motoneuron that runs in the peripheral nerve, the neuromuscular junction, and the muscle fibres innervated by the motor nerve.[8] Diseases that act on the nerve cell bodies or peripheral nerves are termed "neurogenic diseases." These can be subdivided into motoneuron disease which affects the nerve cell body, and peripheral neuropathy which affects the peripheral axon. In contrast, diseases affecting muscles with little damage to motoneurons are called myopathies. Neurogenic diseases include amyotrophic lateral sclerosis, affecting the motoneuron, and Guillain–Barré syndrome, affecting the peripheral nerves. Myopathic diseases include muscular dystrophies and myotonic dystrophy. Both classes of disease result in muscle weakness.

Amyotrophic lateral sclerosis

Amyotrophic lateral sclerosis (ALS) is a form of neurogenic muscle atrophy disease of the corticospinal tracts of the spinal cord. This results in the block of impulse transmission through the axons of the premotor cells from the cortex and brain stem to the spinal cord.[8] This disease results in painless weakness that progresses to muscle wasting and fasciculations. Sensation remains normal, and ultimately this muscle wasting is fatal because of involvement of the muscles of respiration. Decreased levels of acetylcholine occur secondary to a diminished store of choline acetyl-transferase which is found with the degeneration of the anterior horn cells of the spinal cord.[9] This results in an increased sensitivity to the non-depolarising muscle relaxants.[10] Use of a depolarising muscle relaxant may result in severe hyperkalaemia.[11] The clinician when faced with such a patient should carefully titrate small doses of non-depolarising relaxant until a desired state of neuromuscular blockade is achieved. This is facilitated by close observation of the surgical field, coupled with use of a peripheral nerve stimulator.

Muscular dystrophies

Duchenne and Becker muscular dystrophies are two progressive myo-pathies that are inherited as X linked recessive traits. Duchenne muscular dystrophy is more severe and common, with an incidence of one in 3500 live male births.[12] Becker muscular dystrophy has an incidence of about one in 30 000 male births.[13] Both diseases result from a mutation in the gene that codes for the high molecular weight membrane protein, dystrophin.[13] Patients with the more severe Duchenne muscular dystrophy have none of this protein, whereas patients with Becker muscular dystrophy have abnormal amounts or sizes of this protein.[14] The normal function of dystrophin has yet to be clarified. Also the relation of the lack of dystrophin to muscular dystrophy is unclear.[8]

Duchenne muscular dystrophy usually becomes clinically evident in boys between the ages of two and three. Muscle weakness, usually first affecting the proximal limb muscles of the legs, is noted. This progresses until the child is eventually wheelchair bound. Mental handicap and cardiac conduction abnormalities are often associated with Duchenne muscular dystrophy. In contrast, Becker muscular dystrophy appears later in life, and is associated with milder symptoms and slower progression than Duchenne muscular dystrophy. Additionally, mental handicap is less common with Becker muscular dystrophy.

The anaesthetist is presented with multiple concerns when choosing muscle relaxants for patients with muscular dystrophy. First, there is the concern that these patients will be at increased risk for malignant hyperthermia. This is based on the results of muscle biopsies of Duchenne muscular dystrophy patients—found positive for malignant hyperthermia.[15][16] There is a clear association between the use of suxamethonium (succinylcholine) and adverse outcome in patients with muscular dystrophy. The reported events include hyperkalaemia, rhabdomyolysis, myoglobinuria, and cardiac arrest.[17][18] The potential for suxamethonium to trigger massive damage has led the US Food and Drug Administration to recommend against the routine use of this drug in paediatric anaesthetic practice. The response to non-depolarising muscle relaxants can be either normal or prolonged.[19] Again, use of a nerve stimulator should be encouraged.

Myotonias

The myotonias represent the most common form of muscular dystrophy among white people, with an incidence of one in 8000.[13] The myotonias are multisystem diseases which are characterised by muscle weakness, wasting, and myotonia, or delayed muscle relaxation after contraction.[13] This disease is caused by a genetic mutation that leads to the decreased production of myotonin protein kinase mRNA.[20] Increased sensitivity to non-depolarising agents has been reported with myotonias.[21] In contract, suxamethonium may actually trigger a myotonic response, which could lead to the inability to ventilate or intubate an affected patient.[22] Careful titration of non-depolarising relaxants would be the proper approach to muscle relaxation in these patients.

Malignant hyperthermia

Another muscular disease with a genetic basis is malignant hyperthermia. This disease is of special interest to the anaesthetist, because it can be triggered by exposure to depolarising neuromuscular blocking agents and volatile agents. This disease has an incidence of about one in 14 000 episodes of anaesthesia, but the exact prevalence of the disease is unknown, resulting from the fact that some patients are never exposed to a triggering anaesthetic.[23] The genetic inheritance of malignant hyperthermia is probably multifactorial. Up to half of the affected patients demonstrate autosomal dominant inheritance, but other patients appear to have recessive or multifactorial inheritance.[24]

The clinical syndrome of malignant hyperthermia is marked by acute hypermetabolism which progresses to acidosis, tachypnoea, tachycardia, rigidity, fever, cyanosis, and possibly death, if left untreated.[23] This hypermetabolism results from a sudden rise in myoplasmic calcium secondary to an action of the volatile anaesthetics on the sarcoplasmic reticulum.[25] The genetic basis for this disease is thought to be a point mutation of the ryanodyne receptor gene.[26]

Early treatment of a malignant hyperthermia episode is necessary to ensure survival, consisting of the immediate discontinuation of all triggering anaesthetics, aggressive supportive treatment of the metabolic abnormalities, and rapid administration of dantrolene. Dantrolene acts to decrease intracellular calcium content and limit the progression of an episode of malignant hyperthermia.[23]

Myasthenia gravis

Damage at the neuromuscular junction can lead to significant disease. An example is myasthenia gravis. This disease is caused by the autoimmune destruction of acetylcholine receptors of the neuromuscular junction. This causes interference with transmission by reducing the number of functional receptors or by impeding the interaction of acetylcholine with its receptors.[27] Weakness caused by this disease often involves the cranial, as well as limb, muscles; it often waxes and wanes throughout the day and is reversed by anticholinesterase drugs. In addition to the autoimmune changes, the myasthenic patient demonstrates changes in the geometry of the endplate region. The normal infolding of the junctional cleft is reduced, and the junctional cleft itself is enlarged in patients with myasthenia gravis.[28] These changes result in fewer acetylcholine molecules reaching functional receptors to trigger action potentials. All of these changes result in early muscle fatigue and weakness which is most pronounced after repetitive exercise. Diagnosis of the disease is based on clinical symptoms and electromyography which demonstrates fade after repeated nerve stimulation.[29]

Treatment of mysthenia gravis is multifactorial. As there is a clear association between thymomas and myasthenia, thymectomy is often performed. This operation will result in improvement of between 70% and 80% of patients.[30] Additionally, plasmapheresis can be performed to decrease the amount of autoantibodies present in the patient's serum.[31] The mainstay of therapy is treatment with long lasting anticholinesterase agents, such as pyridostigmine. Therapy with these drugs results in an increase in the amount of acetylcholine available at the neuromuscular junction.

Rational anaesthetic management of the myasthenic patient must be based on the pathophysiological changes that occur at the neuromuscular junction. Reports have indicated that the myasthenic patient is more resistant to suxamethonium than normal patients.[32] Great individual variation in response to depolarising agents is, however, possible, so that there should be careful dose titration to clinical effect. Small doses of non-depolarising agents have been successfully used in myasthenic patients. Once again, close monitoring of the patient's response to the drug is required to ensure adequate effect without serious side effects.[33] In all patients with myasthenia, close monitoring of postoperative respiratory status is necessary to avoid the potential of respiratory arrest.

Myasthenic syndrome

Patients with the Eaton–Lambert myasthenic syndrome often complain of proximal limb weakness with more severe involvement of the leg muscles. This disease seems to result from blockade of the calcium channels which results in a reduction in the amount of acetylcholine packets released through the prejunctional membrane.[34] There is a strong association between occurrence of this disease and carcinoma, especially small cell carcinoma of the bronchus. The EMG is useful in diagnosing Eaton–Lambert syndrome. As with myasthenia gravis, there is a reduced muscle response to single nerve stimulus. Unlike myasthenia gravis, after tetanic stimulation, there is a progressive increase in muscle strength as frequency and duration of stimulus is increased. Patients with Eaton–Lambert syndrome are extremely sensitive to both depolarising and non-depolarising agents. Great care should be used in the titration of such drugs.

Nerve degeneration

Progressive nerve degeneration can also lead to disease. As an example, amyotrophic lateral sclerosis is caused by the degeneration of the pyramidal motoneurons that result in secondary change in muscle fibres.[36] Patients with this disease develop progressive muscle weakness that may progress to respiratory failure. There are often muscle fasciculations present in affected patients. Therapy for the disease is supportive only. If muscle relaxants are required in such patients, suxamethonium should be avoided as a result of the possibility of release of potassium after its administration. Non-depolarising relaxants should be given in reduced doses, and the effects of the relaxants must be closely monitored.

Effect of inhalational anaesthetics

The interaction of potent inhalational anaesthetic agents with muscle relaxants is complex and multifactorial. It has been known for many years that the anaesthetic agents may affect muscular activity. This effect was first reported in 1914. The effects of these potent agents can involve both inhibitory or stimulatory actions. It is often difficult to determine the exact actions of the potent anaesthetic agents on the neuromuscular junction, resulting from the need to conduct experiments in preparations where multiple agents are required to provide adequate anaesthesia and haemo-dynamic stability. In spite of experimental difficulty, several conclusions can be drawn. The potent agents have direct effects on neuromuscular transmission which is generally inhibitory. Additionally, indirect effects arise that are caused by anaesthetic induced changes in organ blood flow which could lead to increased duration of action of the neuromuscular blocking agents.

The major direct action of the volatile anaesthetics seems to be a dose related potentiation of the neuromuscular blocking agents. This potentiation appears to result from depressant actions on the postjunctional membrane.[37] A depressant action on acetylcholine release may also be partially responsible for the depression of neuromuscular transmission.[38 39] This dose related depression is also encountered with the use of newer agents, such as desflurane.[40] Regardless of agent chosen, the clinician should expect at least minimal potentiation of the effects of muscle relaxants, and appropriately monitor neuromuscular transmission to avoid overdose.

The human neuromuscular junction is extremely complex, and easily affected by multiple insults. These include both diseases and drugs used in clinical anaesthesia. Avoidance of morbidity requires the clinician to have a working knowledge of the central control of neuromuscular function coupled with an understanding of the pathophysiology of diseases that affect the neuromuscular junction. If this knowledge is appropriately applied, significant morbidity and mortality can be avoided, and the patient will directly benefit from appropriate application of this increased knowledge.

1 King BS, Rampil IJ. Anesthetic depression of spinal motor neurons may contribute to lack of movement in response to noxious stimuli. *Anesthesiology* 1994;**81**:1484–92.
2 Steinbach JH, Ifune C. How many kinds of nicotinic acetylcholine receptors are there. *Trends Neurosci* 1989;**12**:3–6.
3 Chang CC, Lin SO, Hong SJ, *et al.* Neuromuscular block by verapamil and diliatzem and inhibition of acetylcholine release. *Brain Res* 1988;**454**:332.
4 Kuba K. Effects of cathecholamines on the neuromuscular junction in the rat diaphragm. *J Physiol* 1970;**211**:511–70.
5 Clausen T, Flatman JA. The effect of catecholamine on NaK transport and membrane potential in the rat soleus. *J Physiol* 1977;**270**:383–414.
6 New H, Mudge A. Calcitonin gene related peptide regulates muscle acetyl choline receptor synthesis. *Nature* 1986;**323**:809–11.
7 Micevych PE, Kruger L. The status of calcitonin gene-related peptide as an effector peptide. *Ann NY Acad Sci* 1992;**657**:379–96.
8 Rowland LP. Diseases of the motor unit. In: Kandel ER, Swartz JA, Jessel TM, eds, *Principles of neurosciences.* New York: Elsevier, 1981.
9 Mulder DW, Lambert EM, Eaton LM. Myasthenic syndrome in patients with ALS. *Neurology* 1959;**9**:627–31.
10 Rosenbaum KJ, Neigh JT, Strobel GE. Sensitivity to nondepolarizing muscle relaxants in amyotrophic lateral sclerosis. Report of two cases. *Anesthesiology* 1971;**35**:638–4.
11 Beuch TP, Stone WA, Hamelberg W. Circulatory collapse following succinylcholine: report of a patient with diffuse lower motor neuron disease. *Anesth Analg* 1971;**50**:431–7.
12 Moser H. Duchenne muscular dystrophy: pathogenetic aspects and genetic prevention. *Hum Genet* 1984;**66**:17.
13 Cutler RWP, Daras BT. Diseases of the muscle and the neuromuscular junction. In: Rubenstein E, Federman DD, eds, *Scientific american medicine.* New York: Scientific American Inc., 1994.
14 Hoffman EP, Fischbeck KH, Brown RH, *et al.* Characterization of dystrophin in muscle-biopsy specimens from patients with Duchenne's and Becker's muscular dystrophy. *N Engl J Med* 1988;**318**:1363–8.
15 Brownell AKW, Paasuke RT, Elash A. Malignant hyperthermia in Duchenne muscular dystrophy. *Anesthesiology* 1983;**58**:180.
16 Wang JM, Stanley TH. Duchenne muscular dystrophy and malignant hypothermia, two case reports. *Can Anaesth Soc J* 1986;**33**:799.
17 Kelfer HM, Singer WD, Reynolds RN. Malignant hyperthermia in a child with Duchenne muscular dystrophy. *Pediatrics* 1983;**71**:118.
18 Seay AR, Ziter FA, Thompson JA. Cardiac arrest during induction of anesthesia in Duchenne muscular dystrophy. *J Pediatr* 1973;**93**:88.

19 Azar I. The response of patients with neuromuscular disorders to muscle relaxants: A review. *Anesthesiology* 1984;**61**:173.

20 Fu YH, Fridman DL, Richards S, *et al*. Decreased expression of myotonic protein kinase messenger RNA and protein in adult form of myotonic dystrophy. *Science* 1993;**260**:235.

21 Mitchell MM, Ali HH, Savarese JJ. Myotonia and neuromuscular blocking agents. *Anesthesiology* 1978;**49**:44–7.

22 Thiel RE. The myotonic response to suxamethonium. *Br J Anaesth* 1967;**39**:815–20.

23 Muldoon SM, Karan S. Hyperthermia and hypothermia. In: Rogers M, Tinker J, Covino B, Longnecker D, eds, *Principles and practices of anesthesiology*. Mosby: St Louis, 1993.

24 McPherson EW, Yaylor CA. The genetics of malignant hypothermia: Evidence for heterogeneity. *Am J Med Genet* 1982;**11**:273.

25 Nelson TE, Sweo T. Calcium uptake and calcium release by skeletal muscle scarcoplasmic reticulum: different sensitivity to inhalational anesthetics. *Anesthesiology* 1988;**69**:571.

26 Fujii J, Otsu K, Zorzato F. Identification of a mutation in porcine ryanodine receptors associated with malignant hypothermia. *Science* 1991;**233**:48.

27 Rowland LP. Diseases of chemical transmission at the nerve-muscle synapse: myasthenia gravis. In: Kandel ER, Swartz JA, Jesseli TM, eds, *Principles of neurosciences*. New York: Elsevier, 1981:235–43.

28 Drachman DB. Myasthenia gravis: immunobiology of a receptor disorder. *Trends Neurosci* 1993;**6**:446–51.

29 Sanders DB. The electrodiagnosis of myasthenia gravis. *Proc NY Acad Sci* 1987;**505**:825.

30 Mulder DG, Hermann C, Keesky J, *et al*. Thymectomy for myasthenia gravis. *Am J Surg* 1983;**146**:61.

31 Spence PA, Morin JE, Katz M. Role of plasmapheresis in preparing myasthenic patients for thymectomy: initial results. *Can J Surg* 1984;**27**:303.

32 Wainwright AP, Brodrick PM. Suxamethonium in myasthenia gravis. *Anaesthesia* 1987;**42**:50.

33 Hunter JM, Bell CF, Florence AM, *et al*. Vecuronium in the myasthenic patient. *Anaesthesia* 1985;**48**:48.

34 Kim YI. Lambert–Eaton myasthenic syndrome: evidence for calcium channel blockade. *Ann NY Acad Sci* 1987;**505**:377.

35 Miller JD, Lee C. Muscle diseases. In: Katz J, Benumof J, Kadis LB, eds, *Anesthesia and uncommon diseases*, 3rd edn. Philadelphia: Saunders, 1990.

36 Mitsumoto H, Hanson ME, Chad DA. Amyotrophic lateral sclerosis: recent advances in pathogenesis and therapeutic trials. *Arch Neurol* 1988;**45**:189.

37 Auer J, Meltzer SJ. The effect of ether inhalation upon the skeletal motor mechanisms. *J Pharmacol Expl Ther* 1914;**5**:521.

38 Karis JH, Gissen AJ, Nastuk WL. The effects of volatile anesthetic agents on neuromuscular transmission. *Anesthesiology* 1967;**28**:128.

39 Hughes R, Payne JP. Interaction of halothane with non-depolarising neuromuscular blocking drugs in man. *Br J Clin Pharmacol* 1979;**7**:485.

40 Caldwell JE, Laster MJ, Magorian T, *et al*. The neuromuscular effects of desflurane alone and combined with pancuronium and succinylcholine in humans. *Anesthesiology* 1991;**74**:412.

4: Pharmacological interference with neuromuscular transmission

CA SHANKS, IM RAMZAN

Introduction

Drug interactions are inherent in all aspects of anaesthesia. These may be the result of therapy for pre-existing conditions, or drugs administered in the peri-, intra-, or postoperative periods. Some of these are intentional, such as the use of potent inhalational agents during muscle relaxant induced paralysis. Others produce unwanted side effects, a possibility that is likely to be minimised by foreknowledge about potential drug–drug interactions. The clinician venturing to explore the underlying mechanisms of drug interactions involving neuromuscular transmission is immediately confronted with a complex myriad of concepts and challenges. This chapter attempts to outline a survival view of relaxant interactions with other co-administered drugs, with particular emphasis on those with direct clinical relevance.

Basic pharmacology

Drug effects are expressed in terms of intensity and duration of action. For an intravenous bolus dose, these are usually maximal effect and clinically useful duration; for relaxants these might be the "intubating dose," and the "surgical duration," the time interval before return of the fourth response to train-of-four stimulation. Most dose–response relationships for the relaxants are manifested as a sigmoid (Hill type) curve, with emphasis being placed on that dose eliciting 95% depression of the muscle responses to supramaximal nerve stimulation—the ED_{95}. The dose–response curve is based in part on the concentration–effect (pharmacodynamic) relationship, which ordinarily for the relaxants is depicted as

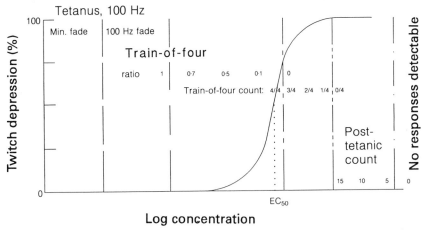

Fig 4.1 The concentration–effect curve for twitch depression with a neuromuscular blocking agent. The thresholds for tetanus, train-of-four, and post-tetanic count have been superimposed

another sigmoid curve. The pharmacokinetics thus characterise the relaxant disposition in the body, usually as a mathematical description of the plasma concentration–time curve. These sigmoid curves are usually shown with log transformations of the dose or concentration (fig 4.1), which makes these curves linear in the 20–80% range of responses. Further transformation of the curve is achieved with probit transformation of the responses, providing linearity from 0·1% to 99·9% response range. This linearity simplifies statistical analysis of the data because linear (rather than non-linear) data fitting procedures can be used, enabling drug–drug comparisons such as relative potency or potential for interactions. Dose–response curves generated for the muscle relaxants, especially those acting via a similar mechanism, are, by and large, parallel to each other.

Drug interactions with the relaxants may alter either their pharmacokinetics or their pharmacodynamics. One example of a pharmacokinetic interaction is the alteration of suxamethonium (succinylcholine) biodegradation by agents that inhibit plasma cholinesterase, resulting in higher plasma concentrations of suxamethonium and hence prolonged neuromuscular blockade. The pharmacodynamic interaction between a non-depolarising relaxant and an inhalational anaesthetic agent at the neuromuscular junction can be depicted as a leftward shift in the concentration–effect curve (fig 4.1).

Several terms are used commonly to describe the extent of such drug interactions. *Addition* is when the half dose (ED_{50}) of relaxant A and the half dose of relaxant B result in a response equivalent to or equi-effective as a full dose of either, and *synergism* is when the result (response or effectiveness) is greater than expected. For agents without particular neuromuscular effect, *antagonism* is the reduction of the relaxant effect, such as with neostigmine, and *potentiation* is the term used for interactions

59

where the intensity of blockade is increased, such as with isoflurane or other agents that also inhibit neuromuscular transmission.

Neuromuscular transmission and neuromuscular blockade

Quantification of relative effectiveness of neuromuscular blockers is difficult, because there is a range of sensitivity in the muscular responses to relaxant induced paralysis, even within the same muscle group. It is the response of those fibres unaffected by the relaxant drugs that we observe in assessment of a train-of-four ratio. Differences in the response of the various muscle groups are considerable: the resistance of the respiratory muscles is well known; and the sensitivity of the ocular muscles is evident in the postanaesthesia recovery room, where diplopia is frequently discovered following apparently adequate reversal of pancuronium.[1]

Relaxants block neuromuscular transmission at the interface of the motor nerve terminals with the striated muscle membrane. The depolarising relaxant, suxamethonium, resembles acetylcholine chemically. As it occupies the receptors for a considerably longer period of time, making them unavailable for further depolarisation, the muscle can no longer respond to the released acetylcholine. The non-depolarising relaxants compete with acetylcholine for the receptors situated either on the nerve terminal (prejunctional) or on the muscle membrane (postjunctional). The all or none response of the anterior horn cell is an electrical response propagated along its axon. This excitation spreads along the terminal nerve branches which end in a specialised region, the neuromuscular junction. Arrival of the nerve impulse results in the coordinated release of acetylcholine into the cleft, where this neurotransmitter (an ester) can combine with its receptors, or be destroyed by true (or acetyl) cholinesterase. The five subunits of the ion channel are arranged like a rosette around the central pore. When the receptor sites of the two α units are both occupied by acetylcholine, the ion channel opens. Although this is an all or none (on/off) response, it forms the basis for biological amplification, generating a total condition of many ion channels in time and space. If the flux of sodium, potassium, and calcium ions reaches a sufficient magnitude, the muscle membrane responds to the depolarisation with its own all or none action potential. Its generation at the sarcomere results in the calcium driven contraction of the muscle fibre. Supramaximal stimulation of a motor nerve results in the combined condition of many muscle fibres, with the transient response recordable with electromyography as a compound action potential. The resultant muscle contraction lasts for much longer, some 200 milliseconds, and is readily used clinically in the assessment of neuromuscular blockade.

Pharmacological interference with neuromuscular transmission can be envisaged at any stage of this process. The sudden complaints of the surgeon commencing traction at peritoneal closure may be diminished by deepening anaesthesia with an agent acting centrally, such as thiopentone (thiopental). With such breakthrough stimulation, an increase in the depth of anaesthesia could result in a reduction in the release of acetylcholine from the motor nerve and an immediate increased surgical relaxation. Many drugs depress electrically excitable membranes, including those of nerve and muscle, directly affecting conduction. Others affect neural synthesis, storage, release, or uptake of acetylcholine at neuromuscular junctions. Acetylcholine is required on both α subunits of the acetylcholine receptor for the ion channel to open; drugs need to occlude only one of these ion channels to make the receptor unresponsive. Other drugs attach themselves to separate binding sites elsewhere on the receptor pentamere, perhaps altering the time period for which the channel remains open. The channel can be blocked internally by a drug molecule obstructing the lumen, or externally by distortion of its walls, when lipid soluble agents cause deformation of the surrounding cell membrane. Other drugs have their action at the nerve ending or the sarcomere by interfering with calcium transport or availability. High concentrations of volatile anaesthetics depress the "excitation–contraction coupling" of the muscle fibres; even higher concentrations directly depress the actin–myosin contractile elements.

Pharmacokinetic interactions

Cholinesterase inhibition

Suxamethonium (succinylcholine) is usually administered in doses some three to five times its ED_{95}, maximising the rate of onset of blockade. Its expected brevity of effect may not occur when the action of pseudocholinesterase is impaired, as occurs with exposure to some of the insecticides. The neuromuscular junctions are then flooded with high suxamethonium concentrations for a longer time than projected. Variable enhancement of the duration of action of suxamethonium is found with anticholinesterases, such as neostigmine and edrophonium. Neostigmine is often successful when used for reversal of desensitising (phase II) neuromuscular blockade. Ecothiophate, administered daily into the eye for the treatment of glaucoma, causes an irreversible inhibition of the enzyme.[2] Agents producing temporary enzyme inhibition, as in the "extension" of suxamethonium paralysis with tetrahydroaminoacridine (THA), have become clinically unfashionable. Bambuterol is a long acting bronchodilator which, because of a selective plasma cholinesterase inhibiting action, is slowly bioconverted into terbutaline. Bambuterol prolonged the duration of action of a single dose of suxamethonium, and produced phase II block in some patients.[3] This prolongation was seen in patients heterozygous for the abnormal form of plasma cholinesterase.[4] The non-depolarising relaxant, mivacurium, is also destroyed by pseudocholinesterase, and the presence of atypical forms of this enzyme has been associated with prolonged paralysis. However, the *cis–cis* isomer of mivacurium does not accumulate in patients with low serum cholinesterase activity.[5] The administration of purified human pseudo (butyryl) cholinesterase to cats resulted in a shift, to the right, of the dose–response curves for mivacurium.[6]

The efficacy of, or even the need or requirement for, reversal of neuromuscular blockade with an anticholinesterase is still under discussion. Administration of edrophonium appears to be associated with an increase in plasma concentrations of mivacurium (DM Fisher, personal communication). When neostigmine, pyridostigmine, or edrophonium was administered before a dose of mivacurium, the maximum block was less intense, and the recovery times were reduced.[7]

Cardiovascular influences

Circulation is an important factor in the speed of onset of neuromuscular blockade. Cardiac failure increases both the arm to arm circulation time, and the interval from injection to the onset of suxamethonium paralysis.[8] Mechanical augmentation of blood flow to muscle decreased the onset time of gallamine but not its rate of recovery.[9] Neither cardiovascular depression with the induction agents (see below) nor altered thenar muscle blood flow with isoflurane appears to produce major changes in the time course of paralysis with vecuronium.[10]

Hepatic and/or renal failure may result in reduced removal of a non-depolarising neuromuscular blocking agent via these organs of elimination; with large or multiple doses, paralysis may be prolonged. Although many therapeutic agents result in reduction of hepatic and renal blood flow, such changes are rarely clinically significant. In those patients whose intravenous anaesthesia was supplemented with isoflurane, rather than with halothane or midazolam, the plasma clearance of atracurium was increased.[11] No clear explanation was offered for this specific effect on atracurium elimination as compared with other neuromuscular blocking agents.

Patients undergoing coronary artery surgery were randomised according to the administration of low dose dopamine.[12] Although this did not alter systemic haemodynamics, low dose dopamine increased the renal elimination of pancuronium by an increase in glomerular filtration rate; the overall pharmacokinetics of pancuronium did not differ between control and dopamine groups.

Pharmacodynamic interactions

Pharmacological interference with neuromuscular transmission can occur at any part of the physiological pathway; enhancement of neuromuscular blockade can take place at more than one site.

Inhalational agents

The potent inhalational agents produce a dose dependent potentiation of the action of the non-depolarising relaxants. Isoflurane and enflurane are more potent in this respect than halothane for equivalent anaesthetic effects (multiples of minimum effective alveolar concentrations or MACs).[13] The converse, an alteration of MAC by the non-depolarising relaxants, has not been confirmed.[14] Enflurane administration was associated with a time dependent increase in sensitivity to the action of the relaxants.[15] Similarly, the interaction between atracurium and enflurane was found to be time dependent.[16] Isoflurane and halothane have no effect on the muscle twitch response when administered in the absence of relaxants.[13] The extent of potentiation by the inhalational agents is variable, but most studies report a reduction in dose requirements of about 40% compared with those observed during balanced (nitrous oxide–opioid) anaesthesia.

Suxamethonium

Desflurane both depresses neuromuscular function and augments the action of suxamethonium.[17] The ED_{50} doses (the mean effective dose, to obtain 50% paralysis) of suxamethonium during desflurane and isoflurane anaesthesia were reduced to 0·13 and 0·12 mg/kg, respectively. Suxamethonium produced more profound block during isoflurane anaesthesia than with halothane.[18] The development of phase II block is related to the total dose of suxamethonium administered. This occurred sooner, and at a lower suxamethonium dose, during enflurane, halothane, and isoflurane anaesthesia.[19–21] Compared with patients anaesthetised with enflurane or halothane, a greater cumulative dose of suxamethonium was required to produce phase II block during fentanyl–nitrous oxide anaesthesia.[22]

Mivacurium

Dose–response relationships of mivacurium in adult patients were compared during nitrous oxide–fentanyl and nitrous oxide–enflurane anaesthesia;[23] the curve generated during enflurane anaesthesia was displaced to the left. Enflurane anaesthesia was also associated with prolongation of blockade. Isoflurane versus balanced anaesthesia had similar results.[24] Enflurane reduces the infusion (maintenance) require-ments: rates, which during balanced anaesthesia averaged 5–8 µg/kg per min, were reduced by about 30%.[25] In children, the dose requirements with balanced anaesthesia are greater than those with nitrous oxide–halothane anaesthesia.[26] Infusion requirements are similarly reduced by halothane,[27] although the doses in paediatric patients are 50% greater than those in adults. Desflurane also potentiates and prolongs the neuromuscular blockade produced by mivacurium.[28]

Atracurium

Although the onset time of atracurium was not affected by the anaesthetic technique, its duration was prolonged more by enflurane than with balanced or halothane anaesthesia.[29] Atracurium infusion require-ments were compared in different groups of children whose anaesthesia was maintained with halothane, isoflurane, or opioids.[30] During balanced anaesthesia an average dose of 9·3 µg/kg per min was required, and the volatile anaesthetics reduced this by 32%. In adults the potency of atracurium did not differ between groups anaesthetised with either halothane or enflurane in nitrous oxide.[31] A retrospective analysis suggested that the dose–response curves were similar to those obtained with nitrous oxide–opioid or nitrous oxide–isoflurane techniques.[31] When a closed loop infusion was used to maintain 90% blockade, dose requirements were reduced from an average of 6·2 µg/kg per min during nitrous oxide–morphine anaesthesia, to 4·9 µg/kg per min with halothane, 3·5 µg/kg per min with enflurane, and 4·1 µg/kg per min with isoflurane.[32] Sevoflurane and isoflurane administered in equipotent concentrations produce similar potentiation of atracurium, vecuronium, and pancuronium.[33] Desflurane 9% is almost equivalent to 1·6% isoflurane in its potentiating effect on atracurium.[34]

Rocuronium

When a closed loop, feedback technique was used to evaluate rocuronium infusion requirements, these were reduced 35–40% during isoflurane anaesthesia, as compared with the intravenous (etomidate, fentanyl, midazolam, propofol, and thiopentone) anaesthetics.[35] In a comparison with total intravenous anaesthesia, the dose–response curves were shifted to the left during anaesthesia with the volatile agents,[36] although the experimental design did not enable full characterisation of the dose–response curves. The neuromuscular effects of rocuronium during halothane anaesthesia were similar to those observed in control patient groups.[37] After two hours of a rocuronium infusion titrated to maintain 95% block, the requirements during nitrous oxide–opioid anaesthesia averaged 9·8 µg/kg per min and were reduced by 40% during anaesthesia with enflurane or isoflurane.[38]

Vecuronium

Vecuronium infusion requirements for 90% twitch depression averaged 0·92 µg/kg per min during fentanyl anaesthesia.[39] Enflurane and isoflurane anaesthesia reduced these requirements by about 70%. Potentiation of vecuronium effect by the volatile agents was greatest with enflurane, followed by isoflurane, and halothane which produced the smallest effect.[40] This potentiation was concentration dependent for 1·2 versus 2·2 MAC. Neither the pharmacodynamics nor the pharmacokinetics of vecuronium in humans differed between groups receiving nitrous oxide–halothane or nitrous oxide–opioid anaesthesia.[41] In contrast, infusion rates of vecuronium to maintain 90% block during nitrous oxide–opioid anaesthesia averaged 1·2 µg/kg per min and was reduced by 36% by halothane.[42] The onset time and duration of action of vecuronium was similar for balanced, halothane, and enflurane anaesthesia.[29] Isoflurane and halothane both potentiate vecuronium's effect in children.[43] The infusion requirements of vecuronium are reduced by 20% in the presence of desflurane, and the duration of action of an intubating dose was greater with desflurane than with isoflurane anaesthesia.[44]

Doxacurium

A dose dependent reduction in the time to reach maximal blockade with doxacurium has been shown; doses should be decreased 20–40% when using enflurane, isoflurane, or halothane together with doxacurium.[45]

Pancuronium

Pancuronium produced more profound block during isoflurane anaesthesia than with halothane.[13] The pancuronium dose–response curve is shifted to the left, in a dose dependent fashion, for both halothane and isoflurane (fig 4.2).[46] Although the onset time of pancuronium was not affected by the anaesthetic regimen, its duration of action was more prolonged by enflurane than with balanced or halothane anaesthesia.[29] Desflurane both depresses neuromuscular function and augments the action of pancuronium.[27] The ED_{50} doses of pancuronium during desflurane and isoflurane anaesthesia were 0·011 and 0·012 mg/kg, respectively.

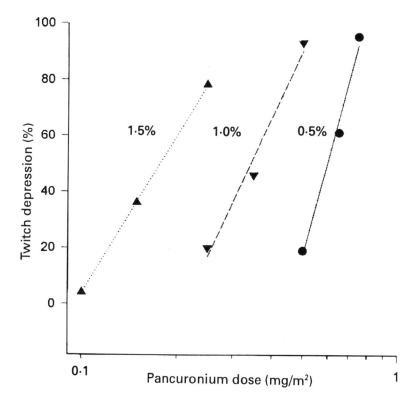

Fig 4.2 Isoflurane (percentages given on the curves) produces a dose dependent shift to the left of the pancuronium dose–response curves. (Data based on Miller *et al.*[46])

Pipecuronium

Although the onset time of pipecuronium was not affected by the anaesthetic technique, its duration of action was prolonged more by enflurane than with balanced or halothane anaesthesia.[29] The dose requirements for pipecuronium during fentanyl–nitrous oxide halothane anaesthesia were similar, but were reduced during isoflurane anaesthesia.[47] Neither halothane nor isoflurane altered the duration of neuromuscular blockade. Children showed similar results to adults. The potentiating effects of halothane and isoflurane on the action of pipecuronium were reflected by the prolongation of the effect following both initial and maintenance doses, compared with the time course of paralysis during balanced anaesthesia.[48]

Other neuromuscular blocking agents

Interactions between the non-depolarising relaxants may be either additive or synergistic. The classic paper examining the underlying theory on this is by Waud and Waud.[49]

Suxamethonium

Many studies have investigated the non-depolarising agents for pre-curarisation, to ameliorate the unwanted affects of suxamethonium. When tubocurarine, alcuronium, pancuronium, gallamine, vecuronium, and a placebo pre-treatment were compared, all drugs were equally effective.[50] Intubating conditions were, however, optimal in the control and pancur-onium groups. Pancuronium prolonged suxamethonium block; the other non-depolarising agents shortened its duration. The dose–response rela-tionship of decamethonium in 12 patients was used as a tool to investigate the effects of vecuronium before use of a depolarising relaxant.[51] When decamethonium was administered after recovery of the single twitch (but not train-of-four) response, the dose–response curve was shifted to the right. The non-parallel shift of this curve from that of decamethonium alone indicates that this is not likely to be a simple agonist–antagonist effect at a single site.

Mivacurium

A larger mivacurium dose is required when given during a partial suxamethonium block compared with when a partial mivacurium block is present.[52] During partial pancuronium blockade there is a marked increase in the duration of action of mivacurium, with a 0·01 mg/kg dose lasting for nearly 30 min.[53] Partial blockade with doxacurium also prolongs the action of a subsequent dose of mivacurium.[54]

Atracurium

Atracurium 0·6 mg/kg and vecuronium 0·1 mg/kg were used alone, or in combinations proportional to their potencies.[55] The half dose combination was more than additive in terms of duration, but onset of blockade was not shortened.

Prior treatment with suxamethonium 1 mg/kg increased the intensity, but not the duration, of atracurium.[56] When the pharmacokinetics and pharmacodynamics of atracurium were compared with and without previous suxamethonium administration, neuromuscular block was more intense, and recovery was slower with prior suxamethonium.[57] Slight increase in the distribution volume was more than compensated for by a decrease in atracurium concentration for a given effect. The interaction between atracurium and suxamethonium was assessed by determining the infusion dose of atracurium needed to maintain a 50% block.[58] The prior administration of suxamethonium did not affect atracurium requirements.

Vecuronium

The prior administration of suxamethonium increased the maximal intensity of blockade induced by vecuronium, and prolonged its duration of action.[59] When increments of vecuronium were administered during spontaneous recovery from pancuronium, the initial increment lasted much longer than subsequent similar doses of the same size.[60] The interactions between pancuronium and vecuronium were studied when 95% blockade was produced in four patient groups by infusing either drug.[61] The same or the other agent was administered at 25% or 50% recovery, in increments, also to produce 95% block. Pancuronium doses required were larger than the vecuronium dose by 15–20%. After pancuronium, both pancuronium and vecuronium had a longer duration of action than after vecuronium; this made the vecuronium increment appear to be longer lasting when it followed pancuronium dosing.

Doxacurium

Neither the intensity nor the duration of doxacurium was altered by prior use of suxamethonium.[62] Doxacurium was administered to groups of patients at either 10% or 95% recovery from suxamethonium, and to a control group; there were no differences between the groups. The paper by Katz *et al*[62] includes an excellent discussion on the interaction between suxamethonium and the non-depolarising relaxants.

Pancuronium

Pre-treatment with pancuronium antagonised and delayed the onset, and increased the duration of action of suxamethonium.[63] Prior administration of suxamethonium did not alter pancuronium's duration of action.[64] Pancuronium–metocurine and pancuronium–tubocurarine combinations were considerably more potent than the additive effects of each of the individual agents given alone.[65] This may have resulted from a combination of both prejunctional and postjunctional blockade. The in vitro plasma binding of tubocurarine or of metocurine was not altered by the addition of pancuronium (and vice versa).[66] Also there was no in vivo displacement of metocurine from non-specific binding sites when pancuronium was administered, because metocurine plasma concentrations did not increase subsequent to pancuronium dosing. The duration of surgical relaxation was shorter with an equipotent combination of pancuronium (0·124 mg/kg) and tubocurarine (0·144 mg/kg) than with either pancuronium 0·07 mg/kg or tubocurarine 0·51 mg/kg administered alone.[67] The dose–response curves for pancuronium and alcuronium, alone and in combination, indicated that their combined effect was purely additive.[68] Following neuromuscular blockade established with pancuronium, the incremental doses of atracurium resembled those of additional pancuronium in terms of duration.[69]

Pipecuronium

The dose–response curves for pipecuronium and vecuronium, alone and in combination, indicated that their individual dose–response relationships were additive.[70] Pipecuronium 10 μm/kg or vecuronium 15 μg/kg was administered as incremental maintenance doses after initial intubating doses of either relaxant.[71] The duration of action of vecuronium after pipecuronium was increased to a similar extent as when pipecuronium was given after pipecuronium.

Premedicants, opioids, and induction agents

Rocuronium infusion requirements were reduced 35–40% during isoflurane anaesthesia, as compared with other intravenous anaesthetics (for example, etomidate, fentanyl, midazolam, propofol, and thiopentone).[35] There was no appreciable interaction between the relaxants and the intravenous anaesthetic agents thiopentone, fentanyl, midazolam, droperidol, or etomidate in cats.[72] Relaxant plasma concentrations associated with 90% block averaged 46% more during anaesthesia maintained with an infusion of thiopentone than during opioid anaesthesia.[73] Propofol anaesthesia did not alter effective relaxant concentrations either. Others have confirmed lack of an interaction between propofol and vecuronium.[74] Propofol at clinically relevant concentrations appears to have minimal neuromuscular blocking or anticholinesterase activity in vitro in rats (Y K Tse and I Ramzan, 1995, unpublished data).

The response to suxamethonium 1 mg/kg was not different in patients receiving either midazolam or thiopentone for induction of anaesthesia.[75] Similarly, the dose–response curves for pancuronium did not differ in these two groups. Propofol potentiated the action of suxamethonium, vecuronium, and pancuronium in rat in vitro preparations.[76] When propofol 2 mg/kg was administered during an infusion of atracurium or vecuronium, the intensity of blockade was increased but the duration of block was not changed.[77]

Patients receiving etomidate for induction of anaesthesia had a shorter onset time after vecuronium 0·1 mg/kg than those receiving either thiopentone or propofol for induction.[78] There was a negative correlation between the onset time to maximal blockade and the maximal change in mean arterial blood pressure. Pipecuronium's effect was unaffected by propofol, etomidate, midazolam, or methohexitone (methohexital).[79]

When the effect of ketamine 2 mg/kg was assessed in halothane anaesthetised monkeys, vecuronium and atracurium effects were potentiated more than those of tubocurarine and pancuronium action.[80] In patients, however, ketamine failed to potentiate either suxamethonium or pancuronium.[81] Others have reported a dose dependent enhancement by ketamine of both phase I and phase II block produced with suxamethonium.[82]

Diazepam 0·16 mg/kg had no effect on the depth of recovery of neuromuscular block produced by suxamethonium or pancuronium.[83] The interactions between intravenous diazepam, lorazepam, lormetazepam, and midazolam, and either atracurium or vecuronium were compared with those in a group receiving thiopentone for the induction of anaesthesia; none of the interactions was clinically significant.[84] Pancuronium infusion requirements were assessed in six patients, using a feedback mechanism which automatically maintained neuromuscular blockade within a narrow range.[85] Diazepam 0·14 mg/kg did not produce consistent changes in the intensity of blockade, effective pancuronium concentrations, or pancuronium requirements.

Premedication with papaveretum and hyoscine (scopolamine) was shown to alter the pharmacodynamics of atracurium, with a 21% reduction in the plasma concentrations associated with 90% block.[86] High concentrations of pethidine in rat in vitro preparations were associated with a slowly developing inhibition of the mechanical twitch response.[87] Morphine infusion did not affect tetanic fade in humans.[88]

Antibiotics

Polymyxin B potentiated pancuronium induced blockade,[89] and neostigmine intensified this potentiation. Recurrence of vecuronium induced block was observed in a patient receiving polymyxin and amikacin as a mediastinal infusion.[90] The interaction of pancuronium with colistin and streptomycin has produced prolonged respiratory depression.[91] Intraoperative administration of gentamicin was examined during infusion of atracurium,[86] and its use was predicted to produce a 25% decrease in plasma concentrations of atracurium associated with 90% block. Tobramycin, gentamicin, and cefazolin were reported to lack clinical neuromuscular blocking or relaxant potentiating effects clinically.[92] Others have reported that gentamicin and tobramycin increased the duration of action of vecuronium, but not that of atracurium.[93] The time course of rocuronium induced blockade was not altered by the concomitant use of netilmicin, cefuroxime, and metronidazole, compared with placebo.[94]

Anticonvulsants

Dose–response relationships of atracurium and vecuronium were compared in 50 patients receiving phenytoin chronically and in 50 control patients.[95] Patients receiving phenytoin were resistant to vecuronium, but not to atracurium. The duration of neuromuscular block with vecuronium was shorter, and recovery was more rapid; the dose–response curve was shifted to the right. As with the longer acting agents, a larger dose of vecuronium was necessary to provide a given intensity of neuromuscular effect when phenytoin was administered chronically. Patients undergoing craniotomy, grouped according to the duration of their phenytoin therapy, were also compared.[96] Those receiving phenytoin acutely, within eight hours of surgery, required an average of 0·06 mg/kg per h of vecuronium; those on chronic phenytoin therapy required 0·16 mg/kg per h. Acute administration of phenytoin in vivo in rats potentiates the action of both alcuronium and suxamethonium; the major metabolite of phenytoin has similar effects to phenytoin.[97] Intubating doses of doxacurium showed accelerated recovery in patients receiving chronic anticonvulsant therapy.[98]

When intravenous phenytoin was used to prevent the fasciculations from suxamethonium, it increased the intensity of suxamethonium block by 50%, but did not alter the duration of action.[99]

Chronic carbamazepine therapy shifts the vecuronium concentration–effect curve to the right.[100] Carbamazepine alone, or in combination with either phenytoin or valproic acid, resulted in resistance to pipecuronium.[101] Unlike previous findings with the intermediate and long acting relaxants, carbamazepine was not found to produce resistance to mivacurium.[102] As with acute administration of phenytoin, acute carbamazepine potentiates the action of both non-depolarising and depolarising agents in vivo in rats (A Nguyen and I Ramzan, 1995, unpublished results).

Antiarrhythmics, antihypertensives, and calcium channel blockers

Verapamil potentiated the twitch depression induced with either suxa-methonium or pancuronium in patients.[103] It had no effect on neuromuscular blockade, however, following α-bungarotoxin.[103] Pancur-onium induced neuromuscular block in vitro in the rat was intensified with nicardipine and verapamil more than with diltiazem.[104] Nifedipine, verapamil, and bepridil did not affect indirectly elicited muscle twitches, but did potentiate the effects of vecuronium in animals;[105] the probable site of the interaction was thought to be the postjunctional muscle membrane. Sodium nitroprusside did not potentiate vecuronium's action. Verapamil and nifedipine both decreased the dose requirements of d-tubocurarine, pancuronium, vecuronium, and atracurium in rats.[106] These effects were reversed only partially by neostigmine or 4-aminopyridine. Neither the onset time nor the duration of clinical relaxation with either atracurium or vecuronium was affected by chronic nifedipine therapy.[107]

A patient undergoing abdominal surgery was given three doses of disopyramide, 10 mg each, for superventricular ectopic beats, followed by an infusion at 25 mg/h.[108] Vecuronium induced paralysis was reversed with neostigmine 2·5 mg, when the twitch height reached 25% of control. In spite of return of the twitch to 100% and train-of-four ratio to 75%, responses to 100 Hz tetanic stimulation remained markedly depressed at 10%.

Calcium and magnesium ions

Eclamptic women in labour who received intravenous magnesium therapy were compared with a control group of non-eclamptic women in labour.[109] Neuromuscular blockade during their surgery was achieved with suxamethonium 1·5 mg/kg and vecuronium 0·025 mg/kg. The intensity and duration of blockade induced by vecuronium were much greater in the group receiving magnesium, and they required fewer incremental doses to maintain satisfactory relaxation. The suxamethonium dose–response relationship was shifted to the right in the presence of magnesium,[110] as assessed by three different techniques in cats. Infusions of calcium resulted in a 7–13% shift in the dose–response curves for atracurium and vecuronium in cats;[111] these interactions were thought to be of minor clinical significance. The dose–response relationship for vecuronium in patients pre-treated with magnesium showed a 25% increase in potency for vecuronium.[112]

Local anaesthetic agents

Ineffective (subanaesthetic) concentrations of local anaesthetics (including cocaine, procaine, and lignocaine) decreased the organ bath concentrations eliciting 50% paralysis (ED_{50}) for *d*-tubocurarine, pancuronium, and suxamethonium.[113] During partial paralysis with nortoxiferine, muscle twitch was depressed 5–8% by all the local anaesthetics tested including mepivacaine, bupivacaine, lignocaine (lidocaine), and prilocaine.[114] This apparently minor potentiation was accompanied by a marked decrease in the tidal volume. Bupivacaine, administered to patients into the epidural space, prolonged the effect of atracurium.[115]

Other

Doxapram

The analeptic agent, doxapram, can be used to stimulate respiration at the conclusion of anaesthesia; the recovery index after vecuronium was longer in the presence of doxapram.[116] No interaction was, however, observed between atracurium and doxapram.[116]

Theophylline, aminophylline, and steroids

An asthmatic man, admitted to the intensive care unit with severe respiratory distress, received large doses of intravenous aminophylline and corticosteroids.[117] Pancuronium was given to facilitate mechanical ventilation, in doses as high as 5 mg/h to a total dose of 800 mg during the two week period. The patient could open his eyes one hour following pancuronium discontinuation. A similar case report suggested that aminophylline produced resistance to pancuronium, but not to vecuronium.[118] In another clinical case, corticosteroids were thought to be the cause of rapid reversal of pancuronium induced blockade.[119]

Azathioprine and cyclosporin

The immunosuppressive agent, cyclosporin (cyclosporine) has been implicated in potentiation of the pancuronium effect in a patient who received a renal transplant and who also received prednisone and azathioprine.[120] The reported antagonistic effects of azathioprine against atracurium, vecuronium, and pancuronium appear to be of negligible clinical significance.[121]

Antihistamines and H_2-receptor antagonists

Neither cimetidine nor ranitidine significantly affected the duration of action of suxamethonium in women in labour.[122] In general surgical patients, however, cimetidine was reported to increase the duration of action of suxamethonium by more than twofold.[123] Others have found that neither cimetidine nor ranitidine changed the duration of action of suxamethonium.[124][125] Although cimetidine pre-treatment prolonged the action of vecuronium, ranitidine failed to produce any such effect.[126] Neither ranitidine nor cimetidine altered the time course of paralysis induced with atracurium. In vivo in rats, both cimetidine and ranitidine have neuromuscular effects producing predominantly a potentiation of paralysis with cimetidine and reversal of paralysis with ranitidine, although the interaction is very much dependent on the H_2 antagonist–relaxant combination.[127-133] Famotidine, however, fails to potentiate either the non-depolarising or depolarising relaxants.[134] In vitro, both cimetidine and ranitidine possess neuromuscular blocking and anticholinesterase activity, but at supratherapeutic concentrations famotidine is devoid of such cholinergic actions.[135]

Anticancer drugs

In a myasthenic patient, given pancuronium 0·5 mg with two increments of 0·25 mg in divided doses, until twitch responses were suppressed,[136] thiotepa (an alkylating agent) was instilled intraperitoneally during spontaneous recovery from paralysis, and the twitch response disappeared immediately. Neostigmine was not effective in reversing this effect, and had even to be continued intramuscularly the next day. A dose of gentamicin resulted in further muscle weakness.

Tamoxifen has been suggested to interact with atracurium in patients.[127]

Cyclophosphamide and some other antineoplastic drugs are pseudo-cholinesterase inhibitors[138] and may affect the duration of action of suxamethonium.

Antiemetics

Metoclopramide acts at the chemoreceptor trigger zone to reduce nausea and vomiting. Its dose dependent prolongation of suxamethonium block is probably via inhibition of plasma cholinesterases.[138] Ondansetron, either 8 or 16 mg, did not alter the time course of paralysis induced with atracurium.[139]

Antirheumatics

Both prostaglandins E_2 and $F_{2\alpha}$ may induce transmitter release at the neuromuscular junction which may be enhanced by indomethacin (and perhaps other non-steroidal anti-inflammatory drugs), thus antagonising non-depolarising blockade induced with d-tubocurarine, and potentiating suxamethonium's effect.[140]

Quinine

The start of intravenous quinine during the postoperative period resulted in good clinical reversal of blockade reverting to marked flaccidity.[141]

Dantrolene

Dantrolene acts principally by interfering with calcium uptake or release at the sarcoplasmic reticulum. Dantrolene and d-tubocurarine produce additive effects at low doses of the relaxant.[142] Recovery time with vecuronium was prolonged, and the rate of recovery was slowed, in a patient receiving oral dantrolene.[143]

Diuretics

Diuretics such as frusemide (furosemide) and mannitol are often used during renal transplantation surgery to induce diuresis in the newly transplanted kidney. In such patients, these diuretics have been reported to augment d-tubocurarine induced blockade, although it was not clear whether both agents were responsible for the interaction.[144] This interaction is of particular significance because renal transplant recipients are already at risk of prolonged neuromuscular blockade as a result of diminished relaxant elimination and/or interaction with antibiotics or immunosuppressants.

Omeprazole

The neuromuscular effects of the newly introduced proton pump inhibitor, omeprazole, have not been evaluated in patients, but in rats in vivo it produces a minor (about 5%) neuromuscular blockade by itself, although potentiating the actions of both atracurium and suxamethonium by 20–70% at intravenous doses ranging between 0·5 and 10 mg/kg.[145] Omeprazole is an optically active drug and it is not known which enantiomer is responsible for this interaction because only the racemic drug is marketed.

Summary

Most drug interactions with the neuromuscular blocking agents involve their potentiation. The increased intensity of paralysis is usually not a problem before the completion of surgery, when blockade cannot be adequately reversed. Given that the shift to the left of the concentration–response curve (see fig 4.1) continues into the postoperative period, the altered pharmacodynamics will be prolonged in time, but once twitch responses can be evoked (for example, train-of-four count returns) the time course of spontaneous recovery thereafter should follow the expected pattern. Conversely, if the factor altering the dynamics can be withdrawn, as with ventilatory removal of isoflurane, then the time course of spontaneous recovery will be shortened.

1 Fragen RJ, Shanks CA. Neuromuscular recovery after laparoscopy. *Anesth Analg* 1984; **63**:51–4.
2 Donati F, Bevan DR. Controlled succinylcholine infusion in a patient receiving echothiophate eye drops. *Can Anaesth Soc J* 1981;**28**:488-90.
3 Fisher DM, Caldwell JE, Sharma M, Wiren JE. The influence of bambuterol (carbamylated terbutaline) on the duration of action of succinylcholine-induced paralysis in humans. *Anesthesiology* 1988;**69**:757–9.
4 Bang U, Viby-Morgensen J, Wiren JE. The effect of bambuterol on plasma cholinesterase activity and suxamethonium-induced neuromuscular blockade in subjects heterozygous for abnormal plasma cholinesterase. *Acta Anaesthesiol Scand* 1990;**34**:600–4.
5 Goudsouzian N, Chakavorti S, Denman W, deBros F, Patel S. Lack of cumulation of the *cis-cis* isomer of mivacurium in patients with low plasma cholinesterase activity. *Anesthesiology* 1994;**81**:A1060.
6 Stout RG, Bownes P, Chiscolm D, Abalos A, Savarese JJ. The attenuation of mivacurium induced neuromuscular blockade by purified human butyryl cholinesterase in cats. *Anesthesiology* 1994;**81**:A1108.
7 Fleming NW, Lewis BK. Cholinesterase inhibitors do not prolong neuromuscular block produced by mivacurium. *Br J Anaesth* 1994;**73**:241–3.
8 Harrison GA, Junius J. The effect of circulation time on the neuromuscular action of suxamethonium. *Anaesth Intens Care* 1972;**1**:33–40.
9 Goat V, Yeung ML, Blakeney C, Feldman SA. The effect of blood flow upon the activity of gallamine triethiodide. *Br J Anaesth* 1976;**48**:69–73.
10 Abdulatif M, Hegazy M. Thenar muscle blood flow and neuromuscular effects of vecuronium in patients receiving balanced or isoflurane anaesthesia. *Br J Anaesth* 1994;**72**:650–3.
11 Parker CJR, Hunter JM, Snowden SL. Effect of age, sex, and anaesthetic technique on the pharmacokinetics of atracurium. *Br J Anaesth* 1992;**69**:439–43.
12 Wierda JMKH, van der Starre PJA, Scag AHJ, Kloppenburg WD, Proost JH, Agoston S. Pharmacokinetics of pancuronium in patients undergoing coronary artery surgery with and without low dose dopamine. *Clin Pharmacokinet* 1990;**19**:491–8.
13 Miller RD, Way WL, Dolan WM, Stevens WC, Elger EI 2d. Comparative neuromuscular effects of pancuronium, gallamine, and succinylcholine during forane and halothane anesthesia in man. *Anesthesiology* 1971;**35**:509–14.
14 Fahey MR, Sessler DI, Cannon JE, Brady K, Stoen R, Miller RD. Atracurium, vecuronium, and pancuronium do not alter the minimum alveolar concentration of halothane in humans. *Anesthesiology* 1989;**71**:53–6.
15 Stanski DR, Ham J, Miller RD, Sheiner LB. Time-dependent increase in sensitivity to *d*-tubocurarine during enflurane anesthesia in man. *Anesthesiology* 1980;**52**:483–7.
16 Withington DE, Donati F, Bevan DR, Varin F. Potentiation of atracurium neuromuscular blockade by enflurane time-course of effect. *Anesth Analg* 1991;**72**:469–73.
17 Caldwell JE, Laster MJ, Magorian T, *et al.* The neuromuscular effects of desflurane, alone and combined with pancuronium or succinylcholine in humans. *Anesthesiology* 1991;**74**:212–18.
18 Miller RD, Eger EI 2d, Way WL, Stevens WL, Dolan WM. Comparative neuromuscular effects of forane and halothane alone and in combination with *d*-tubocurarine in man. *Anesthesiology* 1971;**35**:38–42.
19 Donati F, Bevan DR. Effect of enflurane and fentanyl on the clinical characteristics of long-term succinylcholine infusion. *Can Anaesth Soc J* 1982;**29**:59–64.
20 Lee C, Barnes A, Katz RL. Comparison of the effects of enflurane and halothane on development of phase II neuromuscular block by suxamethonium. *Br J Anaesth* 1976;**48**:930–1.
21 Donati F, Bevan DR. Long-term succinylcholine infusion during isoflurane anesthesia. *Anesthesiology* 1983;**58**:6–10.

22 Hilgenberg JC, Stoelting RK. Characteristics of succinylcholine-produced phase II neuromuscular block during enflurane, halothane, and fentanyl anesthesia. *Anesth Analg* 1981;**60**:192–6.

23 Caldwell JE, Kitts JB, Heier T, Fahey MR, Lynam DP, Miller RD. The dose–response relationship of mivacurium chloride in humans during nitrous oxide–fentanyl or nitrous oxide–enflurane anesthesia. *Anesthesiology* 1989;**70**:31–5.

24 Weber S, Brandom BW, Powers DM, *et al.* Mivacurium chloride (BW B1090U)-induced neuromuscular blockade during nitrous oxide–isoflurane and nitrous oxide–narcotic anesthesia in adult surgical patients. *Anesth Analg* 1988;**67**:495–9.

25 Shanks CA, Fragen RJ, Pemberton D, Katz JA, Risner ME. Mivacurium-induced neuromuscular blockade following single bolus doses and with continuous infusion during either balanced or enflurane anesthesia. *Anesthesiology* 1989;**71**:362–6.

26 Sarner JB, Brandom BW, Woefel SK, *et al.* Clinical pharmacology of mivacurium chloride (BW1090U) in children during nitrous oxide–halothane and nitrous oxide–narcotic anesthesia. *Anesth Analg* 1989;**68**:116–21.

27 Brandom BW, Sarner JB, Woelfel SK, *et al.* Mivacurium infusion requirements in pediatric surgical patients during nitrous oxide–halothane and during oxide–narcotic anesthesia. *Anesth Analg* 1990;**71**:16–22.

28 Tuchy GL, Tuchy E, Bleyberg M, Smith GL, Calvala J. Pharmacodyamics of mivacurium during desflurane anesthesia. *Anesthesiology* 1994;**81**:A1116.

29 Swen J, Rashkovsky OM, Ket JM, Koot HW, Hermans J, Agoston S. Interaction between nondepolarising neuromuscular blocking agents and inhalational anesthetics. *Anesth Analg* 1989;**69**:752–5.

30 Brandom BW, Cook DR, Woefel SK, Rudd GD, Fehr B, Lineberry CG. Atracurium infusion requirements in children during halothane, isoflurane, and narcotic anesthesia. *Anesth Analg* 1985;**64**:471–6.

31 Rupp SM, McChristian JW, Miller RD. Neuromuscular effects of atracurium during halothane–nitrous oxide and enflurane–nitrous oxide anesthesia in humans. *Anesthesiology* 1985;**63**:16–19.

32 O'Hara DA, Derbyshire GJ, Overdyk FJ, Bogen DK, Marshall BE. Closed-loop infusion of atracurium with four different anesthetic techniques. *Anesthesiology* 1991;**74**:258–63.

33 Vanlinthout LEH, de Wolff MH, van Egmond J, Booij LHDJ, Robertson EN. The effect of isoflurane and sevoflurane on the potency and the recovery of neuromuscular blockade by vecuronium, pancuronium, and atracurium. *Anesthesiology* 1984;**81**:A1113.

34 Lee C, Tsai SK, Kwan WF, Chen BJ, Cheng ML. Desflurane potentiates atracurium in humans. A comparative study with isoflurane. *J Clin Anesth* 1992;**4**:448–54.

35 Olkkola KT, Tammisto T. Quantifying the interaction of rocuronium (Org 9426) with etomidate, fentanyl, midazolam, propofol, thiopental, and isoflurane using closed-loop feedback control of rocuronium infusion. *Anesth Analg* 1994;**78**:691–6.

36 Oris B, Crul JF, Vendermeesch E, Van Aken H, Van Egmond J, Sabbe MB. Muscle paralysis by rocuronium during halothane, enflurane, isoflurane, and total intravenous anesthesia. *Anesth Analg* 1993;**77**:570–3.

37 Cooper RA, Mirakhur RK, Maddineni VR. Neuromuscular effects of rocuronium bromide (Org 9426) during fentanyl and halothane anesthesia. *Anaesthesia* 1993;**48**:103–5.

38 Shanks CA, Fragen RJ, Ling D. Continuous intravenous infusion of rocuronium (ORG 9426) in patients receiving balanced enflurane or isoflurane anesthesia. *Anesthesiology* 1993;**78**:649–51.

39 Cannon JE, Fahey MR, Castagnoli KP, *et al.* Continuous infusion of vecuronium. The effect of anesthetic agents. *Anesthesiology* 1987;**67**:503–6.

40 Rupp SM, Miller RD, Gencarelli PJ. Vecuronium-induced neuromuscular blockade during enflurane, isoflurane, and halothane anesthesia in humans. *Anesthesiology* 1984;**60**:102–5.

41 Shanks CA, Avram MJ, Fragen RJ, O'Hara DA. Pharmacokinetics and pharmaco-dynamics of vecuronium administered by bolus and infusion during halothane or balanced anesthesia. *Clin Pharmacol Ther* 1987;**42**:459–64.

42 Swen J, Gencarelli PJ, Koot HW. Vecuronium infusion dose requirements during fentanyl and halothane anesthesia in humans. *Anesth Analg* 1985;**64**:411–14.

43 Wright PMC, Hart PS, Lau M, Brown R, Fisher DM. Potentiation of vecuronium by desflurane vs. isoflurane. *Anesthesiology* 1994;**81**:A1114.

44 Pittet JF, Melis A, Rouge JC, Morel DR, Gemperle G, Tassonyi E. Effect of volatile anesthetics on vecuronium-induced neuromuscular blockade in children. *Anesth Analg* 1990;**70**:248–52.

45 Katz JA, Fragen RJ, Shanks CA, Dunn K, McNulty B, Rudd GD. Dose–response relationships of doxacurium chloride in humans during anesthesia with nitrous oxide and fentanyl, enflurane, isoflurane, or halothane. *Anesthesiology* 1989;**70**:432–6.

46 Miller RD, Way WL, Dolan WM, Stevens WC, Eger II EI. The dependence of pancuronium- and d-tubocurarine-induced neuromuscular blockades on alveolar concentrations of halothane and forane. *Anesthesiology* 1972;**37**:573–81.

47 Pittet JF, Tassonyi E, Morel DR, Gemperle G, Richter M, Rouge JC. Pipecuronium-induced neuromuscular blockade during nitrous oxide–fentanyl, isoflurane, and halothane anesthesia in adults and children. *Anesthesiology* 1989;**71**:210–13.

48 Wierda JM, Richardson FJ, Agoston S. Dose–response relation and time course of action of pipecuronium bromide in humans anesthetized with nitrous oxide and isoflurane, halothane, or droperidol and fentanyl. *Anesth Analg* 1989;**68**:208–13.

49 Waud BE, Waud DR. Internation among agents that block end-plate depolarization competitively. *Anesthesiology* 1985;**63**:4–15.

50 Erkola O, Salmenpera A, Kuoppamaki R. Five non-depolarizing muscle relaxants in precurarization. *Acta Anaesthesiol Scand* 1983;**27**:427–32.

51 Campkin NT, Hood JR, Feldman SA. Resistance to decamethonium neuromuscular block after prior administration of vecuronium. *Anesth Analg* 1993;**77**:78–80.

52 Belmont MR, Lien CA, Abalos A, Eppich LM, Savarese JJ. Mivacurium block with and without prior administration of succinylcholine. *Anesthesiology* 1994;**81**:A1059.

53 Erkola O, Rautoma P, Meretoja OA. Pancuronium makes mivacurium a long-acting muscle relaxant. *Anesthesiology* 1994;**81**:A1061.

54 Patel R, Katz R, Chung A, Foster S, Calmes S. The effect of mivacurium on a preestablished doxacurium or mivacurium block. *Anesthesiology* 1994;**81**:A1068.

55 Gibbs NM, Rung GW, Braunegg PW, Martin DE. The onset and duration of neuromuscular blockade using combinations of atracurium and vecuronium. *Anaesth Intens Care* 1991;**19**:96–100.

56 Stirt JA, Katz RL, Murray AL, Schehl DL, Lee C. Modification of atrucurium blockade by halothane and by suxamethonium. A review of clinical experience. *Br J Anaesth* 1983;**55**:71S–5S.

57 Donati F, Gill SS, Bevan DR, Ducharme J, Theoret Y, Varin F. Pharmacokinetics and pharmacodynamics of atracurium with and without previous suxamethonium administration. *Br J Anaesth* 1991;**66**:557–61.

58 Olkkola KT, Tammisto T. Assessment of the interaction betwen atracurium and suxamethonium at 50% neuromuscular block using closed-loop feedback control of infusion of atracurium. *Br J Anaesth* 1994;**73**:199–203.

59 Krieg N, Hendrickx HH, Crul JF. Influence of suxamethonium on the potency of ORG NC 45 in anaesthetized patients. *Br J Anaesth* 1981;**53**:259–62.

60 Kay B, Chestnut RJ, Sum-Ping JS, Healy TE. Economy in the use of muscle relaxants. Vecuronium after pancuronium. *Anaesthesia* 1987;**42**:277–80.

61 Rashkovsky OM, Agoston S, Ket JM. Interaction between pancuronium bromide and vecuronium bromide. *Br J Anaesth* 1985;**57**:1063–6.

62 Katz JA, Fragen RJ, Shanks CA, Dunn K, McNulty B, Rudd GD. The effects of succinylcholine on doxacurium-induced neuromuscular blockade. *Anesthesiology* 1988;**69**:604–6.

63 Ivankovich AD, Sidell N, Cairoli VJ, Dietz AA, Albrecht RF. Dual action of pancuronium on succinylcholine block. *Can Anaesth Soc J* 1977;**24**:228–42.

64 Walts LF, Rusin WD. The influence of succinylcholine on the duration of pancuronium neuromuscular blockade. *Anesth Analg* 1977;**56**:22–5.

65 Lebowitz PW, Ramsey FM, Savarese JJ, Ali HH. Potentiation of neuromuscular blockade in man produced by combinations of pancuronium and metocurine or pancuronium and d-tubocurarine. *Anesth Analg* 1980;**59**:604–9.

66 Martyn JA, Leibel WS, Matteo RS. Competitive nonspecific binding does not explain the potentiating effects of muscle relaxant combinations. *Anesth Analg* 1983;**62**:160–3.

67 Mirakhur RK, Pandit SK, Ferres CJ, Gibson FM. Time course of muscle relaxation with a combination of pancuronium and tubocurarine. *Anesth Analg* 1984;**63**:437–40.

68 Shanks CA. Dose–response curves for alcuronium and pancuronium alone and in combination. *Anaesth Intensive Care* 1982;**10**:248–51.

69 Whalley DG, Lewis B, Bedocs NM. Recovery of neuromuscular function after atracurium and pancuronium maintenance of pancuronium block. *Can J Anaesth* 1994;**41**:31–5.

70 Naguib M, Abdulatif M. Isobolographic and dose–response analysis of the interaction between pipecuronium and vecuronium. *Br J Anaesth* 1993;**71**:556–60.

71 Smith I, White PF. Pipecuronium-induced prolongation of vecuronium neuromuscular block. *Br J Anaesth* 1993;**70**:446–8.

72 Khuenl-Brady KS, Agoston S, Miller RD. Interaction of ORG 9426 and some of the clinically used intravenous anaesthetic agents in the cat. *Acta Anaesthesiol Scand* 1992;**36**:260–3.

73 Beemer GH, Bjorksten AR, Crankshaw DP. Pharmacodynamics of atracurium during propofol, thiopentone and opioid anaesthesia. *Br J Anaesth* 1990;**65**:675–83.

74 McCarthy GJ, Mirakhur RK, Pandit SK. Lack of interaction between propofol and vecuronium. *Anesth Analg* 1992;**75**:536–8.

75 Cronnelly R, Morris RB. Comparison of thiopental and midazolam on the neuromuscular responses to succinylcholine or pancuronium in humans. *Anesth Analg* 1983;**62**:75–7.

76 Fragen RJ, Booij LH, van der Pol F, Robertson EN, Crul JF. Interactions of diisopropyl pheno (ICI 35868) with suxamethonium, vecuronium and pancuronium *in vitro. Br J Anaesth* 1983;**55**:433–6.

77 Robertson EN, Fragen RJ, Booij LH, van Egmond J, Crul JF. Some effects of diisopropyl phenol (ICI 35868) on the pharmacodynamics of atracurium and vecuronium in anaesthetized man. *Br J Anaesth* 1983;**55**:723–8.

78 Gill RS, Scott RP. Etomidate shortens the onset time of neuromuscular block. *Br J Anaesth* 1992;**69**:444–6.

79 Dutre P, Rolly G, Vermeulen H. Effect of intravenous hypnotics on the actions of pipecuronium. *Eur J Anaesthesiol* 1992;**9**:313–17.

80 Tsai SK, Lee C. Ketamine potentiates nondepolarizing neuromuscular relaxants in a primate. *Anesth Analg* 1989;**68**:5–8.

81 Johnston RR, Miller RD, Way WL. The interaction of ketamine with d-tubocurarine, pancuronium, and succinylcholine in man. *Anesth Analg* 1974;**53**:496–501.

82 Tsai SK, Lee CM, Tran B. Ketamine enhances phase I and phase II neuromuscular block of succinylcholine. *Can J Anaesth* 1989; **36**:120–3.

83 Bradhsaw EG, Maddison S. Effect of diazepam at the neuromuscular junction. A clinical study. *Br J Anaesth* 1979;**51**:955–60.

84 Driessen JJ, Crul JF, Vree TB, van Egmond J, Booij LH. Benzodiazepines and neuromuscular blocking drugs in patients. *Acta Anaesthesiol Scand* 1986;**30**:642–6.

85 Asbury AJ, Henderson PD, Brown BH, Turner DJ, Linkens DA. Effect of diazepam on pancuronium-induced neuromuscular blockade maintained by a feedback system. *Br J Anaesth* 1981;**53**:859–63.

86 Beemer GH, Bjorksten AR. Pharmacodynamics of atracurium in clinical practice. Effect of plasma potassium patient demographics and concurrent medication. *Anesth Analg* 1993;**76**:1288–95.

87 Boros M, Chaudhry IA, Nagashima H, Duncalf RM, Sherman EH, Foldes FF. Myoneural effects of pethidine and droperidol. *Br J Anaesth* 1984;**56**:195–202.

88 Duke PC, Johns CH, Pinsky C, Goertzen P. The effect of morphine on human neuromuscular transmission. *Can Anaesth Soc J* 1979;**26**:201–5.

89 Van Nyhuis LS, Miller RD, Fogdall RP. The interaction between d-tubocurarine, pancuronium, polymyxin B, and neostigmine on neuromuscular function. *Anesth Analg* 1976;**55**:224–8.

90 Kronenfeld MA, Thomas SJ, Turndorf H. Recurrence of neuromuscular blockade after reversal of vecuronium in a patient receiving polymyxin/amikacin sternal irrigation. *Anesthesiology* 1986;**65**:93–4.

91 Giala MM, Paradelis AG. Two cases of prolonged respiratory depression due to interaction of pancuronium with colistin and streptomycin. *J Antimicrob Chemother* 1979;**5**:234–5.

92 Lippmann M, Yang E, Au E, Lee C. Neuromuscular blocking effects of tobramycin, gentamicin, and cefazolin. *Anesth Analg* 1982;**61**:767–70.

93 Dupuis JY, Martin R, Tetrault JP. Atracurium and vecuronium interaction with gentamicin and tobramycin. *Can J Anaesth* 1989;**36**:407–11.

94 Cooper R, Maddineni VR, Mirakhur RK. Clinical study of interaction between

rocuronium and some commonly used antimicrobial agents. *Eur J Anaesthesiol* 1993;**10**:331–5.

95 Ornstein E, Matteo RS, Schwartz AE, Silverberg PA, Young WL, Diaz J. The effect of phenytoin on the magnitude and duration of neuromuscular block following atracurium or vecuronium. *Anesthesiology* 1987;**67**:191–6.

96 Baumgardner JE, Bagshaw R. Acute versus chronic phenytoin therapy and neuromuscular blockade. *Anaesthesia* 1990;**45**:493–4.

97 Heffernan D, Ramzan I. Acute *in vivo* pharmacodynamic interaction of phenytoin and its metabolite, p-HPPH with neuromuscular blockers in rats. *Pharmaceutical and Pharmacological Letters* 1994;**3**:209–12.

98 Ornstein E, Matteo RS, Weinstein JA, Halevy JD, Young WL, Abou-Donia MM. Accelerated recovery from doxacurium-induced neuromuscular blockade in patients receiving chronic anticonvulsant therapy. *J Clin Anesth* 1991;**3**:108–11.

99 Hartman GS, Fiamengo SA, Riker Jr WF. Succinylcholine mechanism of fasciculations and their prevention by d-tubocurarine or diphenylhydantoin. *Anesthesiology* 1986;**65**:405–13.

100 Alloul K, Varin F, Chutway F, Ebrahim Z, Whalley D. Carbamazepine effect on pharmacokinetic-pharmacodynamic modeling in anesthetized patients. *Anesthesiology* 1994;**81**:A414.

101 Jellish WS, Modica PA, Tempelhoff R. Accelerated recovery from pipecuronium in patients treated with chronic anticonvulsant therapy. *J Clin Anesth* 1993;**5**:105–8.

102 Spacek A, Neiger FX, Katz RL, Watkins WD, Spiss CK. The influence of chronic anticonvulsant therapy with carbamazepine on mivacurium-induced neuromuscular blockade. *Anesthesiology* 1994;**81**:A1063.

103 Durant NN, Nguyen N, Katz RL. Potentiation of neuromuscular blockade by verapamil. *Anesthesiology* 1984;**60**:298–303.

104 Salvador A, del-Pozo E, Carlos R, Baeyens JM. Differential effects of calcium channel blocking agents on pancuronium- and suxamethonium-induced neuromuscular blockade. *Br J Anaesth* 1988;**60**:495–9.

105 Anderson KA, Marshall RJ. Interactions between calcium entry blockers and vecuronium bromide in anaesthetized cats. *Br J Anaesth* 1985;**57**:775–81.

106 Bikhazi GB, Leung I, Flores C, Mikati HM, Foldes FF. Potentiation of neuromuscular blocking agents by calcium channel blockers in rats. *Anesth Analg* 1988;**67**:1–8.

107 Bell PF, Mirakhur RK, Elliott P. Onset and duration of clinical relaxation of atracurium and vecuronium in patients on chronic nifedipine therapy. *Eur J Anaesthesiol* 1989;**6**:343–6.

108 Baurain M, Barvais L, d'Hollander A, Hennart D. Impairment of the antagonism of vecuronium-induced paralysis and intra-operative disopyramide administration. *Anaesthesia* 1989;**44**:34–6.

109 Baraka A, Yazigi A. Neuromuscular interaction of magnesium with succinylcholine–vecuronium sequence in the eclamptic parturient. *Anesthesiology* 1987;**67**:806–8.

110 Tsai SK, Huang SW, Lee TY. Neuromuscular interactions between suxamethonium and magnesium sulphate in the cat. *Br J Anaesth* 1994;**72**:674–8.

111 Gramstad L, Hysing ES. Effect of ionized calcium on the neuromuscular blocking actions of atracurium and vecuronium in the cat. *Br J Anaesth* 1990;**64**:199–206.

112 Fuchs-Buder T, Wilder-Smith OHG, Tassonyi E. Dose–response relationship for vecuronium with and without magnesium sulphate pretreatment. *Anesthesiology* 1994;**81**:A1118.

113 Telivuo L, Katz RL. The effects of modern intravenous local analgesics on respiration during partial neuromuscular block in man. *Anaesthesia* 1970;**25**:305.

114 Toft P, Kirkegaard-Nielsen H, Severinsen I, Helbo-Hansen HS. Effect of epidurally administered bupivacaine on atracurium-induced neuromuscular blockade. *Acta Anaesthesiol Scand* 1990;**34**:649–52.

115 Cooper R, McCarthy G, Mirakhur RK, Maddineni VR. Effect of doxapram on the rate of recovery from atracurium and vecuronium neuromuscular block. *Br J Anaesth* 1992;**68**:527–8.

116 Azar I, Kumar D, Betcher AM. Resistance to pancuronium in an asthmatic patient treated with aminophylline and steroids. *Can Anaesth Soc J* 1982;**29**:280–2.

117 Daller JA, Erstad B, Rosado L, Otto C, Putnam CW. Aminophylline antagonizes the neuromuscular blockade of pancuronium but not vecuronium. *Crit Care Med* 1991;**19**:983–5.

118 Laflin MF. Interaction of pancuronium and corticosteroids. *Anesthesiology* 1977;**47**: 471–2.
119 Crosby E, Robblee JA. Cyclosporine–pancuronium interaction in a patient with a renal allograft. *Can J Anaesth* 1988;**35**:300–2.
120 Gramstad L. Atracurium, vecuronium and pancuronium in end-stage renal failure. Dose–response properties and interactions with azathioprine. *Br J Anaesth* 1987; **59**:995–1003.
121 Bogod DG, Oh TE, The effect of H₂ antagonists on duration of action of suxamethonium in the parturient. *Anaesthesia* 1989;**44**:591–3.
122 Kambam RJ, Dymond R, Krestow M. Effect of cimetidine on duration of action of succinylcholine. *Anesth Analg* 1987:**6**:191–2.
123 Woodworth GE, Sears DH, Grove TM, ruff RH, Kosek PS, Katz RL. The effect of cimetidine and ranitidine on the duration of action of succinylcholine. *Anesth Analg* 1989;**68**:295–7.
124 Stirt JA, Sperry RJ, DiFazio CA. Cimetidine and succinylcholine. Potential interaction and effect on neuromuscular blockade in man. *Anesthesiology* 1988;**69**:607–8.
125 McCarthy G, Mirakhur RK, Elliot P, Wright J. Effect of H₂-receptor antagonist pretreatment on vecuronium- and atracurium-induced neuromuscular block. *Br J Anaesth* 1991;**66**:713–15.
126 Mishra Y, Ramzan I. Interaction between succinylcholine and cimetidine in rats. *Can J Anaesth* 1992;**39**:370–4.
127 Law SC, Ramzan I, Brandom B, Cook DR. Intravenous ranitidine antagonizes intense atracurium-induced neuromuscular blockade in rats. *Anesth Analg* 1989;**69**:611–13.
128 Mishra Y, Ramzan I. Enhancement of neuromuscular paralysis induced with atracurium in rats. *Arch Int Pharmacodyn Ther* 1992;**318**:97–106.
129 Mishra Y, Ramzan I. Potentiation of gallamine-induced neuromuscular paralysis *in vivo* in rats by intravenous cimetidine. *Clin Expl Pharmacol Physiol* 1992;**19**:803–7.
130 Mishra Y, Ramzan I. Influence of cimetidine and ranitidine on gallamine disposition and neuromuscular pharmacodynamics in rats. *Pharmaceutical and Pharmacological Letters* 1992;**2**:169–72.
131 Mishra Y, Ramzan I. Interaction between succinylcholine and ranitidine in rats. *Can J Anaesth* 1993;**40**:32–7.
132 Mishra Y, Ramzan I. Ranitidine reverses gallamine paralysis in rats. *Anesth Analg* 1993; **76**:627–30.
133 Mishra Y, Ramzan I. Interaction between famotidine and neuromuscular blockers. *Anesth Analg* 1993;**77**:780–3.
134 Mishra Y, Torda T, Ramzan I, Graham G. *In vitro* interaction between H₂-antagonists and vecuronium. *J Pharm Pharmacol* 1994;**146**:205–8.
135 Bennett EJ, Schmidt GB, Patel KP, Grundy EM. Muscle relaxants, myasthenia, and mustards? *Anesthesiology* 1977;**46**:220–1.
136 Naguib M, Gyasi HK. Antiestrogenic drugs and atracurium—a possible interaction. *Can Anaesth Soc J* 1986;**33**:682–3.
137 Chung F. Cancer, chemotherapy, and anaesthesia. *Can J Anaesth* 1982;**29**:364–71.
138 Kao YJ, Turner DR. Prolongation of succinylcholine block by metoclopramide. *Anesthesiology* 1989;**70**:905–8.
139 Lien CA, Gadalla F, Kudlak TT, Embree PB, Sharp GJ, Savarese JJ. The effect of ondansetron on atracurium-induced neuromuscular blockade. *J Clin Anesth* 1993;**5**:399–403.
140 Hill GE, Wong KC. Effects of prostaglandins and indomethacin on neuromuscular blocking agents. *Can Anaesth Soc J* 1980;**27**:146–9.
141 Sher MH, Mathews PA. Recurarization with quinine administration after reversal from anaesthesia. *Anaesth Intensive Care* 1983;**11**:241–3.
142 Flewellen EH, Nelson TE, Bee DE. Effect of dantrolene on neuromuscular block by d-tubocurarine and subsequent antagonism by neostigmine in the rabbit. *Anesthesiology* 1980;**52**:126–30.
143 Driessen JJ, Wuis EW, Gielen MJ. Prolonged vecuronium neuromuscular blockade in a patient receiving orally administered dantrolene. *Anesthesiology* 1985;**62**:523–4.
144 Miller RD, Sohn YJ, Matteo RS. Enhancement of d-tubocurarine neuromuscular blockade by diuretics in man. *Anesthesiology* 1976;**45**:442–5.
145 Fu C, Mishra Y, Ramzan I. Omeprazole potentiates atracurium and succinylcholine paralysis *in vivo* in rats. *Anesth Analg* 1994;**78**:527–30.

5: Suxamethonium in clinical practice

DAVID R BEVAN, FRANÇOIS DONATI

> Except when used for emergency tracheal intubation or in instances where immediate securing of the airway is necessary, succinylcholine is contraindicated in children and adolescent patients.

In October 1993, a letter from Burroughs Wellcome Inc. containing this statement was sent to all anaesthetists in Canada and the United States of America. This was followed, particularly in Canada, with a storm of protest so great that the company, with the approval of the Health Protection Branch in Ottawa, replaced the contraindication with a warning of the "rare possibility of inducing life-threatening hyperkalaemia in infants and children with undiagnosed myopathies." Not for the first time was the risk of severe side effects of suxamethonium (succinylcholine) (hyperkalaemia, malignant hyperthermia, anaphylaxis) brought to the attention of practising anaesthetists. No other drug used during anaesthesia is associated with such a high incidence of complications, and yet continues to be used 45 years after its introduction. Although all recognise and are aware of the problems, its continued use is a reflection of the failure of the pharmaceutical industry to introduce a replacement that will produce intense neuromuscular block as rapidly and the effects of which will dissipate as quickly. Several possible alternatives have been introduced which may meet some of these goals.

The purpose of this chapter is to review the current place of suxamethonium in clinical practice, to examine its therapeutic and toxic profile, and to determine the situations in which the recently introduced agents, such as mivacurium and rocuronium, might be adequate substitutes.

Pharmacology

Suxamethonium was introduced into clinical anaesthesia in 1949 as a depolarising neuromuscular blocking agent.[1] The ED_{50} (the dose eliciting

50% of the response) of suxamethonium at the adductor pollicis during oxygen–opioid anaesthesia is 0·3 mg/kg,[2] which is reduced to 0·15–0·2 mg/kg in the presence of nitrous oxide.[3] After a defasciculating dose of *d*-tubocurarine these values are doubled. Suxamethonium is metabolised rapidly by plasma cholinesterase and, with an estimated plasma half life of about two minutes,[4] return of neuromuscular activity occurs quickly. After doses used to facilitate tracheal intubation ($4 \times ED_{50}$:1 mg/kg), the clinical duration of block is about eight minutes. The rapid clearance is also responsible for the quick onset because the acute decrease in plasma concentration allows only a brief time for equilibration at the neuromuscular junction.[5] In patients homozygous for atypical plasma cholinesterase, in whom suxamethonium is cleared slowly and has a prolonged effect, the onset of action is much slower.[3]

Continued neuromuscular blockade can be maintained with suxamethonium using either repeated bolus injections (whose effects are short lived) or a continuous infusion. Although, when using a continuous infusion, requirements for suxamethonium tend to change as the characteristics of the block alter (phase II), the technique was very valuable when the only alternative was a long acting relaxant such as *d*-tubocurarine or pancuronium. The introduction of intermediate acting blocking drugs— atracurium and vecuronium—and more recently of mivacurium and rocuronium has, however, made the additional manipulation required with suxamethonium infusions unnecessary.[6]

The neuromuscular blocking action of suxamethonium is probably a result of desensitisation. As an agonist, the continuous presence of suxamethonium at the receptor decreases the receptor's responsiveness.[7] Another possible mechanism of action is the inactivation of Na^+ channels in the perijunctional area. In addition to its neuromuscular blocking action suxamethonium produces in some muscles, particularly the masseter but also to some extent at the abductor pollicis, a sustained increase in muscle tension.[8 9] The cause of this increased tone is uncertain, but it can be prevented with large amounts of non-depolarising relaxants,[10] which suggests that it is mediated via the neuromuscular junction. The increased tone may be responsible for the inadequate intubating conditions which are occasionally encountered.[11] Also, the "masseter spasm" which is associated with malignant hyperthermia is an exaggerated form of this response.

Complications

Most of the complications of suxamethonium are mild and cause inconvenience rather than major injury. Some, such as severe hyperkalaemia, anaphylaxis, and malignant hyperthermia, are life threatening. Many, such as fasciculations and myalgias are the result of agonist activity (table 5.1). Others concern the changing nature of the block (phase II), or its duration (atypical plasma cholinesterase).

Table 5.1   Complications of suxamethonium

Common	Rare and serious
Hyperkalaemia*	Severe hyperkalaemia
Increased intraocular pressure*	Malignant hyperthermia
Increased intracranial pressure*	Anaphylaxis
Increased intragastric pressure*	
Fasciculations*	
Myalgias*	
Myoglobinaemia*	
Masseter spasm	
Atypical plasma cholinesterase	
Phase II block	
Bradycardia	
Sympathetic stimulation	

*Complications resulting from initial agonist activity.

Life threatening complications

Severe hyperkalaemia

Usually, serum potassium concentration increases by less than 0·5 mmol/l after suxamethonium. Occasionally, severe hyperkalaemia producing arrhythmias occurs. This was first observed in severely burned patients, but is also seen in several other conditions, including multiple trauma, sepsis, and neurological disease, after suxamethonium:

- Burns
- Cold injury
- Duchenne dystrophy
- Metabolic acidosis
- Paraplegia
- Radiation
- Brachial plexus injury
- Denervation
- Hemiplegia
- Metastatic rhabdomyosarcoma
- Parkinson's disease
- Trauma
- Closed head injury
- Disuse atrophy
- Infection
- Myelomeningocele
- Polyneuropathy
- Hypovolaemic acidosis.

The response does not occur for several days after the predisposing event and is thought to result from multiplication of immature extrajunctional receptors producing upregulation of the receptor. Urgent treatment is with calcium chloride and sodium bicarbonate to encourage intracellular potassium shift. There have been several reports of hyperkalaemia following the use of suxamethonium in young boys, who were later shown to have Duchenne type muscular dystrophy, and it has been estimated that suxamethonium is responsible for four to six deaths from this cause each year in North America.[12] The source of the potassium that has been observed in the presence of hypovolaemic acidosis is more likely to be the liver than the muscle.[13]

Anaphylaxis

Muscle relaxants are responsible for up to 80% of the acute hypersensitivity reactions during anaesthesia, and suxamethonium is the most common offender.[14] Most reactions are not immunologically mediated, although IgE related reactions have been reported to all muscle relaxants.[15] The cause of severe reactions (skin flushing, bronchospasm, hypotension) can only be determined by skin testing, which demonstrates that most are the result of anaphylactoid and not anaphylactic reactions. Treatment of the acute, severe reaction is urgent and should be with adrenaline (epinephrine), fluids, and the usual resuscitation procedures.

Malignant hyperthermia

Malignant hyperthermia is an inherited human skeletal muscle disorder which is triggered by suxamethonium and all anaesthetic vapours. It is characterised by accelerated metabolism, hyperthermia, hypercapnia, and, occasionally, muscle rigidity. The incidence in children is about 1:12 000 and in adults 1:40 000. Although some studies[16 17] have suggested a single genetic locus on chromosome 19 (near the ryanodine gene), a more recent investigation has demonstrated possible linkages to at least three sites.[18] The primary defect in malignant hyperthermia is considered to lie in abnormal calcium regulation, perhaps in the calcium release channel (the ryanodine receptor, *RYDR*) of the sarcoplasmic reticulum. Diagnosis of malignant hyperthermia is by the caffeine–halothane contracture test performed on muscle biopsy specimens.

Clinically, malignant hyperthermia presents with signs of hypermetabolism—tachycardia, hypercapnia, increased oxygen consumption, ventricular tachyarrhythmia, unstable blood pressure, cyanosis, and hyperthermia. Occasionally these may be preceded by muscle rigidity. The presentation is complicated by electrolyte abnormalities, myoglobinuria, creatinine kinase elevation, renal failure, acidosis, impaired coagulation, and pulmonary oedema. A recent retrospective review has shown that previous uneventful anaesthesia (20%) and an absence of family history (76%) were common.[19] Since 1985, the overall mortality rate has declined to less than 10%, largely as a result of dantrolene therapy. Congenital defects and musculoskeletal surgical procedures were associated with malignant hyperthermia which was described more frequently in the paediatric and male surgical population.

Although definitive diagnosis of malignant hyperthermia requires laboratory testing of skeletal muscle to caffeine, a clinical grading scale based upon the clinical history (rigidity, hypercapnia—$Paco_2 > 55$ mm Hg (7·3 kPa), hyperthermia—$> 38·8°C$, tachycardia), biochemical tests (creatinine kinase $> 20\ 000$ IU/l, metabolic acidosis), and a family history may enable more reliable diagnosis.[20]

Consequences of agonist activity

Initial stimulation by suxamethonium results in generalised muscle contractions visible as fine fasciculations starting in the facial muscles. They may be followed by severe myalgias. The uncoordinated contractions lead to the release of some intracellular constituents to produce mild hyperkalaemia and, particularly in children, myoglobinaemia and myoglobinuria. There are small increases in intraocular, intragastric, and intracranial pressures, but their importance has been exaggerated. Clinical studies have failed to detect any adverse effects when suxamethonium is used in the patient with an open eye injury[18] and the increase in intragastric pressure is matched by an increase in oesophagogastric sphincter tone,[19] so that the risk of regurgitation is probably not increased if the oesophagogastric junction is intact.

Fasciculations and myalgias can be reduced by pre-treatment, defasciculation, with many drugs including non-depolarising relaxants, lignocaine, and benzodiazepines, but d-tubocurarine, 0·05 mg/kg three minutes before suxamethonium, seems to be the most effective.[23] Pre-treatment is ineffective in reducing the increase in potassium concentration or intraocular pressure.

Characteristics of the block

Phase II block

Prolonged administration of suxamethonium, for example, by infusion, leads to a change in the nature of the block. The rate of suxamethonium infusion, required to maintain the same degree of block, gradually increases during the first 90 min of infusion (fig 5.1), and, using train-of-four stimulation, fade in the response develops after about 7–10 mg/kg.[24] The phase II block is associated with slow spontaneous recovery but this can be accelerated with edrophonium or neostigmine. A similar appearance is seen during recovery from suxamethonium in the presence of atypical plasma cholinesterase, but this cannot be antagonised with anticholinesterase.

Atypical plasma cholinesterase

There are several atypical forms of cholinesterase which lead to a very prolonged block (2–3 hours) in homozygous subjects. The complete amino acid sequence of plasma cholinesterase has now been determined using molecular genetics techniques.[25] The cholinesterase gene is located on chromosome 3 at q26,[26] and more than 20 mutations in the coding region of the plasma cholinergic gene have been identified. The concentration of plasma cholinesterase may be decreased in several conditions including

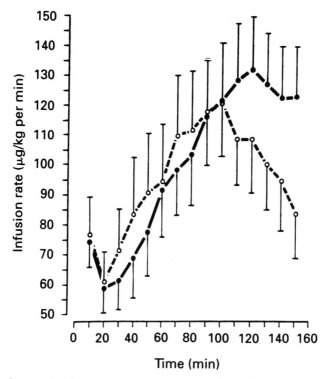

Fig 5.1 Suxamethonium requirement to maintain 90% neuromuscular block during halothane (●—●; $n=8$) and fentanyl (○—○; $n=9$) anaesthesia. (Reproduced, with permission, from Futter et al[24])

pregnancy, hepatic disease, malnutrition, and treatment with pancuronium, anticholinesterases (particularly neostigmine[27]), and ecothiopate eye drops, all of which may lead to decreased suxamethonium metabolism and modest degrees of prolonged block.

Drug interactions

The duration of action of suxamethonium is reduced after defasciculating doses of *d*-tubocurarine so that intubating doses need to be increased from 1 to 2 mg/kg. Suxamethonium tends to antagonise the action of non-depolarising drugs.

Inadequate relaxation

It is now clear that, in several situations, suxamethonium does not produce the anticipated excellent intubating conditions. Spasm of the masseter muscles which may be the first sign of malignant hyperthermia may make intubation impossible. The increase in masseteric tone, which is probably always present to some degree, may lead to imperfect intubating conditions and is the probable reason for the poor conditions seen in 5% of paediatric patients described by Hanallah et al.[11] More subtle measurements of the force on the laryngoscope blade necessary to achieve the best view of the vocal folds suggest that experienced anaesthetists use more force after suxamethonium than after vecuronium.[28] Thus, there are several reasons to look for a replacement for suxamethonium—avoidance of complications and production of better intubating conditions.

Arrhythmias

Bracycardia frequently occurs after suxamethonium especially in children and, particularly, if a repeated dose is given. Thus, it is usual for atropine to be given before suxamethonium in paediatric practice. Bradycardia is a consequence of muscarinic stimulation. In addition, stimulation of the nicotinic endings in sympathetic and parasympathetic ganglia may lead to hypertension, tachycardia, and ventricular arrhythmias.

Alternatives to suxamethonium

Much of the current neuromuscular drug development programmes are concerned with the search for a replacement for suxamethonium. As a result of the intrinsic complications associated with depolarising drugs, it is likely that the compound will be non-depolarising. During the development of the aminosteroids (pancuronium, vecuronium, pipecuronium, rocuronium) and benzylisoquinolinium compounds (atracurium, doxacurium, mivacurium), many of the relationships between molecular structure and activity (structure–activity relationships) were established. In particular, those parts of the molecule responsible for the cardiovascular effects of pancuronium were identified in the production of vecuronium, and the physical properties concerned with speed of onset and rate of recovery were established. It is unlikely that any future neuromuscular blocking drug will be introduced into clinical practice unless it is relatively free from cardiovascular activity. In the search for a replacement for suxamethonium, the onset and recovery characteristics are important.

Onset

It is now realised that the onset of non-depolarising relaxants is inversely proportional to their potency. Thus, of the four recently introduced relaxants—doxacurium, mivacurium, pipecuronium, rocuronium—the most potent, doxacurium ($ED_{50} = 0.015$ mg/kg), has the slowest onset (10–15 min) and the least potent, rocuronium ($ED_{50} = 0.15$ mg/kg), the most rapid (1·5–2·5 min). Thus, doxacurium is most unsuitable to facilitate tracheal intubation for which rocuronium seems to be nearly as rapid as suxamethonium[29] (table 5.2). The rapid onset of suxamethonium is related to its very rapid metabolism and plasma clearance. When metabolism is impaired, that is, in the presence of atypical cholinesterase, the onset is also slower.[3] Large doses of non-depolarising relaxants, by producing a relative overdose, will produce good intubating conditions more rapidly, but at the cost of prolonged block.

The onset of action of suxamethonium is more rapid at the laryngeal

Table 5.2 Onset and duration of neuromuscular block: a comparison of suxamethonium, rocuronium, vecuronium, atracurium, and mivacurium

	Dose (mg/kg)	Onset—t_1 (s)	Duration—t_{25} (min)	RI—$t_{1(25-75\%)}$ (min)
Suxamethonium[31]	1·0	50±17	9±2	2±1
Rocuronium[29]	0·6	89±33	37±15	14±8
Vecuronium[29]	0·1	144±39	41±19	20±18
Atracurium[30]	0·5	150±30	46±8	14±3
Mivacurium[31]	0·2	144±24	21±6	9±3

RI, recovery index.

adductor muscles (important for intubating conditions) than at the adductor pollicis[32] (muscle usually monitored clinically) (fig 5.2). The extent of the block is, however, similar at the two muscles which is different from vecuronium after which blockade at the laryngeal muscles is less intense than at the thumb.[33] The reason for the different time course and intensity of block is multifactorial and probably includes differences in perfusion as well as different sensitivities of different muscle fibres to relaxants. The clinical application of this information suggests that neuromuscular monitoring of the ulnar nerve–adductor pollicis would be a poor guide to the optimal intubating conditions which may have passed if intubation is delayed until maximal effect of suxamethonium at the thumb is achieved.

Duration

The ideal relaxant to facilitate intubation would have a rapid recovery so that, if intubation were impossible, spontaneous respiration would be

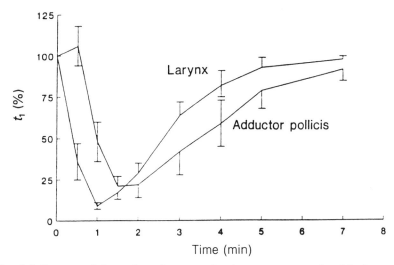

Fig 5.2 Onset and intensity of suxamethonium neuromuscular block at the adductor pollicis and laryngeal adductor muscles. (Reproduced, with permission, from Meistelman *et al*[32])

resumed promptly. All the non-depolarising relaxants have a longer duration of action than suxamethonium, although mivacurium, which is also metabolised by plasma cholinesterase, is the most rapid. Its recovery index is half that of atracurium or vecuronium (table 5.2). However, the onset of action of mivacurium is no more rapid than that of atracurium and in the usual recommended doses intubation conditions do not approach those produced by suxamethonium.[30][31] The duration of action of the non-depolarising relaxants is dependent upon plasma clearance by redistribution (vecuronium, rocuronium), metabolism (atracurium, mivacurium), or excretion (pancuronium, d-tubocurarine, doxacurium, pipecuronium).

Clinical use

Indications

The single absolute indication for suxamethonium is to provide rapid and intense neuromuscular block to facilitate tracheal intubation in emergency situations. These will include emergency surgery in patients suspected of having a full stomach, for example, trauma, acute abdominal surgery, caesarean section, as well as in the relief of acute laryngospasm. Good to excellent intubating conditions can be expected in 60–90 s after a dose of 1 mg/kg which should be increased to 1·5 mg/kg when preceded by defasciculating doses of d-tubocurarine (3 mg, 0·04 mg/kg).

The routine use of suxamethonium to facilitate intubation, followed by a non-depolarising relaxant for maintenance of relaxation, is gradually being replaced by intermediate (atracurium, vecuronium, rocuronium) or short acting (mivacurium) non-depolarising relaxants. Similarly, there is no place for suxamethonium infusions in the provision of longer lasting relaxation. Again, intermediate and short acting agents produce the same effect, more reliably and easily with fewer complications. Although suxamethonium is cheap, this should not be used as a reason to persist with the use of an agent with so many unwanted effects.

Contraindications

The large number of serious unwanted effects from suxamethonium has produced the following growing list of contraindications:

- Burns
- Stroke
- Sepsis
- Multiple trauma
- Hypovolaemic acidosis
- Myopathy
- Muscle dystrophy
- Peripheral neuropathy
- Previous anaphylaxis

- Malignant hyperthermia
- Hypokalaemia
- Open eye injury
- Atypical plasma cholinesterase.

In particular, the poor outcome following severe hyperkalaemia makes those predisposing conditions the most frequent contraindication.

Summary

For 45 years, suxamethonium has been the principal drug with which anaesthetists have produced intense paralysis of rapid onset and brief duration. The development of shorter and more rapidly acting non-depolarising agents is, however, gradually eliminating it from clinical practice. Premature obituaries for suxamethonium have been written frequently. Suxamethonium is not dead, but its role is now reduced to providing intense paralysis to facilitate tracheal intubation in emergency patients with the risk of gastric regurgitation and pulmonary aspiration. Few drugs can boast continuous widespread use for nearly half a century.

1 Mayrhofer OK. Self-experiments with succinylcholine chloride: a new ultra-short-acting muscle relaxant. *BMJ* 1952;2:1332–4.
2 Smith CE, Donati F, Bevan DR. Dose–response curves for succinylcholine: single versus cumulative techniques. *Anesthesiology* 1988;**69**:338–42.
3 Szalados JE, Donati F, Bevan DR. Effect of d-tubocurarine pretreatment on succinylcholine twitch augmentation and neuromuscular blockade. *Anesth Analg* 1990;**71**:55–9.
4 Cook DR, Wingard LB, Taylor FH. Pharmacokinetics of succinylcholine in infants, children, and adults. *Clin Pharmacol Ther* 1976;**20**:493–8.
5 Bevan DR, Donati F. Muscle relaxants of the future. *Semin Anesth* 1992; **11**:123–30.
6 Hickey DR, O'Connor JP, Donati F. Comparison of atracurium and succinylcholine for electroconvulsive therapy in a patient with atypical plasma cholinesterase. *Can J Anaesth* 1987;**34**:280–3.
7 Waud DR. The nature of "depolarization block". *Anesthesiology* 1968;**29**: 1014–24.
8 Plumley MH, Bevan JC, Saddler JM, Donati F, Bevan DR. Dose-related effects of succinylcholine on the adductor pollicis and masseter muscles in children. *Can J Anaesth* 1990;**37**:15–20.
9 Storella RJ, Keykhah MM, Rosenberg H. Halothane and temperature interact to increase succinylcholine-induced jaw contraction in the rat. *Anesthesiology* 1993;**79**:1261–5.
10 Smith CE, Saddler JM, Bevan JC, Donati F, Bevan DR. Pretreatment with non-depolarizing neuromuscular blocking agents and suxamethonium-induced increases in resting jaw tension in children. *Br J Anaesth* 1990;**64**:577–81.
11 Hanallah RS, Kaplan RF. Jaw relaxation after a halothane/succinylcholine sequence in children. *Anesthesiology* 1994;**81**:99–103.
12 Rosenberg H, Gronert G. Intractable cardiac arrest in children given succinylcholine. (Letter). *Anesthesiology* 1992;77:1054.
13 Antognini JF. Splanchnic release of potassium after hemorrhage and succinylcholine in rabbits. *Anesth Analg* 1994;**78**:678–90.
14 Laxenaire MC, Moneret-Vauterin DA, Widmer S, Mouton C, Gueant JL, Bonnet M. Anesthetics responsible for anaphylactic shock. A French multi-centre study. *Ann Fr Anesth Reanim* 1990;**9**:501–6.
15 Kumar AS, Thys J, Van Aken HK, Stevens E, Crul JF. Severe anaphylactic shock after atracurium. *Anesth Analg* 1993;**76**:423–5.
16 MacLennan DH, Duff C, Zorzato F, *et al.* Ryanodine receptor gene is a candidate for predispostiion to malignant hyperthermia. *Nature* 1990; **343**:559–61.

17 McCarthy TV, Healey JMS, Heffron JJA, *et al.* Localization of the malignant hyperthermia susceptibility locus to human chromosome 19q12-13.2. *Nature* 1990;**343**:562–4.

18 Levitt RC, Olckers A, Meyers S, *et al.* Evidence for the localization of a malignant hyperthermia susceptibility locus (MHS2) to human chromosome 17q. *Genomics* 1992;**14**:562–6.

19 Strazis KP, Fox AW. Malignant hyperthermia: a review of published cases. *Anesth Analg* 1993;**77**:297–304.

20 Larach MG, Localio AR, Allen GC, *et al.* A clinical grading scale to predict malignant hyperthermia susceptibility. *Anesthesiology* 1994;**80**:771–9.

21 Libonati MM, Leahy JJ, Ellison N. The use of succinylcholine in open eye surgery. *Anesthesiology* 1985;**62**:637–40.

22 Smith G, Dalling R, Williams TIR. Gastro-oesophageal pressure gradient changes produced by induction of anaesthesia and suxamethonium. *Br J Anaesth* 1978;**50**:1137–43.

23 Erkola O, Salmenpera A, Kuoppamaki, R. Five nondepolarizing muscle relaxants in precurization. *Acta Anaesthesiol Scand* 1983;**27**:427–32.

24 Futter ME, Donati F, Bevan DR. Prolonged suxamethonium infusion during nitrous oxide anaesthesia supplemented with halothane or fentanyl. *Br J Anaesth* 1983;**55**:974–53.

25 Lockridge O, Bartels CF, Vaughan TA, *et al.* Complete amino acid sequence of human plasma cholinesterase. *J Biol Chem* 1987;**262**:549–57.

26 Allerdice PW, Gardner HAR, Galutira D, *et al.* The cloned butyrylcholinesterase (BCHE) gene maps to a single chromosome site 3q26. *Genomics* 1991; **11**:452–4.

27 Mirakhur RK, Lavery TD, Briggs LP, Clarke RSJ. Effects of neostigmine and pyridostigmine on serum cholinesterase activity. *Can Anaesth Soc J* 1982; **29**:55–8.

28 Bucx MJL, Van Geel RTM, Meursing AEE, Stijnen T, Scheck PAE. Forces applied during laryngoscopy in children. Are volatile anaesthetics essential for suxamethonium induced muscle rigidity? *Acta Anaesthesiol Scand* 1994;**38**:448–52.

29 Magorian T, Flannery KB, Miller RD. Comparison of rocuronium, succinylcholine, and vecuronium for rapid-sequence induction of anaesthesia in adult patients. *Anesthesiology* 1993;**79**:913–18.

30 Caldwell JE, Heier T, Kitts JB, Lynam DP, Fahey MR, Miller RD. Comparison of the neuromuscular block induced by mivacurium, suxamethonium or atracurium during nitrous oxide–fentanyl anaesthesia. *Br J Anaesth* 1989; **63**:393–9.

31 Maddineni VR, Mirakhur RK, McCoy EP, Fee JPH, Clarke RSJ. Neuromuscular effects and intubating conditions following mivacurium: a comparison with suxamethonium. *Anaesthesia* 1993;**48**:940–5.

32 Meistelman C, Plaud B, Donati F. Neuromuscular effects of succinylcholine on the vocal cords and adductor pollicis muscles. *Anesth Analg* 1991;**73**:278–82.

33 Donati F, Plaud B, Meistelman C. Vecuronium neuromuscular blockade at the adductor pollicis muscles of the larynx and adductor pollicis. *Anesthesiology* 1991;**74**:833–7.

6: Clinical use of non-depolarising muscle relaxants

ERIC N ROBERTSON, LEO HDJ BOOIJ

Introduction

The development of clinically useful muscle relaxants started with the examination of the arrow poison produced from the plants *Chondodendron* and *Strychnos* spp. This poison was used by some Indian tribes in the northern part of South America. From this poison alkaloids (respectively chondocurine and toxiferine I) were extracted which served as the basis for the development of the benzylisoquinoline type relaxants.[1] In Africa poisons were extracted from *Malouetia bequaertiana*, which was found to cause paralysis. From these poisons, malouétine was extracted, and this served as the basis for the steroidal relaxants.[2]

Brodie, in 1812, demonstrated that rabbits paralysed by curare could be kept alive with artificial respiration.[3] Curare was further studied in frogs in 1850 by Claude Bernard, who demonstrated its effect to be on the neuromuscular junction.[4] In 1857, Lewis Albert Sayre advocated its use to relieve the spasms of tetanus.[5] Curarine was extracted from the calabash curare in 1897 by Boehm.[6] It took until 1912, however, before curarine was administered to a patient for the first time in conjunction with anaesthesia by Läwen.[7] Bennett used curare in 1938 for the prevention of trauma in convulsive shock therapy.[8] In 1939 Francis Sibson attempted to treat patients with rabies with curare. In 1935 King isolated tubocurarine from curare.[9]

The introduction of muscle relaxants into clinical anaesthesia in 1942 by Griffith and Johnson[10] has changed the practice of anaesthesia and increased the surgical possibilities to the benefit of humankind. In 1943, Cullen described the benefits of curare administration during laparotomy under inhalational anaesthesia.[11]

Nowadays, relaxants are part of the standard armamentarium of the anaesthetist. Operations, which until 1942 could only be dreamed of, were suddenly feasible, while the safety of anaesthesia improved because lighter levels of anaesthesia could be used in conjunction with pharmacological muscle relaxation. Shortly after the introduction of muscle relaxation, it became apparent that muscle relaxants also had side effects, can cause adverse effects, and are potentially dangerous drugs that must be administered with extreme caution.[12] Soon it was also realised that numerous factors, related to the physical condition of the patient and to the pharmacological properties of the relaxant, contribute to the deleterious effects observed after the administration of such compounds.[13]

Non-depolarising muscle relaxants are now used routinely in clinical anaesthesia and in intensive care. A wide variety of such compounds has been introduced, for example, d-tubocurarine (1942), gallamine (1947),[14] alcuronium (1961),[15] pancuronium (1967),[16] metocurine (1948 and reintroduced in 1972),[17] dioxonium (1972),[18] fazadinium (1974),[19] vecuronium (1980),[20 21] pipecuronium (1980),[22] atracurium (1981),[23 24] doxacurium 1988),[25] mivacurium (1988),[26] and rocuronium (1991).[27] Although the newer relaxants are nearer to the "ideal" requirements (see box) of a neuromuscular blocker, and provide more flexibility than the older ones, there is still no single compound that can be used in all circumstances. A large number of experimental relaxants have been studied in animals and in a small number of patients but have not come into routine clinical use, for example, tropanyl esters,[28] bulky esters dioxonium, diadonium, anatruxonium, cyclobutonium, and truxilonium,[29] the steroidal relaxants chandonium,[30] Org 6368,[31] Org 7617,[32 33] Org 8764,[34] Org 9991,[35] and Org 9616,[32] and the benzylisoquinolines such as BW 252C64[36] and BW 403C65.

Requirements for the ideal muscle relaxant

Non-depolarising mechanism of action
Rapid onset
Appropriate duration
Rapid recovery
Non-cumulative
No serious cardiovascular side effects
No histamine release
Reversible effect
Lack of drug interaction
Pharmacologically inactive metabolites
Independent of organ excretion (liver, kidney)
Absence of nervous system effects (use in intensive care unit)
Absence of muscular effects (use in intensive care unit)
Stable in solution/ready for use formulation

Mechanism of action of non-depolarising relaxants

The non-depolarising muscle relaxants act by competing with acetylcholine for binding to postjunctional nicotinic acetylcholine receptors in the motor endplate.[37] About 75% of the receptors have to be occupied with a non-depolarising relaxant before muscle relaxation occurs.[38] Such receptor binding is characterised by a constant association and dissociation of the relaxant or acetylcholine.[39] The rates of receptor association (association constant) and dissociation (dissociation constant) determine receptor affinity, and thus are important factors in the "onset" and "offset" of the neuromuscular blockade. As long as there is relaxant in the vicinity of the receptor, it can be occupied again by relaxant, and thus neuromuscular blockade will be maintained. The duration of neuromuscular blockade thus depends on the concentration of receptor in the receptor compartment (biophase). The concentration in the biophase is determined by the plasma concentration and the physicochemical characteristics of the relaxant. There is, therefore, a relationship between the plasma concentration of the relaxant and receptor occupation.[40-43]

The plasma concentration of the relaxant is determined by the pharmacokinetic behaviour of the drug. Contrary to depolarising relaxants, non-depolarising relaxants have no agonistic effect on the receptor (no intrinsic activity); they also bind to prejunctional receptors, which normally keep up acetylcholine release during high frequency stimulation.[44] This receptor blockade thus decreases prejunctional acetylcholine release in a feedback mechanism,[45-47] whereas binding to postjunctional receptors prevents depolarisation of the postjunctional membrane (see chapter 2). Decrease in prejunctional acetylcholine release results in fade in the responses to tetanic or train-of-four stimulation. The amount of fade produced by different non-depolarising drugs varies, and so, presumably, does the effect on the nerve terminal.[48]

Characteristics of a non-depolarising neuromuscular blockade

As the non-depolarising relaxants have no intrinsic activity, depolarisation of the postjunctional membrane is not seen. The clinical effects of neuromuscular blocking agents in patients is characterised by a wide interindividual variability, in both the intensity and the time course of action.[49] Besides anatomical and physiological reasons, such as variability in body size and composition, muscular maturity (age), gender, and variability in plasma cholinesterase activity, many other factors are important. These factors include interaction of relaxants with concurrent medication (see chapter 4), and the physical status of the patient (see chapter 7). A variety of diseases, such as hepatic and renal failure, acid–base imbalance, electrolyte shift, and neuromuscular disorders, can cause pharmacodynamic or pharmacokinetic change in the properties of the relaxant administered. Muscle relaxants themselves have physiological and pharmacological effects, and may interfere with concurrent diseases and co-administered drugs.

The degree of muscle relaxation produced by muscle relaxants and the time course of blockade can be monitored using nerve stimulation and measurement of the resulting muscle response. A non-depolarising block is characterised by decreased contraction force on single twitch stimulation (T1), fade in the response to tetanic (TET) and train-of-four (TOF) stimulation, and in post-tetanic facilitation (see chapter 8).

Pharmacodynamic characteristics of neuromuscular blockade

The effect of muscle relaxants is usually described using a number of parameters: potency (degree of blockade produced by a given dose), latency or lag time (time from injection to first visible effect), onset (time from injection until maximal effect), clinical duration or duration$_{25}$ (time from injection until 25% T1 recovery), total duration or duration$_{90}$ or TOF$_{0.75}$ (time from injection until 90% T1 recovery, or time from injection until a train-of-four ratio of 0·75), and recovery (index) rate (time from 25% to 75% T1 recovery). As these pharmacokinetic parameters depend on the dose administered, they are in general related to a dose causing 95% block of T1 (ED$_{95}$). For endotracheal intubation, a dose equal to two times this ED$_{95}$ is generally used.

Potency, latency time, and onset

With non-depolarising neuromuscular blockers, a correlation between potency and rate of onset appears to exist—the less potent the compound, the faster the onset.[50 51] With low potency non-depolarising muscle relaxants, recovery is fast, whereas with high potency drugs it is slow.[52] This may be related to a high receptor association rate, making dissociation from the receptor more "difficult" (low dissociation constant). This effect may, however, be masked if the relaxant remains in the vicinity of the receptor, that is, if the plasma concentration is not decreasing rapidly.[53] For short duration of action, low affinity of the molecules to the receptor is necessary. This automatically implies low potency. This has recently been confirmed as applicable for the offset of effect of all non-depolarising relaxants, giving, in humans, the following sequence:[52 54] gallamine < rocuronium < d-tubocurarine < atracurium < pancuronium < vecuronium < doxacurium. Some studies have suggested that the rate of diffusion from the plasma to the receptor was more important than the rate and affinity of drug–receptor association.[55] This agrees with clinical data obtained for fazadinium, pancuronium, tubocurarine, and suxamethonium (succinylcholine).[56]

Theoretical considerations indicate that onset time must have a limit, because it cannot be shorter than the circulation time. The circulation time is the shortest latency time possible. The latency time is furthermore determined by the receptor association rate and the amount of relaxant present in the biophase. As about 90% of receptors must be blocked for full relaxation, and thus an equal number of relaxant molecules must be administered, this means that potency is also limited. The probable non-depolarising equivalent to suxamethonium would have, compared with other compounds in the same chemical group of substances, low potency.

A variety of methods to decrease the onset of relaxants, and thus to decrease the delay between administration of the relaxant and endotracheal intubation, has been used with the currently available relaxants. The onset time of an individual compound decreases with an increase in the dose, as has been demonstrated for atracurium[57] and vecuronium.[58] This has also been seen with other relaxants, but this leads to a marked increase in duration of action and side effects. With the longer acting relaxants, the duration of action can become extremely long and unpredictable. When larger dosages of relaxants are administered, there is a frequent need to antagonise the block produced. In a clinical study, the administration of, respectively, 100, 200, 300, and 400 µg/kg vecuronium in 10 patients each demonstrated a decrease in onset time with an increase in duration and recovery rate. Side effects were not seen, however.[59] These results were confirmed in another study in which the onset time of vecuronium halved when 0·3 mg/kg was administered instead of 0·1 mg/kg.[60] The duration of action was, however, increased markedly with the higher doses.

With the "priming principle" technique, one third of the calculated dose of relaxant is administered 3–5 min before induction of anaesthesia, then the remainder is administered immediately after induction. Although it has been demonstrated that the "priming principle" decreases the onset time, there are a number of unwanted side effects. In one study, the onset times after priming with vecuronium, atracurium, and pancuronium were compared with that after suxamethonium. The optimal dose for priming with vecuronium was 0·012 mg/kg, pancuronium 0·015 mg/kg, and atracurium 0·09 mg/kg. The optimal time interval between the doses of relaxant was 3–5 min.[61] With all these relaxants, however, double vision, difficulty with breathing, and swallowing occurred frequently. This has been confirmed in other studies.[62 63] The side effects of priming vary with the interindividual variability in sensitivity for relaxants.

The administration of combinations of particular relaxants, for example, pancuronium and metocurine, gallamine and metocurine, and tubocurarine and pancuronium, can lead to a faster onset of action, but can also lead to a potentiation or prolongation of effect.[64] This can be difficult to predict because of the large interindividual variability in response to relaxants. The mechanism of such an interaction is probably caused by the differences in the mechanism of the various relaxants. As some relaxants have a more pronounced prejunctional effect than others, and some cause more ion channel plugging than others, and as some depend more on redistribution and others more on metabolism to terminate their effects (different pharmacokinetic behaviour), marked interactions are possible. Although this technique of combined administration has been advocated in the past, further studies are necessary before it can be considered safe for routine use. In one such study, it was demonstrated that rocuronium and mivacurium potentiate each other. Not only was the duration of the combination longer, but also the onset was shorter. Interestingly, a combination of rocuronium 150 μg/kg + mivacurium 37·5 μg/kg produced a blockade with a rapid onset (114 s) and short duration (14·7 min); a combination of rocuronium 300 μg/kg + mivacurium 75 μg/kg produced a shorter onset (69 s) and a longer duration (34 min); a combination of rocuronium 600 μg/kg + mivacurium 150 μg/kg did not produce a faster onset, but did lead to a significantly prolonged duration (55·2 min).[65]

The onset time is not necessarily the same as the intubation time. With most relaxants, it is possible to intubate the trachea under excellent conditions when the neuromuscular blockade, measured at the adductor pollicis muscle, is 70–80%. This results from the fact that the pharmacodynamic profile of the relaxants varies with the different muscles. Intubation with rocuronium, for example, is possible with excellent conditions, comparable to those after suxamethonium, within 60–90 seconds of administration of a dose that is two times the ED_{95}.

Duration of action and recovery rate

The duration of action of a relaxant depends on its dissociation rate from the receptor and the amount of relaxant in the vicinity of the receptor. This amount depends on the dose administered, the rate of metabolism, and the rate of (re)distribution and elimination. Most relaxants depend on redistribution for termination of effect. Some are rapidly inactivated in the biophase, or have a built in self antagonistic action, whereas others are metabolised in the plasma or by enzymatic processes in the liver, or excreted unchanged by the kidneys. The recovery rate also depends on the speed with which the acetylcholine receptors are freed from the relaxant. If there is a high receptor affinity (that is, high potency), then the relaxant binds again to the receptor. With a lower affinity, it may diffuse away or be metabolised. The recovery rate is, however, independent of the degree of neuromuscular blockade.[52] Depending on the pharmacokinetic characteristics of each relaxant, organ failure can lead to a change in the pharmacokinetic behaviour of the relaxant. This can alter the pharmacodynamic profile of the relaxant.

Physicochemical and general pharmacokinetic properties of relaxants

All non-depolarising muscle relaxants contain at least two nitrogen structures with an interion distance of 0·9–1·4 nm. At least one or both of these nitrogen atoms are quaternised, and cause the relaxant molecule to be positively charged (ionised) at body temperature. In general, bisquaternary compounds are more potent than monoquaternary compounds. As a result of the ionisation, the relaxants are highly water soluble and relatively insoluble in fat. They are, for instance, poorly absorbed from the gut. Although relaxants are mainly administered intravenously, in some circumstances other routes of administration can be used. When administered intramuscularly, the actual absorption rate is dependent on the site of intramuscular administration. The onset is slower than after intravenous administration.[66] As a result of ionisation, relaxants are often excreted in the urine. There is, however, a wide variability in this excretion between compounds. For example, gallamine is completely excreted in the urine, whereas mivacurium is practically not excreted. Also liver uptake, metabolism, and excretion vary widely among the agents, with extremes of gallamine, which is not eliminated by the liver at all, and vecuronium, which is eliminated mainly by the liver.

The pharmacokinetics of the currently used relaxants can be described in a two or three compartment model, with a rapid distribution phase (distributional clearance) in which they distribute from the central compartment (VD_c) into a peripheral compartment. This is followed by one or two slower elimination phases, consisting of biotransformation and excretion (metabolic clearance). For most relaxants, a two compartment model is suitable and thus two half life times can be determined: the half life of distribution ($t_{\frac{1}{2}\alpha}$) and the half life of elimination ($t_{\frac{1}{2}\beta}$).

As a result of the high water solubility, the volume of distribution of relaxants is small. After intravenous administration, the initial volume of distribution can vary from 80 to 150 ml/kg, and the subsequent volume of distribution (central plus peripheral compartment, VD_{area} or VD_{ss}) from 200 to 450 ml/kg. This is somewhere between the volume of the extracellular water compartment and the total body water in humans. VD_c governs the peak plasma concentration after a rapid bolus injection, and VD_{ss}, the tissue penetration of the compound. These distribution volumes and the clearances of relaxants can be markedly affected by disease states, such as hepatic and renal failure, and cardiovascular disturbances. In hepatic and renal diseases, but also in other diseases, the metabolism and excretion of drugs may be affected, leading to changes in plasma clearance (Cl_p) and $t_{\frac{1}{2}\beta}$. They can also change the volumes of distribution. Disease states are thus frequently connected with changes in the pharmacokinetic behaviour and the pharmacodynamic profile of relaxants (see chapter 7). As drug distribution in the tissues depends on tissue perfusion, the cardiac output is an important factor in the pharmacokinetics of relaxants. Reduction in cardiac output usually leads to a redistribution with lengthening of the $t_{\frac{1}{2}\alpha}$, and a slower onset of action and a greater effect. With increased cardiac output, tissue perfusion is elevated. This means more rapid and widespread distribution. A higher dose is, therefore, needed for the same effect. In hypovolaemic shock, the VD_c is smaller, and thus a higher peak concentration occurs. This leads to a greater clinical effect.

In patients with oedema, the volume of distribution of water soluble drugs is increased. Plasma concentrations of drugs are, therefore, smaller and their effect is decreased.

If the plasma concentration at which a particular neuromuscular block exists is known, the single bolus dose or the rate of continuous infusion, to reach that degree of blockade, can be calculated.[67]

Table 6.1 Pharmacokinetic data in "normal patients" for clinically used non-depolarising muscle relaxants

Relaxant	VD_c (l/kg)	VD_{ss} (l/kg)	Cl_p (ml/kg per min)	$t_{\frac{1}{2}\beta}$ (min)	Percentage protein binding
Alcuronium	0·15	0·35	1·34	143	75
Atracurium	0·05	0·20	6·6	21	80
Doxacurium		0·22	2·76	99	30–35
Gallamine	0·10	0·20	1·2	134	15
Metocurine	0·05	0·57	1·2	360	30–45
Mivacurium		0·11	70	18	
Pancuronium	0·10	0·26	1·8	132	85
Pipecuronium	0·11	0·31	2·3	137	25
Rocuronium	0·04	0·21	3·7	97	
Tubocurarine	0·03	0·25	2·4	84	35–55
Vecuronium	0·07	0·27	5·2	71	70

* Values are rounded up or down.

As surgically optimal neuromuscular blockade is present when 95% T1 block exists, the plasma concentration at which this occurs (C_{ss95}) is of clinical importance.

Protein binding of muscle relaxants varies between 30% and 85%, and is another important factor in their pharmacokinetic behaviour (table 6.1).[68] Both changes in the protein concentration in disease states and binding of concurrently administered drugs to proteins influences the protein binding of relaxants. This binding can alter the volume of distribution, metabolism, and the excretion of the relaxants. Protein binding also plays an important role in maternal–fetal drug equilibration during pregnancy.

Relationships between pharmacodynamic and pharmacokinetic characteristics

A variety of factors determines the pharmacodynamic profile (onset, duration, and recovery) of relaxants in individual patients. Among them are the type and depth of the anaesthetic administered, interactions with concurrently administered drugs, and the age and physical status of the patient. Some of the alterations in the pharmacodynamics can be explained by changes in the pharmacokinetic behaviour of the drug in that particular patient.

Various authors have demonstrated a direct relationship between the plasma concentration of non-depolarising relaxants and the degree of neuromuscular blockade.[40][69] There is, however, a time lag between the plasma concentration change and its clinical effect. The magnitude of this time lag depends on the muscle blood perfusion, the rate of drug diffusion from blood to receptor, the blood–biophase partition coefficient for the drug, and the drug–receptor association/dissociation constants. This means that, assuming muscle perfusion to be equal in all experiments, the physicochemical properties of the compounds determine their pharmacodynamic profile. Onset of action, then, is optimally fast when the drug has a fast diffusion rate, a low partition coefficient, a high receptor affinity, and a fast receptor association. The duration of action is short when the drug–receptor dissociation rate is fast, the drug–receptor affinity low, and the elimination of the drug from the biophase rapid (that is, a rapid decrease in biophase and plasma concentration). In general, relaxants that depend mainly on renal excretion for their elimination have a long duration of action (gallamine, d-tubocurarine, metocurine, alcuronium, pancuronium), those depending partly on renal excretion and partly on metabolism, an intermediate duration (atracurium, vecuronium, rocuronium), and those depending mainly on metabolism (suxamethonium, mivacurium) a shorter duration of action.

Characteristics of individual non-depolarising relaxants

It was originally thought that the basic structure of non-depolarising muscle relaxants required a bisquaternary ammonium compound (pancuronium, pipecuronium). Later it was recognised that a combination of monoquatenary (vecuronium, rocuronium, tubocurarine) and trisquaternary amides (gallamine) can also be muscle relaxants. Many muscle relaxants have been synthesised, and many of them have been clinically tested, but only a limited number are still in clinical use. They mainly belong to two groups: the benzylisoquinolines and the steroids.

Benzylisoquinolines

These compounds contain, like tubocurarine, two benzylisoquinoline groups. In the newer compounds, they are separated by an ester bridge. The benzylisoquinoline molecular structure is such that compounds exist in different isomeric forms, for example, there are 10 isomers of atracurium and three of mivacurium. The benzylisoquinolines are, with the exceptions of d-tubocurarine and metocurine, often metabolised by ester hydrolysis. Common characteristics of this group of compounds are a lack of a vagolytic effect, dose related histamine release, and reversibility by anticholinesterases.

d-Tubocurarine and metocurine

d-Tubocurarine, a monoquaternary compound, is the oldest representative of the isoquinoline type muscle relaxants. It is excreted unchanged in the urine, with the liver as a secondary pathway. A portion of the injected drug is stored in body tissues for a longer period, then slowly mobilised and excreted.[70] The onset of action of d-tubocurarine is slow, its duration is long, and its recovery is slow (table 6.2). The usual intubating dose is 0·5–0·6 mg/kg, maintenance doses are 0·1–0·2 mg/kg. The pharmacokinetic behaviour of d-tubocurarine has been studied extensively (see table 6.1). In burn patients, and in patients with hepatic or renal failure, the duration of action of d-tubocurarine is prolonged. With d-tubocurarine,

Table 6.2 Pharmacodynamic profile of non-depolarising relaxants

Relaxant	ED_{90} (mg/kg)	Onset (min)	$Duration_{25}$ (min)	$Duration_{90}$ (min)	Recorded rate (min)
Alcuronium	0·25	6·0	30	65	30
Atracurium	0·25	6·5	20	35	10
BW 51W89	0·05	7·5	20	40	10
Doxacurium	0·03	7·5	85	120	40
Gallamine	2·50	6·0	50	90	45
Metocurine	0·30	7·0	60	95	35
Mivacurium	0·10	4·0	15	25	5
Pancuronium	0·05	5·0	35	75	35
Pipecuronium	0·05	6·5	60	80	30
Rocuronium	0·40	4·0	15	30	10
Tubocurarine	0·45	10·0	35	95	60
Vecuronium	0·05	4·5	10	25	10

*Values have been rounded up or down.

marked histamine release and ganglion blockade lead to hypotension and reflex tachycardia. Flushing and bronchoconstriction can be observed. Following suxamethonium, a *d*-tubocurarine block is prolonged.

Metocurine is a methylated derivative of *d*-tubocurarine. The ED_{95} is 0·30 mg/kg, and the maintenance dose 0·05–0·1 mg/kg. Its pharmacokinetic behaviour is similar to *d*-tubocurarine, although there is more dependence on renal excretion. It has fewer cardiovascular side effects and causes less histamine release than *d*-tubocurarine.

In the clinic, both compounds are nowadays replaced almost completely by other non-depolarising relaxants. Metocurine is not available in Europe.

Atracurium

Atracurium consists of a racemic mixture of 10 stereoisomers, most of which are pharmacologically active.[71] All isomers, however, have a pharmacodynamic profile and pharmacokinetic behaviour that are different from each other.[72 73] After administration of the ED_{90} dose (0·19 mg/kg), the onset of action is 6·7 min, the clinical duration is 17·1 min, and the total duration is 32·0 min (table 6.2). The recovery rate is 12·0 min.[74] After an initial (intubating) dose of atracurium 0·4–0·5 mg/kg, either intermittent bolus (0·1–0·15 mg/kg every 20–30 min) or continuous infusion (0·3–0·6 mg/kg per hour) can be used to maintain the neuromuscular blockade. Even in intensive care patients there is easy control of the blockade.[75] Compared with other non-depolarising relaxants, atracurium has a short elimination half life (see table 6.1).

One of the main disadvantages of atracurium is that it causes histamine release at higher clinical doses in about 30% of the patients. Slow administration and avoiding high doses largely overcome this problem, which can lead to skin flushing, hypotension, tachycardia, and bronchoconstriction.

It was initially thought that the metabolism of atracurium was by temperature and pH dependent Hofmann degradation into laudanosine, an acrylate, and a monoquaternary ester, which was further degraded to a second laudanosine molecule and an acrylate ester.[76][77] The plasma concentration of laudanosine, in both younger and elderly patients, is, however, highest immediately after injection of atracurium.[78] This is incompatible with spontaneous (Hofmann) degradation of atracurium, therefore another rapid but limited metabolism, proportional to the dose of atracurium administered, must also be present.[79] Thus a large fraction of injected atracurium is degraded rapidly, a small part causes the neuro-muscular block, and leads to a long lasting, slow production of laudanosine. It has also been suggested that non-specific ester hydrolysis plays an important role in the metabolism of atracurium.[73] Neither true cholinester-ase nor plasma cholinesterase has any effect on the metabolism or effects of atracurium. The metabolite laudanosine may cumulate especially if high doses are administered. Laudanosine can cause excitatory effects on the central nervous system in such situations. Atracurium has a slower onset and prolonged effect during hypothermic cardiopulmonary bypass.[80]

Atracurium is suitable for continuous infusion at a rate of 7–8 μg/kg per min.

Mivacurium (BW B1090U)

Mivacurium is a bisquaternary relaxant ($ED_{95} = 70$ μg/kg) which resem-bles atracurium in its structure, has a slow onset, but a short duration of action (see table 6.2).[26] The ED_{95} ($0·07$–$0·08$ mg/kg) dose of mivacurium has, during balanced anaesthesia, an onset of 3–5 min, a clinical duration of 15 min, a total duration of 25–30 min, and a recovery rate of 5–7 min.[26] The short duration of action of mivacurium can be explained by a rapid plasma clearance (see table 6.1). The intubating dose is $0·15$–$0·2$ mg/kg. Mivacurium consists of three stereoisomers, one of which is inactive.[81] Pharmacokinetically, the isomers behave differently from each other.[82] In clinical dosages, mivacurium has no cardiovascular effects.[83] At high doses, there is minor histamine release and some decrease in arterial pressure can occur, with an increase in heart rate. Pre-treatment with mivacurium before suxamethonium administration leads to a marked antagonistic effect on the development of the suxamethonium induced block. Administration of suxamethonium does not, however, influence the effect of mivacurium administered thereafter.

Mivacurium is metabolised by plasma cholinesterase, at a rate of 60–80% that of suxamethonium, into a pharmacologically inactive quaternary monoester, a quaternary amino alcohol, and a dicarboxylic acid.[85] Duration of action thus varies with plasma cholinesterase activity, and a number of such cases showing prolonged mivacurium effects have been published.[86–92] Although during and after cardiopulmonary bypass a 60% decrease in cholinesterase activity is observed, the effect of mivacurium during and after this procedure in normothermic conditions is not prolonged.[93] A case has been reported where a young patient with dermatomyositis and low plasma cholinesterase activity had prolonged paralysis after mivacurium, although the blockade could not be reversed with edrophonium.[94] As edrophonium, unlike neostigmine, does not inhibit plasma cholinesterase, it was expected that edrophonium would be more suitable for reversal of mivacurium induced neuromuscular block. In a prospective study, it was demonstrated, however, that edrophonium is not effective in the reversal of mivacurium.[95] In contrast, another author found edrophonium to be a reliable reversing agent during intense mivacurium induced blockade.[96] A patient with end stage renal failure, and presumably a low cholinesterase activity, had a prolonged effect after mivacurium, although the blockade could not be reversed with neostigmine.[97] This is most probably caused by the fact that the reversal agent inhibits cholinesterases and thus slows down the metabolism of mivacurium. Two recent case reports describe the successful use of purified human cholinesterase to antagonise profound mivacurium induced neuromuscular blockade.[98]

The compound is suitable for continuous infusion.[99] An appropriate rate of infusion is 5–10 μg/kg per min. With such doses there does not appear to be accumulation. Increase in single dose causes a disproportionally small increase in the duration of action, and has no effect on recovery rate; cardiovascular effects may, however, appear. After rapid, but not on slow, injection of larger bolus doses (two to three times ED_{95}), a transient decrease in arterial pressure may occur. This is accompanied by facial flushing and an increase in serum histamine concentration.[100] This occurs in 30% of the cases when 0·2 mg/kg mivacurium is administered.[101]

Mivacurium consists of three isomers (*trans–trans, cis–trans, cis–cis*), of which the *cis–cis* is largely inactive, but contributes largely to the long elimination half life of the mixture. Differences in the pharmacokinetics of the isomers may lead to discrepancy between the pharmacokinetic and pharmacodynamic behaviour of the chiral mixture.[102] The volumes of distribution of mivacurium are comparable with those for other non-depolarising relaxants but the clearance is significantly faster.

Doxacurium (BW A938U)

This bisquaternary compound is the most potent relaxant presently available ($ED_{95}=30$ μg/kg); however, its onset is slow (10–13 min), its duration of action is long (clinical 57–80 min, total 74–128 min), and its recovery rate is slow (32–50 min) (see table 6.2).[25 103 104] Good intubation conditions exist five minutes after administration of two times the ED_{95}.[105] The pharmacodynamic profile is highly variable, and is related to age, obesity, and type of anaesthetic.[106] Proper maintenance doses are 0·005–0·01 mg/kg. The pharmacokinetic behaviour of doxacurium has been studied (see table 6.1). Doxacurium consists of three stereoisomers, is hydrolysed by plasma cholinesterase at a rate of 6% that of suxamethonium, and 40% is excreted unchanged in the urine with small amounts in the bile. The speed of its antagonism by neostigmine is also highly variable. Doxacurium lacks cardiovascular effects, even at high doses.[107 108] Although doxacurium is not associated with histamine release, a case in which cutaneous flush and hypotension occurred has been described.[109] The solution contains 0·9 vol % benzylalcohol as a preservative.

cis-Atracurium (BW 51W89)

Recently, studies have started on cis-atracurium (BW 51W89), one of the 10 stereoisomers of atracurium, with a potency ($ED_{95} = 50$ µg/kg) three to four times greater than atracurium, and a similar time course of neuromuscular blocking activity.[110] This isomer constitutes 15% of the commercial atracurium mixture. Its onset of action is slower than that of atracurium,[111] and is paralleled with less favourable intubating conditions, making higher ED_{95} multiples necessary for intubation.[112] The compound causes an increase in plasma histamine concentration in some patients,[113] but does not lead to clinical signs of histamine release or related cardiovascular effects. cis-Atracurium is metabolised by the Hofmann degradation and ester hydrolysis. Its pharmacokinetics are similar to those of atracurium.[114]

cis-Atracurium can be used by continuous infusion; an infusion rate of 1.4 µg/kg per min is appropriate to maintain a 95% neuromuscular blockade.

Steroids

This group includes the relaxants pancuronium, pipecuronium, vecuronium, and rocuronium. A large number of other steroidal compounds have been studied, but were rejected after clinical testing.

Ever since the discovery of the muscle relaxing effect of the natural substance malouétine in 1960, and the subsequent design in 1964 and introduction of pancuronium as a steroidal non-depolarising neuromuscular transmission blocker into clinical anaesthesia in 1967–70, the steroidal skeleton has played a role in the development of new relaxants. The steroidal skeleton offers a relatively fixed geometry and accommodates high levels of asymmetry and stereospecificity.

The basic structure of the steroidal non-depolarising muscle relaxants contains an androstane skeleton, with 1,2-amino alcohol functions stereoselectively introduced into the steroidal nucleus. This results in two acetylcholine like moieties, which are important for the interaction with the acetylcholine receptors.[115] In pancuronium, acetylcholine like moieties are present in both the A and D rings. Vecuronium has such a moiety only in the D ring.[116] It has been demonstrated that this difference is responsible for the lack of cardiovascular side effects of vecuronium.[117 118] The acetylcholine like moiety at the D ring is apparently responsible for binding the molecule to the nicotinic acetylcholine receptor at the neuromuscular junction sites, and the acetylcholine like moiety at the A ring for binding to muscarinic receptors at other sites. For high potency, it is probably essential to have two nitrogen atoms in the molecule, with at least one of them quaternised. Bowman et al[50] demonstrated a relationship between potency and onset in anaesthetised cats, based on this structure–activity relationship. Compounds with a low potency were demonstrated to have a faster onset of action than relaxants with a higher potency. Combinations of steroidal relaxants interact in an additive manner.[119]

Pancuronium

This is one of the most frequently used non-depolarising muscle relaxants, in both anaesthesia and intensive care. After administration of the ED_{90} (0·06 mg/kg) the onset is 4·9 min, the clinical duration 34·4 min, the total duration 73·2 min, and the recovery rate 31·9 min (see table 6.2).[120] The intubating dose is 0·08–0·1 mg/kg. For repeated administration, doses of 0·01–0·05 mg/kg every hour are used. With continuous infusion an infusion rate of 0·06–0·1 mg/kg per hour is used.

Pancuronium is metabolised mainly by deacetylation in the liver, and thereafter excreted in the urine. The 3-hydroxy-, 17-hydroxy, and 3,17-dihydroxy metabolites are considerably less potent as relaxants.[121] As their concentrations are also low and their pharmacokinetics are comparable to those of pancuronium, they contribute little to the neuromuscular blocking effect. About 40–60% of pancuronium is excreted in the urine and 11% in the bile.

Pancuronium increases heart rate, arterial pressure, and cardiac output. This is a sympathomimetic and anticholinergic effect. It can lead to increased myocardial oxygen consumption and a decrease in myocardial oxygen supply. The sympathomimetic effect may also alter pulmonary circulation and result in pulmonary vasoconstriction, and thus in ventilation–perfusion mismatch. This has especially been noted in neonates.[122] Pancuronium causes no histamine release.

Pancuronium inhibits plasma cholinesterase and thus prolongs the effect of suxamethonium and possibly mivacurium.

Vecuronium

This is a monoquaternary non-depolarising neuromuscular blocking agent, which when administered at an ED_{95} dose (50 μg/kg), results in an onset of 4·5 min, a clinical duration of 11·6 min, a total duration of 24·9 min, and a recovery rate of 9·7 min (see table 6.2). After an initial (intubating) dose, usually of 0·08–0·15 mg/kg, the blockade can be maintained by intermittent doses (0·01–0·04 mg/kg every 20–30 min) or continuous infusion (0·075–0·10 mg/kg per hour). The pharmacokinetic data on vecuronium are given in table 6.1.

Even at high doses, vecuronium does not release histamine and has no effects on the cardiovascular system. The frequently observed bradycardia at induction of anaesthesia is the result of the bradycardiac effect of other drugs, for example, opioids and intravenous anaesthetics.

Hepatic uptake lowers the blood concentration of vecuronium, which subsequently is metabolised in the liver by deacetylation into three possible metabolites: 3-hydroxy-, 17-hydroxy-, and 3,17-dihydroxyvecuronium.[123] [124] The 3-hydroxy metabolite has neuromuscular blocking effects, but is only produced in small amounts. When, however, vecuronium is administered for a long period of time or in large doses, this metabolite may contribute to the blockade.[125] This is seen as accumulation, for example, increase in recovery time. About 30% of vecuronium is excreted unchanged in the urine. The duration of vecuronium induced neuromuscular block is dependent on hepatic function and less on renal function. Its effect can thus be prolonged in patients with hepatic failure and also, to some extent, in patients with renal dysfunction. This can be explained pharmacokinetically.

Vecuronium is suitable for continuous infusion at a rate of 1–2 µg/kg per min.

Pipecuronium

Pipecuronium is a bisquaternary relaxant ($ED_{95} = 45$ µg/kg) with a slow onset and a long duration of action, similar to pancuronium (see table 6.2).[22 126–128] Increasing the dose shortens the onset, but prolongs the duration. There is wide interindividual variability in the response to pipecuronium. Intubation with a dose that is twice the ED_{95} is possible after two minutes. The pharmacokinetic profile of pipecuronium is slightly different from that of pancuronium, with a greater plasma clearance and a larger VD_{ss} (see table 6.1). Once some spontaneous recovery of neuromuscular block is visible, the blockade can be adequately reversed with neostigmine. Edrophonium, however, is an unreliable antagonist for pipecuronium.[129] Pipecuronium has no histamine release or relevant cardiovascular effects.[130–133]

About 40% of the dose administered is excreted via the kidneys and thus the effect is prolonged in renal failure.[134 135] The remainder of the drug is slowly deacetylated in the liver and then excreted in the bile.

Rocuronium (Org 9426)

Rocuronium is a new monoquaternary muscle relaxant with a pharmacodynamic profile similar to that of vecuronium and atracurium (see table 6.2). It is stable in solution. The ED_{90} of 0·3–0·4 mg/kg results in an onset of 1·5–4 min, a clinical duration of 18·8 min, a total duration of 32·1 min, and a recovery time of 8–12 min.[27] When an intubating dose of rocuronium 0·6 mg/kg (twice the ED_{90}) is used, the intubating conditions at one minute were comparable to those after suxamethonium in 95% of patients.[136–140] Rocuronium is generally free from cardiovascular effects or histamine release.[141 142] Higher doses of rocuronium can, however, cause a slight increase in heart rate and a significant rise in blood pressure, presumably through a vagolytic mechanism.[143 144]

Rocuronium can be used in continuous infusion to maintain neuromuscular blockade. Under nitrous–opioid anaesthesia, 10 µg/kg per min is needed, under enflurane anaesthesia 7 µg/kg per min, and under isoflurane anaesthesia 6 µg/kg per min.[145] The recovery, after stopping the infusion in isoflurane anaesthesia, is slower when compared with enflurane, which, in turn, is slower compared with balanced anaesthesia. Inhalational anaesthetics thus potentiate the effects of rocuronium.[146–148]

Rocuronium can be reversed by both edrophonium and neostigmine; however, neostigmine is more efficient.[149]

The pharmacokinetic behaviour of rocuronium is similar to that of vecuronium, but with smaller volumes of distribution (see table 6.1).[150] Although rocuronium is taken up in the liver, and mainly excreted in the bile,[151 152] the kidneys seem to play an important role in the pharmaco-kinetics of rocuronium because, in normal patients, 33% of rocuronium was found excreted unchanged in the urine.[153] In spite of this, renal failure does not appear to influence the pharmacodynamics of rocuronium.

Rocuronium is suitable for continuous infusion at a rate of 8–15 μg/kg per min.

Org 9487

This compound is presently undergoing clinical investigation. It is characterised by a rapid onset and intermediate duration. Its main advantage is its easy reversibility, even at deep degrees of neuromuscular blockade.

Other structures

Some of the older relaxants have a structure unrelated to benzylisoquino-lines or steroids. Their clinical use is, as a result of the major side effects, decreasing.

Alcuronium

Alcuronium, a synthetic derivative of the natural product toxiferine, is a bisquaternary compound, which is not metabolised but excreted 80–85% unchanged in the urine, with the rest in the bile. The pharmacodynamics of alcuronium are similar to those of pancuronium, pipecuronium, and doxacurium, with a slow onset and a long duration of action (see table 6.2). The intubating dose of alcuronum is 0·20–0·25 mg/kg. Its pharmacokinetics have been studied (see table 6.1).[154] It causes some vagolysis and has minimal effect on the blood pressure. It also causes mild histamine release.

Continuous infusion for maintenance of 95% decrease in contraction force of the adductor pollicis muscle has been described with 0·001 mg/kg per min.

Gallamine

Gallamine is a completely synthesised trisquaternary compound, charac-terised by a strong vagolytic effect. The intubating dose of gallamine is 2·2–2·4 mg/kg. As a result of the vagolysis and the slight sympathomimetic effect, gallamine is currently almost solely used as a precurarising agent before the use of suxamethonium. Gallamine's pharmacokinetics are described in a two compartment model.[155] It is almost entirely excreted by the kidneys.[156] Gallamine is contraindicated in patients with an iodine allergy, because it is an iodine salt.

Side effects of non-depolarising relaxants

The presently clinically available muscle relaxants all have side effects. Muscle relaxants seem to be responsible for 50% of the adverse reactions during anaesthesia.[157] Residual curarisation can contribute to postoperative respiratory depression.[158]

In one study, the use of non-depolarising muscle relaxants increased the risk of a cardiopulmonary complication postoperatively.[159] In another study of 433 patients, it was demonstrated that 30% (133) of the patients admitted to a post anaesthetic care unit experienced one or more complications, with 58% (77) of those having had a muscle relaxant.[160] In 23 patients, a tachyarrhythmia developed; 20 of these patients had received a relaxant. Of the 13 patients who developed postoperative hypertension, 11 had received a relaxant. Of the 33 patients who developed hypotension, 12 had had a relaxant. Muscle relaxants may then contribute to postoperative morbidity.

Many compounds of both the benzylisoquinoline and steroidal group have cardiovascular effects through a number of mechanisms. Some of the effects are mediated by an effect of the relaxants on muscarinic acetylcholine receptors in the parasympathetic nervous system or through ganglionic nicotinic acetylcholine receptors (table 6.3).[161] For example, pancuronium and gallamine cause tachycardia and hypertension by noradrenaline (norepinephrine) reuptake block and vagolysis respectively. Atracurium and d-tubocurarine can exert cardiovascular responses through histamine release. Tubocurarine causes marked ganglion blockade in doses similar to those producing neuromuscular block. It has a simultaneous sympathomimetic effect. Rocuronium in higher doses, because of its slight vagolytic effect, occasionally causes tachycardia and hypertension. Vecuronium, pipecuronium, and apparently doxacurium are free from cardiovascular effects. Alcuronium causes slight hypotension and tachycardia.

The benzylisoquinolines are potential histamine releasers. This is related to the dose and the speed of administration.[162] Tubocurarine and, to a lesser

Table 6·3   Autonomic nervous system effects and histamine release

Relaxant	Autonomic ganglia	Cardiac muscarinic receptors	Histamine release	Neuromuscular block: vagal ratio
Alcuronium	Weak	None	Slight	5
Atracurium	None	None	Moderate	25
Doxacurium	None	None	Slight	300
Gallamine	None	Strong block	None	0·5
Metocurine	Weak block	None	Slight	17
Mivacurium	None	None	Mild	100
Pancuronium	None	Weak block	None	3
Pipecuronium	None	None	None	25
Rocuronium	None	None	None	5
Tubocurarine	Block	None	Strong	1·5
Vecuronium	None	None	None	50

degree, atracurium are the strongest histamine releasers, followed by metocurine and mivacurium. Histamine release after doxacurium and *cis*-atracurium is minimal. The steroidal relaxants are all free from histamine releasing properties (table 6.3).[163]

The use of non-depolarising relaxants in the extremes of age

With age, many physiological functions are altered, including hepatic and renal function. The pharmacokinetic behaviour of relaxants can change with age. This can ultimately lead to altered pharmacodynamics.

Use in children and neonates

Shortly after birth, neuromuscular transmission has not yet matured. Less acetylcholine is released from the prejunctional membrane than in adults. This is seen as spontaneous fade after tetanic and train-of-four stimulation. The postjunctional acetylcholine receptors have a different structure, with more receptors located at the extrajunctional membrane. These morphological differences have an effect on the action of the neuromuscular blocking agents.

Pharmacokinetic behaviour of muscle relaxants is different in the various age groups. In neonates and infants, there is frequently a decreased plasma clearance and prolonged elimination half life of neuromuscular blocking agents (table 6.4). This can lead to prolonged paralysis. The initial volume of distribution in children is larger than in neonates and infants, leading to resistance to relaxants (table 6.5). This has been demonstrated for *d*-tubocurarine and atracurium.[164–166] With *d*-tubocurarine the VD$_{ss}$ is higher in neonates. This correlates with the larger extracellular volume in neonates. Neonates and infants have a increased plasma clearance and prolonged

Table 6.4   Pharmacokinetic data on muscle relaxants in relation to age

Relaxants	VD$_{ss}$ (l/kg) in			Cl$_p$ (ml/kg per min) in			$t_{\frac{1}{2}elim}$ (min) in		
	Adult	Infant	Elderly person	Adult	Infant	Elderly person	Adult	Infant	Elderly person
Alcuronium	0·32	0·32	0·37	1·3		0·53	200		440
Atracurium	0·20	0·21	0·10	6·6	7·7	5·30	21	20	22
Doxacurium	0·13	0·22	0·22	2·2		3·66	86		96
Gallamine	0·20			1·2			134		
Metocurine	0·45		0·28	1·1		0·36	269		530
Mivacurium	0·11			18·7		16·9	18		
Pancuronium	0·20	0·21	0·32	1·8	1·7	1·19	150	103	170
Pipecuronium	0·31		0·39	2·5		2·4	154		181
Rocuronium	0·21	0·24	0·31	5·8	3·1	3·4	56	50	137
Tubocurarine	0·37	0·47	0·28	1·7	1·6	0·79	164	306	268
Vecuronium	0·27	0·32	0·18	5·2	5·7	3·6	71	65	58

Table 6.5 ED_{95} of non-depolarising relaxants in infants, children, and adults

Relaxant	Infant ED_{90} (mg/kg)	Children ED_{90} (mg/kg)	Adult ED_{90} (mg/kg)	Maintenance infusion rate (mg/kg per h)
Alcuronium	0·195	0·270	0·220	0·110
Atracurium	0·240	0·330	0·210	0·530
Doxacurium	0·025	0·050	0·040	
Mivacurium	0·130	0·140	0·080	0·950
Pancuronium	0·065	0·090	0·065	0·060
Pipecuronium	0·040	0·055	0·040	0·040
Rocuronium	0·255	0·400	0·350	0·595
Tubocurarine	0·410	0·500	0·480	
Vecuronium	0·045	0·80	0·045	0·155

Infusion rate for maintenance of 95% block. All values are as rounded figures.

elimination half life of d-tubocurarine. Part of this may be caused by immature renal function in neonates and small infants. The duration of action is not different.

Although there is a decrease in both volume of distribution and plasma clearance in children, in one study, the elimination half life of atracurium was similar for infants, children, and adults.[167] In another study, however, the same group found a prolonged elimination half life and increased volume of distribution of atracurium in children.[168] In children, the onset of doxacurium is more rapid, the duration is shorter, and there is a need for relatively higher doses of doxacurium than in adults.[169 170] In children mivacurium is less potent (ED_{95} 0·10–0·11 µg/kg).[171] The pharmacokinetics of vecuronium are similar in children and adults.[172] Children are slightly more sensitive to pipecuronium than adults; in infants, its duration is shorter than in both children and adults.[173] For rocuronium, plasma clearance decreases with weight and age, and the VD_{ss} is similar in infants and adults.[174]

Use in elderly people

There are a number of reasons why the pharmacokinetic behaviour of muscle relaxants is altered in elderly patients compared with younger adults (table 6.6). This includes impaired liver and kidney function, altered body composition, and diminished cardiovascular function.

In general, in elderly people, there is an increase in total body water, lean body mass, and protein binding, resulting in alteration of the volume of distribution and/or the plasma clearance of most relaxants. Pharmacodynamically increased sensitivity to neuromuscular blocking agents and prolonged effects are seen.[175–181] Also the number of motor units per muscle is decreased in elderly people, and muscular atrophy occurs. This reduces the number and density of acetylcholine receptors in the muscles.

A decrease in cardiac output and increased circulation time lead to a delay in the onset of drugs, including muscle relaxants. Decrease in plasma

Table 6.6 Pharmacokinetic parameters for muscle relaxants in younger and older adults

Drug	Young patients	Elderly people	p
Alcuronium			
$t_{1\beta}$ (h)	2.39 ± 0.99	7.31 ± 2.85	<0.005
Cl (1/70 kg/h)	5.63 ± 1.50	2.23 ± 0.97	<0.001
VD_{auc} (1/70 kg)	24.40 ± 6.2	26.00 ± 5.60	NS
Atracurium			
$t_{1\beta}$ (h)	0.36 ± 0.05	0.26 ± 0.04	NS
Cl (1/70 kg/h)	27.30 ± 4.63	22.26 ± 3.78	NS
VD_{auc} (1/70 kg)	13.16 ± 4.27	6.86 ± 1.61	<0.05
Doxacurium			
$t_{1\beta}$ (h)	1.43 ± 0.83	1.60 ± 0.33	NS
Cl (1/70 kg/h)	9.30 ± 4.60	10.37 ± 2.89	NS
VD_{auc} (1/70 kg)	10.50 ± 2.80	15.40 ± 5.60	<0.05
Metocurine			
$t_{1\beta}$ (h)	4.48 ± 0.90	8.83 ± 1.45	<0.025
Cl (1/70 kg/h)	4.62 ± 0.67	1.51 ± 0.33	<0.01
VD_{auc} (1/70 kg)	31.22 ± 2.94	19.46 ± 2.38	<0.01
Pancuronium			
$t_{1\beta}$ (h)	1.78 ± 0.40	3.35 ± 1.20	<0.005
Cl (1/70 kg/h)	7.60 ± 2.00	5.00 ± 2.00	<0.005
VD_{auc} (1/70 kg)	19.30 ± 4.00	22.40 ± 7.00	NS
Pipecuronium			
$t_{1\beta}$ (h)	2.70 ± 1.00	3.00 ± 1.10	NS
Cl (1/70 kg/h)	10.50 ± 2.90	10.10 ± 4.20	NS
VD_{auc} (1/70 kg)	22.00 ± 4.64	27.50 ± 9.20	NS
Rocuronium			
$t_{1\beta}$ (h)	1.37 ± 0.70	1.63 ± 1.15	NS
Cl (1/70 kg/h)	21.10 ± 6.30	15.41 ± 4.20	<0.05
VD_{auc} (1/70 kg)	38.70 ± 19.50	27.96 ± 8.54	<0.05
Tubocurarine			
$t_{1\beta}$ (h)	2.88 ± 0.63	4.47 ± 0.85	<0.05
Cl (1/70 kg/h)	7.18 ± 0.13	3.32 ± 0.76	<0.025
VD_{auc} (1/70 kg)	29.75 ± 4.20	19.67 ± 2.80	<0.01
Vecuronium			
$t_{1\beta}$ (h)	1.18 ± 0.33	0.97 ± 0.17	NS
Cl (1/70 kg/h)	21.80 ± 2.90	15.50 ± 4.20	<0.05
VD_{auc} (1/70 kg)	18.90 ± 2.80	12.40 ± 2.10	<0.05

elimination of the relaxants from decreased liver and kidney function can lead to a prolonged duration of action. Dehydration and change in body composition result in an apparently increased sensitivity to relaxants. The plasma concentration at which pancuronium, vecuronium, metocurine, d-tubocurarine, doxacurium, and atracurium cause a certain degree of neuromuscular blockade does not, however, differ between younger and elderly patients.[182–184] This indicates that the increased sensitivity is only virtual and that there is no difference in receptor affinity for the relaxants.[185] It merely indicates that the plasma concentration of a relaxant, after administration of a particular dose, is higher in elderly than in younger patients. In pharmacokinetic studies this has been explained by a reduced central volume of distribution.[168 175–178 186–188]

For example, the dose–response relationship of rocuronium is not different in elderly and younger patients.[189] The blockade, however, can last longer and there is a slower onset compared with younger patients.[190] Many of these changes are the result of altered pharmacokinetics.

After administration of atracurium in elderly patients, a high concentration of laudanosine, the major metabolite, is present; the elimination half life of laudanosine is prolonged, and the clearance reduced in elderly people. This can lead to accumulation of laudanosine. The plasma concentration of laudanosine is highest immediately after injection of atracurium in young and old patients.[191] There is no difference in the pharmacodynamics of an atracurium induced muscle relaxation between older and younger adults.[192]

In a study of elderly patients, it was demonstrated that doxacurium had a significantly higher volume of distribution, but a similar elimination half life and clearance, to those in younger adults. Others, however, have found a prolonged elimination half life with a decrease in plasma clearance in elderly people, although the volume of distribution was the same as in younger patients.[193] The pharmacokinetics of doxacurium are similar in young adults and elderly patients;[178] however, elderly patients are about 25% more sensitive to doxacurium induced blockade.[194] The pharmacokinetics of pipecuronium seem to be unaffected by age.[187 195 196]

Age has only a slight effect on the clearance of vecuronium, but VD_{ss} decreases with age; the mean residence time is, therefore, longer.[197 198]

In a study of alcuronium, it was concluded that, in elderly patients, a decreased plasma clearance and prolonged elimination half life exists compared with in younger adults.[177]

Use of non-depolarising relaxants during pregnancy

During pregnancy there is, among other things, an increase in total body water, and a fall in protein concentration and plasma cholinesterase activity. Liver and kidney function are also changed. This has an effect on the pharmacokinetics and pharmacodynamics of the non-depolarising relaxants. In a pregnant woman, the plasma clearance of pancuronium is larger and the elimination half life shorter than in a non-pregnant woman.[199 120] During pregnancy there is transfer of muscle relaxants administered to the mother across the placenta to the fetus. Transplacental transfer can be expressed as a ratio between the maternal and umbilical vein concentration.[201–203] Suxamethonium has a fetal:maternal ratio of 0·3, the transfer ratio of non-depolarisers being smaller (table 6.7). As neonates are more resistant to relaxants than adults, the concentration of relaxants in the fetus has no detectable effects when normal clinical doses are administered to the mother.

Table 6.7 Transplacental transfer of muscle relaxants

Relaxant	UV:MV
Alcuronium	0·26
Atracurium	0·12
Metocurine	0·21
Pancuronium	0·21
Rocuronium	0·16
Vecuronium	0·11

UV = umbilical vein concentration,
MV = maternal venous concentration

Use of non-depolarising relaxants in the intensive care unit

Chronic administration of non-depolarising relaxants has been shown to cause upregulation (increase in number) of acetylcholine receptors in rats, and hence to decrease sensitivity to non-depolarising relaxants.[204] Muscle relaxants were originally developed and tested for relatively short duration administration. Nowadays, relaxants are sometimes used for several weeks in the intensive care unit. Recently, muscle areflexia, atrophy, and sensory impairment in patients with multiorgan failure have been attributed to the prolonged administration of muscle relaxants.[205-208] Muscle weakness may delay weaning from artificial ventilation, and can last for several months. In one study 50% of the patients in the intensive care unit developed polyneuropathy after long duration administration of vecuronium.[209]

Signs of polyneuropathy have, however, also been observed in critically ill patients who have not received muscle relaxants (critical illness neuropathy).[210] In one study, up to 70% of all intensive care patients with sepsis and multiple organ failure had symptoms of this syndrome.[211 212] In 50% of the patients with the syndrome, muscle fibre necrosis has been seen, suggesting that there is also myopathy.[213] Besides motor function deficits, sensory deficits can occur. Electromyographic (EMG) readings in patients with critical illness neuropathy do not demonstrate neuromuscular transmission disorders.[214] This suggests that the problem is more a myopathy than a neuropathy.

The neuropathy after administration of relaxants in intensive care patients is a different entity. It is usually symmetrical, and does not involve the sensory system. Neuromuscular transmission is also affected. EMG readings frequently resemble those changes seen in a Guillain–Barré syndrome or myonecrosis, but can also resemble readings resulting from residual neuromuscular blockade. Furthermore, about 50% of patients receiving vecuronium over a long period of time developed prolonged paralysis. All these patients had renal insufficiency, and about half also had hepatic dysfunction. Most patients developing prolonged paralysis were women and they had a metabolic acidosis. All had a higher plasma concentration of 3-desacetylvecuronium compared with the patients not experiencing prolonged paralysis.[215] This compound does have a significant neuromuscular blocking effect which may have contributed to the blockade in these patients. Other drugs, for example, aminoglycosides, polypeptides, and lincosamines, which are often administered to this type of patient, can lead to neuromuscular and muscular abnormalities. The long term administration of corticosteroids may also potentiate the problem of long term muscle weakness.[216] The muscle weakness usually resolves slowly over weeks or even months after stopping the relaxants. Prolonged weakness after long term relaxant administration has been confirmed by others.[217] Further studies are needed to evaluate these neuropathic and myopathic effects.

The combination of steroidal based relaxants and corticosteroids, especially in patients with renal failure, appears to increase the chance of prolonged block.[218 219] It must be realised, however, that the steroid based relaxants are more frequently used in the intensive care unit than the benzylisoquinolines.

Prolonged administration of atracurium can also lead to prolonged muscle weakness.[220] In intensive care patients, laudanosine, the major metabolite of atracurium, may accumulate both in plasma and in cerebrospinal fluid.[221] This metabolite is also seen at higher concentrations in patients with renal and hepatic disease. In animal experiments, laudanosine causes seizures. This, however, has not been shown in patients.[222] In vitro studies in isolated rat hepatocytes have demonstrated that another metabolite of atracurium, a monoacrylate, causes cell damage through alkylation of endogenous nucleophiles.[223] This effect seems to be negligible in humans. Long term use of atracurium in intensive care patients does seem to be safe, but care is needed when using high doses for a long time.

In contrast to prolonged weakness, cases have been reported where resistance to pancuronium,[224] vecuronium,[225] and atracurium,[226] during their long term administration, has developed. This may be related to increased extrajunctional sensitivity to acetylcholine and/or receptor up-regulation as a result of prolonged neuromuscular blockade.

There is a possibility that muscle relaxants, after long administration, can reach considerable concentrations in the brain and may interfere with cerebral acetylcholine receptors. This is especially possible in patients with disturbed blood–brain barriers (either from disease or the administration of mannitol and other hyperosmolar fluids). It is well known that non-depolarising relaxants do have an excitatory central nervous system effect leading to myotonia, convulsions, and autonomic changes.[227 228] The presence of relaxants in the cerebrospinal fluid has been demonstrated after administration of large doses to patients.[229]

Conclusions

Non-depolarising neuromuscular blocking agents are frequently used by anaesthetists. They can largely be divided into benzylisoquinolines and steroid based groups. Although, within both groups, common characteristics are present, each individual relaxant has its own pharmacological profile. Safe and appropriate administration of neuromuscular blocking agents requires knowledge of these properties. Several (patho)-physiological states and drugs can alter the effects of the relaxants. In each situation, the anaesthetist must make a choice for the best relaxant for that particular situation.

1 Wintersteiner O, Dutcher JD. Curare alkaloids from *Chondodendron tomentosum*. *Science* 1943;**97**:467–70.
2 Huu-Lainé FK, Pinto-Scognamiglio W. Activité curarisante du dichlorure de 3β-20α bistrimethylammonium 5α-prégnane (malouétine) et de ses stéréoisomères. *Arch Int Pharmacodyn Ther* 1974;**147**:209–19.
3 Brodie B. Further experiments and observations on the action of poisons on the animal system. *Phil Trans R Soc Lond* 1812;**1**:205–27.
4 Bernard C. Action de curare et de nicotine sur le système nerveux et sur les systèmes musculaires. *Compte Rendu de la Société de Biologie* 1850;**2**:195.
5 Bevan DR, Bevan JC, Donati F. The arrival of curare in Montreal. In: Bevan DR, Bevan JC, Donati F, eds, *Muscle relaxants in clinical anaesthesia*. Chicago: Year Book Medical Publishers, 1988:1–12.
6 Boehm R. Über Curare und Curarealkaloide. *Arch Pharmacol Berlin* 1897;**235**:660–84.
7 Läwen A. Über die Verbindung Lokalanästhesie mit der Narkose, über hohe Extraduralanesthesie und peridurale Injektionen anästhesierender Lösungen bei tabetischen Magenkriesen. *Beitr Klin Chir* 1912;**80**:168–9.
8 Bennett AE. Curare; a preventative of traumatic complications in convulsive shock therapy. *Am J Psychol* 1941;**97**:1040–60.
9 King H. Curare alkaloids, Part I: Tubocurarine. *J Chem Soc* 1935;**2**:1381–9.
10 Griffith HR, Johnston GE. The use of curare in general anesthesia. *Anesthesiology* 1942;**3**:418–20.
11 Cullen SC. The use of curare for the improvement of abdominal muscle relaxation during inhalation anesthesia. *Surgery* 1943;**14**:261–6.
12 Beecher HK, Todd DP. A study of the deaths associated with anesthesia and surgery. *Ann Surg* 1954;**140**:2–34.
13 Foldes FF. Factors which alter the effects of muscle relaxants. *Anesthesiology* 1959; **20**:464–504.
14 Bovet D, Depoierre F, Lestange Y. Proprietes curasisantes des ethers phenoliques a fonctions ammonium quaternaires. *Comptes Rendus Hebdomadaires des Sceances de l'Academie des Sciences* 1947;**225**:74–6.
15 Lund I, Stovner J. Experimental and clinical experiences with a new muscle relaxant RO 4-3816, diallyl-nor-toxiferine. *Acta Anaesthesiol Scand* 1962;**62**:85–97.
16 Baird WLM, Reid AM. The neuromuscular blocking properties of a new steroid compound, pancuronium bromide. *Br J Anaesth* 1967;**39**:755–80.
17 Sobell HM. Sakore TD, Tavale SS, *et al.* Stereochemistry of curare alkaloid: *O,O', N*-trimethyl-*d*-tubocurarine. *Proc Natl Acad Sci USA* 1972;**69**:2212–15.
18 Kimenis A, Klusha VE, Ginters YA. Pharmacology of Dioxonium, a new myorelaxant. *Farmakologiya i toxicologiya* 1972;**35**:172.
19 Simpson BR, Strunin L, Savege TM, *et al.* An azobis-arylimidazo-pyridinium derivative. A rapidly acting non-depolarising muscle-relaxant. *Lancet* 1972;**1**:516–19.
20 Marshall IG, Agoston S, Booij LHDJ, Durant NN, Foldes FF. Pharmacology of Org NC45 compared with other nondepolarizing neuromuscular blocking drugs. *Br J Anaesth* 1980;**52**:11S–19S.
21 Crul JF, Booij LHDJ. First clinical experiences with Org NC45. *Br J Anaesth* 1980; **52**(suppl):S49–52.
22 Wierda JMKH, Richardson FJ, Agoston S. Dose response relation and time course of action of pipecuronium bromide in humans anesthetized with nitrous oxide and isoflurane, halothane, or droperidol/fentanyl. *Anesth Analg* 1989;**68**:208–13.
23 Payne JP, Hughes R. Evaluation of atracurium in anaesthetized man. *Br J Anaesth* 1981;**53**:45–54.

24 Basta SJ, Ali HH, Savarese JJ, Sunder N, et al. Clinical pharmacology of atracurium besylate (BW 33A): A new non-depolarizing muscle relaxant. Anesth Analg 1982; 61:723–9.

25 Basta SWJ, Savarese JJ, Ali HH, et al. Clinical pharmacology of doxacurium chloride. Anesthesiology 1988;69:478–86.

26 Savarese JJ, Ali HH, Basta SJ, et al. The clinical neuromuscular pharmacology of mivacurium chloride (BW 1090U): A short acting ester neuromuscular blocking drug. Anesthesiology 1988;68:723–32.

27 Booij LHDJ, Knape JTA. The neuromuscular blocking effect of Org 9426. Anaesthesia 1991;46:341–3.

28 Gyermek L, Nguyen N, Lee C. G1-64, a new, rapidly acting nondepolarizing neuromuscular blocking agent. Anesthesiology 1990;73:A862.

29 Kharkevich DA. New curare-like agents. J Pharm Pharmacol 1974;26:153–65.

30 Gandiha A, Marshall IG, Paul D, Rodger IW, Scott W, Singh H. Some actions of chandonium iodide, a new muscle relaxant in anesthetized cats and on isolated muscle preparations. Clin Expl Pharmacol Physiol 1975;2:150–70.

31 Baird WLM. Initial studies in man with a new myoneural blocking agent (Org 6368). Br J Anaesth 1974;46:658–61.

32 Booij LHDJ, Crul JF, van der Pol F. Cardiovascular and neuromuscular blocking effects of four new muscle relaxants in anaesthetized Beagle dogs. Eur J Anaesthesiol 1988;6:70.

33 Muir AW, Houston J, Marshall RJ, Bowman WC, Marshall IG. A comparison of the neuromuscular blocking and autonomic effects of two new short-acting muscle relaxants with those of succinylcholine in the anesthetized cat and pig. Anesthesiology 1989; 70:533–40.

34 Gilly H, Hirtschl MM, Steinbereithner K. Pharmacodynamics of Org 8764, atracurium and vecuronium: a comparison of vocal cord, diaphragm and tibial muscle relaxation. Anesthesiology 1988;69:A481.

35 Muir AW, Anderson K, Marshall RJ, et al. The effects of a 16-N-homopiperidino analogue of vecuronium on neuromuscular transmission in anaesthetized cats, pigs, dogs and monkeys, and in isolated preparations. Acta Anaesthesiol Scand 1991;35:85–90.

36 Hughes R. Evaluation of the neuromuscular blocking properties and side-effects of the two new isoquinolinium bisquaternary compounds (BW 252C64 and BW 403C65). Br J Anaesth 1972;44:27–42.

37 Dreyer F. Acetylcholine receptor. Br J Anaesth 1982;54:115–30.

38 Paton WD, Waud DR. The margin of safety of neuromuscular transmission. J Physiol (London) 1967;191:59–90.

39 Bowman WC. Physiology and pharmacology of neuromuscular transmission, with special reference to the possible consequences of prolonged blockade. Intensive Care Med 1993;19:S45–53.

40 Shanks CA, Somogyi AA, Triggs EJ. Dose–response and plasma concentration–response relationship of pancuronium in man. Anesthesiology 1979;51:111–18.

41 Agoston S, Feldman SA, Miller RD. Plasma concentrations of pancuronium and neuromuscular blockade after injection into isolated arm, bolus injection, and continuous infusion. Anesthesiology 1979;51:119–22.

42 Shanks CA, Somogyi AA, Triggs EJ. Plasma concentrations of pancuronium during pre-determined intensities of neuromuscular blockade. Br J Anaesth 1978;50:235–8.

43 Stanski DR, Sheiner LB. Pharmacokinetics and dynamics of muscle relaxants. Anesthesiology 1979;51:103–5.

44 Prior C, Tian L, Dempster J, Marshall IG. Prejunctional actions of muscle relaxants: synaptic vesicles and transmitter mobilization as sites of action. Gen Pharmacol 1995;26:659–66.

45 Bowman WC. Prejunctional and postjunctional cholinoceptors at the neuromuscular junction. Anesth Analg 1980;59:935–43.

46 Foldes FF, Chaudhry IA, Kinjo M, Nagashima H. Inhibition of mobilization of acetylcholine. Anesthesiology 1989;71:218–23.

47 Bowman WC, Prior C, Marshall IG. Presynaptic receptors in the neuromuscular junction. Ann NY Acad Sci 1990;604:69–81.

48 Williams NE, Webb SN, Calvey TN. Differential effects of myoneural blocking drugs on neuromuscular transmission. Br J Anaesth 1980;52:1111–14.

49 Katz RL. Neuromuscular effects of d-tubocurarine, edrophonium and neostigmine in man. Anesthesiology 1967;28:327–36.

50 Bowman WC, Rodger IW, Houston J, Marshall RJ, McIndewar I. Structure:action relationships among some desacetoxy analogues of pancuronium and vecuronium in the anesthetized cat. *Anesthesiology* 1988;**69**:57–62.

51 Maehr RB, Wastila WB. Comparative pharmacology of atracurium and six isomers in cats. *Anesthesiology* 1993;**79**:A946.

52 Law Min JC, Bakavac I, Glavinovic MI, Donati F, Bevan DR. Iontophoretic study of speed of action of various muscle relaxants. *Anesthesiology* 1992;**77**:351–6.

53 Kim SY, Hwang KH, Ok SY, Kim SI, Kim SC, Park W. Discrepancy of recovery times related to potency between atracurium and mivacurium simultaneously administered in isolated forearms. *Anaesthesia* 1995;**50**:507–9.

54 Kopman AF. Pancuronium, gallamine and d-tubocurarine compared: is speed of onset inversely related to drug potency? *Anesthesiology* 1989;**70**:915–20.

55 Ramzan IM. Molecular weight of cation as a determinant of speed of onset of neuromuscular blockade. *Anesthesiology* 1982;**57**:247–8.

56 Blackburn CL, Morgan M. Comparison of speed of onset of fazadinium, pancuronium, tubocurarine and suxamethonium. *Br J Anaesth* 1978;**50**:361–4.

57 Mirakhur RK, Lavery GG, Clarke RSJ, Gibson FM, McAtees A. Atracurium in clinical anaesthesia: effect of dosage on onset, duration and conditions for tracheal intubation. *Anaesthesia* 1985;**40**:801–5.

58 Feldman S, Fauvel N, Harrop-Griffiths W. The onset of neuromuscular blockade. In: Bowman WC, Denissen PAF, Feldman S, eds, *Neuromuscular blocking agents: past, present and future*. Amsterdam: Excerpta Medica, 1990:44–51.

59 Ginsberg B, Glass PS, Quili T, Shafron D, Ossey KD. Onset and duration of neuromuscular blockade following high-dose vecuronium administration. *Anesthesiology* 1989;**71**:201–5.

60 Tullock WC, Diana P, Cook DR, *et al.* Neuromuscular and cardiovascular effects of high-dose vecuronium. *Anesth Analg* 1990;**70**:86–90.

61 Glass PSA, Wilson W, Mace JA, Wagoner R. Is the priming principle both effective and safe? *Anesth Analg* 1989;**68**:127–34.

62 Mirakhur RF, Lavery GG, Gibson FM, Clarke RS. Intubating conditions after vecorunium and atracurium given in divided doses (the priming principle). *Acta Anaesthesiol Scand* 1986;**30**:347–50.

63 Sosis M, Stiner A, Larijari GE, Marr AT. An evaluation of priming with vecuronium. *Br J Anaesth* 1987;**59**:1236–9.

64 Waud BE, Waud DR. Quantitative examination of the interaction of competitive neuromuscular blocking agents on the indirectly elicited twitch. *Anesthesiology* 1984;**61**:420–7.

65 Naguib M. Neuromuscular effects of rocuronium bromide and mivacurium chloride administered alone and in combination. *Anesthesiology* 1994;**81**:388–95.

66 Iwasaki H, Namiki A, Onote T, Omote K. Neuromuscular effects of subcutaneous administration of pancuronium. *Anesthesiology* 1992;**76**:1049–51.

67 Mitenko PA, Ogilvie RI. Rapidly achieved plasma concentration plateaus, with observations on theophylline kinetics. *Clin Pharmacol Ther* 1972;**13**:329–35.

68 Wood M. Plasma drug binding: implications for anesthesiologists. *Anesth Analg* 1986;**65**:786–804.

69 Agoston S, Feldman SA, Miller RD. Plasma concentratations of pancuronium and neuromuscular blockade after injection into isolated arm, bolus injection, and continuous infusion. *Anesthesiology* 1979;**51**:119–22.

70 Matteo RS, Nishitateno K, Pua EK, Spector S. Pharmacokinetics of d-tubocurarine in man: effect of an osmotic diuretic on urinary excretion. *Anesthesiology* 1980;**52**:335–8.

71 Amaki Y, Waud BE, Waud DR. Atracurium-receptor kinetics: simple behaviour from a mixture. *Anesth Analg* 1985;**64**:777–80.

72 Sternlake JB, Waigh RD, Dewar GH, *et al.* Biodegradable neuromuscular blocking agents. Part 6: Stereochemical studies on atracurium and related polyalkylene diesters. *Eur J Med Chem* 1984;**19**:441–50.

73 Tsui D, Graham GG, Torda TA. The pharmacokinetics of atracurium isomers in vitro and in humans. *Anesthesiology* 1987;**677**:722–8.

74 Robertson EN, Booij LHDJ, Fragen RJ, Crul JF. A clinical comparison of atracurium and vecuronium (Org NC45). *Br J Anaesth* 1983;**55**:125–30.

75 Griffiths RB, Hunter JM, Jones RM. Atracurium infusions in patients with renal failure on an ITU. *Anaesthesia* 1986;**41**:375–81.

76 Hughes R, Chapple DJ. The pharmacology of atracurium: a new competitive neuro-muscular blocking agent. *Br J Anaesth* 1981;53:31–44.

77 Stenlake JB, Waigh RD, Dewar GH. Biodegradable neuromuscular blocking agents part 4: atracurium besylate and related polyalkylene di-esters. *Eur J Med Chem* 1981; 16:515–24.

78 Kent AP, Parker CJR, Hunter JM. Pharmacokinetics of atracurium and laudanosine in the elderly. *Br J Anaesth* 1989;63:661–6.

79 Nigrovic V, Banoub M. Pharmacokinetic modelling of a parent drug and its metabolite. Atracurium and laudanosine. *Clin Pharmacokinet* 1992;22:396–408.

80 Diefenbach C, Abel M, Buzello W. Greater neuromuscular blocking potency of atracurium during hypothermic than during normothermic cardiopulmonary bypass. *Anesth Analg* 1992;75:675–8.

81 Maehr RB, Belmont MR, Wray DL, Savarese JJ, Wastila WB. Autonomic and neuromuscular effects of mivacurium and isomers in cats. *Anesthesiology* 1991;75:A772.

82 Head-Rapson AG, Devlin JC, Parker CJR, Hunter JM. Pharmacokinetics and pharmaco-dynamics of the three isomers of mivacurium in health, in end-stage renal failure and in patients with impaired renal function. *Br J Anaesth* 1995;75:31–6.

83 Stoops CM, Curtis CA, Kovach DA, *et al.* Hemodynamic effects of Mivacurium chloride administered to patients during oxygen-sufentanil anesthesia for coronary artery bypass grafting or valve replacement. *Anesth Analg* 1989;68:333–9.

84 Naguib M, Abdulatif M, Selim M, Al-Ghamdi A. Dose–response studies of the interaction between mivacurium and suxamethonium. *Br J Anaesth* 1995;74:26–30.

85 Cook DR, Stiller RL, Weakly JN, Chakravorti S, Brandom BW, Welch RM. In vitro metabolism of Mivacurium chloride (BW B1090U) and succinylcholine. *Anesth Analg* 1989;68:452–6.

86 Ostergaard D, Jensen FS, Jensen E, Viby-Mogensen J. Influence of plasma cholinesterase activity on recovery from mivacurium-induced neuromuscular blockade. *Acta Anaesthesiol Scand* 1989;33(suppl 191):164.

87 Ostergaard D, Janden E, Jensen FS, Viby-Morgensen J. The duration of action of mivacurium induced neuromuscular block in patients homozygous for the atypical plasma cholinesterase gene. *Anesthesiology* 1991;75:A774.

88 Ostergaard D, Jensen FS, Jensen E, Skovgaard LT, Viby-Morgensen J. Influence of plasma cholinesterase activity on recovery from mivacurium-induced neuromuscular blockade in phenotypically normal patients. *Acta Anaesthesiol Scand* 1992;36:702–6.

89 Goudsouzian NG, d'Hollander AA, Vigy-Morgensen J. Prolonged neuromuscular block from mivacurium in two patients with cholinesterase deficiency. *Anesth Analg* 1993;77:183–5.

90 Maddineni VR, Mirakhur RK. Prolonged neuromuscular block following mivacurium. *Anesthesiology* 1993;71:227–31.

91 Sockalingam I, Green DW. Mivacurium-induced prolonged neuromuscular block. *Br J Anaesth* 1995;74:234–6.

92 Fox MW, Hunt PCW. Prolonged neuromuscular block associated with mivacurium. *Br J Anaesth* 1995;74:237–8.

93 Diefenbach C, Abel M, Rump AFE, Grond S, Korb H, Buzello W. Changes in plasma cholinesterase activity and mivacurium neuromuscular block in response to normo-thermic cardiopulmonary bypass. *Anesth Analg* 1995;80:1088–91.

94 Petersen RS, Bailey PL, Kalameghan R, Ashwood ER. Prolonged neuromuscular block after mivacurium. *Anesth Analg* 1993;76:194–6.

95 Hart PS, Wright PC, Brown R, *et al.* Endophonium increases mivacurium concentrations during constant mivacurium infusion, and large doses minimally antagonize paralysis. *Anesthesiology* 1995;82:912–18.

96 Abdulatif M. Recovery characteristics after early administration of anticholinesterases during intense mivacurium-induced neuromuscular block. *Br J Anaesth* 1995;74:20–5.

97 Mangar D, Kirchloff GT, Rose PL, Castellano FC. Prolonged neuromuscular block after mivacurium in a patient with end-stage renal disease. *Anesth Analg* 1993;76:866–7.

98 Naguib M, El-Grammal M, Daoud W, Ammar A, Moukhtar H, Turkistani A. Human plasma cholinesterase for antagonism of prolonged mivacurium-induced neuromuscular blockade. *Anesthesiology* 1995;82:1288–92.

99 Shanks CA, Fragen RJ, Pemberton D, Katz JA, Rizner ME. Mivacurium induced neuromuscular blockade following single bolus doses and with continuous infusion during either balanced or enflurane anesthesia. *Anesthesiology* 1989;71:362–6.

100 Savarese JJ, Ali HH, Basta SJ, et al. The cardiovascular effects of mivacurium chloride (BW B1090U) in patients receiving oxide-opiate-barbiturate anesthesia. Anesthesiology 1989;70:386–94.

101 Goldhill DR, Whitehead JP, Emmott RS, Griffith AP, Bracey BJ, Flynn PJ. Neuromuscular and clinical effects of mivacurium chloride in healthy adult patients during nitrous oxide–enflurane anaesthesia. Br J Anaesth 1991;67:289–95.

102 Head-Rapson AG, Devlin JC, Parker CJR, Hunter JM. Pharmacokinetics of the three isomers of mivacurium and pharmacodynamics of the chiral mixture in hepatic cirrhosis. Br J Anaesth 1994;73:613–18.

103 Maddineni VR, Cooper R, Stanley JC, Mirakhur RK, Clarke RSJ. Clinical evaluation of doxacurium chloride. Anaesthesia 1992;47:554–7.

104 Murray DJ, Mehta MP, Choi WW, et al. The neuromuscular blocking and cardiovascular effects of Doxacurium chloride in patients receiving nitrous oxide narcotic anesthesia. Anesthesiology 1988;69:472–7.

105 Lennon RL, Hosking MP, Houck PC, et al. Doxacurium chloride for neuromuscular blockade before tracheal intubation and surgery during nitrous oxide–oxygen–narcotic–enflurane anesthesia. Anesth Analg 1989;68:255–60.

106 Schmith VD, Fiedler-Kelly J, Abou-Donia M, Huffman CS, Grasela TH Jr. Population pharmacodynamics of doxacurium. Clin Pharmacol Ther 1992;52:528–36.

107 Emmott RS, Bracey DJ, Goldhill DR, Yate PM, Flynn PJ. Cardiovascular effects of doxacurium, pancuronium, and vecuronium in anaesthetised patients presenting for coronary artery bypass surgery. Br J Anaesth 1990;65:480–6.

108 Stoops CM, Curtis CA, Kovach DA, et al. Hemodynamic effects of doxacurium chloride in patients receiving oxygen–sufentanil anesthesia for coronary artery bypass grafting or valve replacement. Anesthesiology 1988;69:365–70.

109 Reich DL. Transient systemic hypotension and cutaneous flushing in response to doxacurium chloride. Anesthesiology 1989;71:783–5.

110 Meretoja OA, Taivaninen T, Wirtavuori K. Pharmacodynamic effects of 51W89, an isomer of atracurium, in children under halothane anaesthesia. Br J Anaesth 1995; 74:6–11.

111 Belmont MR, Lien CA, Quessy S, et al. The clinical neuromuscular pharmacology of 51W89 in patients receiving nitrous oxide/opioid/barbiturate anesthesia. Anesthesiology 1995;82:1139–45.

112 Littlejohn IH, Abhay K, El Sayed A, Broomhead CJ, Duvaldestin P, Flynn PJ. Intubating conditions following 1R CIS, 1'R CIS atracurium (51W89). Anaesthesia 1995;50: 499–502.

113 Lien CA, Belmont MR, Abalos A, et al. The cardiovascular effects and histamine-releasing properties of 51W89 in patients receiving nitrous oxide/opioid/barbiturate anesthesia. Anesthesiology 1995;82:1131–8.

114 Lien CA, Schmith VD, Belmont MR, Kisor D, Savarese JJ. Pharmacokinetics/dynamics of 51W89 in healthy patients during opioid anesthesia. Anesthesiology 1994;81:A1082.

115 Buckett WR, Hewet CL, Savage DS. Pancuronium bromide and other steroidal neuromuscular blocking agents containing acetylcholine fragments. J Med Chem 1973; 16:1116–24.

116 Savage DS, Sleigh T, Carlyle IC. The emergency of Org.NC45 1-[(2,3, 5,16,17) - 3,17 - bis(acetyloxy) - 2(1-piperydinyl) - androstan - 16 -YL] - 1 - methylpiperi - dinium bromide, from the pancuronium series. Br J Anaesth 1980;52:3S–9S.

117 Durant NN, Marshall IG, Savage DS, Nelson DJ, Sleigh T, Carlyle IC. The neuromuscular and autonomic blocking activities of pancuronium, Org. NC45, and other pancuronium analogues, in the cat. J Pharm Pharmacol 1979;31:831–7.

118 Marshall IG, Agoston S, Booij LDHJ, Durant NN, Foldes FF. Comparison of the cardiovascular actions of Org.NC45 with those produced by other non-depolarizing neuromuscular blocking agents in experimental animals. Br J Anaesth 1980;52:21S–32S.

119 Naguib M, Samarkandi AH, Bakhamees HS, Magboul MA, El-Bakry AK. Comparative potency of steroidal neuromuscular blocking drugs and isobolographic analysis of the interaction between rocuronium and other aminosteroids. Br J Anaesth 1995;75:37–42.

120 Krieg N, Crul JF, Booij LHDJ. Relative potency of Org NC45, pancuronium, alcuronium and tubocurarine in anaesthetized man. Br J Anaesth 1980;52:783–8.

121 Miller RD, Agoston S, Booij LHDJ, Kersten UW, Crul JF, Ham J. The comparative potency and pharmacokinetics of pancuronium and its metabolites in anesthetized man. J Pharmacol Expl Ther 1978;207:539–43.

118

122 Bergin AM, Clarke TA, Matthews TG. Problems with pancuronium in the neonatal intensive care unit. *Irish Med J* 1988;**81**:39–40.

123 Fahey MR, Morris RB, Miller RD, Nguyen TL, Upton RA. Pharmacokinetics of Org NC45 (Norcuron) in patients with and without renal failure. *Br J Anaesth* 1981; **53**:1049–53.

124 Bencinin AF, Scaf AHJ, Sohn YJ, *et al*. Disposition and urinary excretion of vecorunium bromide in anesthetized patients with normal renal function or renal failure. *Anesth Analg* 1986;**65**:245–51.

125 Wright PMC, Hart P, Lau M, Sharma ML, Gruneke L, Fisher DM. Cumulative characteristics of atracurium and vecuronium. *Anesthesiology* 1994;**81**:59–68.

126 Stanley JC, Mirakhur RJ. Comparative potency of pipecuronium bromide and pancuronium bromide. *Br J Anaesth* 1989;**63**:754–55.

127 Fitzal S, Ilias W, Kalina K, Schwarz S, Foldes FF, Steinbereitner K. Neuromuskulare und kardiovaskulare Effekte von Duador, einem neuen kurz wirksamen nicht depolarisierenden Muskelrelaxans. *Anaesthesist* 1982;**32**:674–9.

128 Dubois MY, Fleming NW, Lea DE. Effects of succinylcholine on the pharmacodynamics of pipecuronium and pancuronium. *Anesth Analg* 1991;**72**:364–8.

129 Abdulatif M, Naguib M. Neostigmine and edrophonium for reversal of pipecuronium neuromuscular blockade. *Can J Anaesth* 1991;**38**:159–63.

130 Stanley JC, Carson IW, Gibson FM, *et al*. Comparison of the haemodynamic effects of pipecuronium and pancuronium during fentanyl anesthesia. *Acta Anaesthesiol Scand* 1991;**35**:262–6.

131 Tassonyi E, Neidhart P, Pittet JF, Morel DR, Gemperle M. Cardiovascular effects of pipecuronium and pancuronium in patients undergoing coronary artery bypass grafting. *Anesthesiology* 1988;**69**:793–6.

132 Barankay A. Circulatory effects of pipecuronium bromide during anesthesia of patients with severe valvular and ischaemic heart disease. *Drug Res* 1980;**30**:386–9.

133 Wierda JMKH, Karliczek GF, Vandenbrom RHG, *et al*. Pharmacokinetics and cardiovascular dynamics of pipecuronium bromide during coronary artery surgery. *Can J Anaesth* 1990;**37**:183–91.

134 Caldwell JE, Canfell PC, Castagnoli KP, *et al*. The influence of renal failure on the pharmacokinetics and duration of action of pipecuronium bromide. *Anesthesiology* 1987;**67**:A612.

135 Wierda JMKH, Szenohradszky J, de Wit APM, *et al*. The pharmacokinetics, urinary and biliary excretion of pipecuronium bromide (Adruan). *Eur J Anaesthesiol* 1991;**8**:451–7.

136 Lapreye G, Dubois M, Lea D, Kataria B, Tram D. Effects of 3 intubating doses of Org 9426 in humans. *Anesthesiology* 1990;**73**:A906.

137 Foldes FF, Nagashima H, Nguyen HD, Schiller WS, Mason MM, Ohta Y. The neuromuscular effects of Org 9426 in patients receiving balanced anesthesia. *Anesthesiology* 1991;**75**:191–5.

138 Cooper R, Mirakhur RK, Clarke RSJ, Boules ZS. Comparison of intubating conditions after administration of Org 9426 (rocuronium) and suxamethonium. *Br J Anaesth* 1992;**69**:269–73.

139 Huizenga ACT, Vandenbrom RHG, Wierda JMKH, Hommes FDM, Hennis PJ. Intubating conditions and onset of neuromuscular block of rocuronium (ORG 9426); a comparison with suxamethonium. *Acta Anaesthesiol Scand* 1992;**36**:463–8.

140 Pühringer FK, Khuenl-Brady K, Koller J, Mitterschiffthaler G. Evaluation of the endotracheal intubating conditions of rocuronium (ORG 9426) and succinylcholine in outpatient surgery. *Anesth Analg* 1992;**75**:37–40.

141 Wierda JMKH, de Wit APM, Kuizinga K, Agoston S. Clinical observations on the neuromuscular blocking action of Org 9426, a new steroidal non-depolarizing agent. *Br J Anaesth* 1990;**64**:521–3.

142 Davis GK, Sziam F, Lowdon JD, Levy JH. Evaluation of histamine release following Org 9426 administration using a new radioimmunoassay. *Anesthesiology* 1991;**75**:A818.

143 Robertson EN, Hull JM, Verbeek AM, Booij LHDJ. A comparison of rocuronium and vecuronium: the pharmacodynamic, cardiovascular and intra-ocular effects. *Eur J Anaesthesiol* 1994;**11**(suppl 9):116–21.

144 McCoy EP, Maddineni VR, Elliot P, Mirakhur RK, Caroon IW, Cooper RA. Haemodynamic effects of rocuronium during fentanyl anaesthesia: comparison with vecuronium. *Can J Anaesth* 1993;**408**:703–8.

145 Shanks CA, Fragen RJ, Ling D. Continuous intravenous infusion of rocuronium (Org 9426) in patients receiving balanced, enflurane, or isoflurane anesthesia. *Anesthesiology* 1993;78:649–51.

146 Quil TJ, Begin M, Glass PSA, Ginsberg B, Gorback MS. Clinical responses to Org 9426 during isoflurane anesthesia. *Anesth Analg* 1991;72:203–6.

147 Dubois M, Kataria B, Lea D, Lapeyre G. Neuromuscular effects of Org 9426 in humans during general anaesthesia with and without enflurane. *Anesth Analg* 1991;72:S57.

148 Cooper RA, Mirakhur RK, Maddineni VR. Neuromuscular effects of rocuronium bromide (Org 9426) during fentanyl and halothane anaesthesia. *Anaesthesia* 1993;48: 103–5.

149 Naguib M, Abdulatif M, Al-Ghamdi A. Dose–response relationships for edrophonium and neostigmine antagonism of rocuronium bromide (ORG 9426)-induced neuro-muscular blockade. *Anesthesiology* 1993;79:739–45.

150 Wierda JMKH, Kleef UW, Lambalk LM, Kloppenburg WD, Agoston S. The pharmaco-dynamics and pharmacokinetics of Org 9426, a new non-depolarizing neuromuscular blocking agent, in patients anaesthetized with nitrous oxide, halothane and fentanyl. *Can J Anaesth* 1991;38:430–5.

151 Magorian T, Wood P, Caldwell JE, *et al*. Pharmacokinetics, onset, and duration of action of rocuronium in humans: normal vs hepatic dysfunction. *Anesthesiology* 1991;75:A1069.

152 Khuenyl-Brady K, Castagnoli KP, Canfell C, Caldwell JE, Agoston S, Miller RD. The neuromuscular blocking effect and pharmacokinetics of Org 9426 and Org 9616 in the cat. *Anesthesiology* 1990;72:669–74.

153 Szenohradszky J, Fisher DM, Segredo V, Caldwell JE, Bragg P, Sharma ML. Pharmacokinetics of rocuronium bromide (Org 9426) in patients with normal renal function or patients undergoing cadaver renal transplantation. *Anesthesiology* 1992;77: 899–904.

154 Walker J, Shanks CA, Triggs EJ. Clinical pharmacokinetics of alcuronium chloride in man. *Eur J Clin Phamacol* 1990;17:449–57.

155 Ramzan MI, Triggs EJ, Shanks CA. Pharmacokinetic studies in man with gallamine triethiodide. I. Single and multiple clinical doses. *Eur J Clin Pharmacol* 1980;17:135–43.

156 Ramzan MI, Shanks CA, Triggs EJ. Gallamine disposition in surgical patients with chronic renal failure. *Br J Clin Pharmacol* 1981;12:141–7.

157 Vervloet D. Allergy to muscle relaxants and related compounds. *Clin Allergy* 1985; 15:501–8.

158 Shorten GD. Postoperative residual curisation: incidence, aetiology and associated morbidity. *Anaesth Intens Care* 1993;21:782–9.

159 Pedersen T, Eliasen K, Henriksen E. A prospective study of risk factors and cardiopulmonary complications associated with anaesthesia and surgery: risk indicators of cardiopulmonary morbidity. *Acta Anaesthesiol Scand* 1990;34:144-55.

160 Zelcer J, Wells DG. Anaesthetic-related recovery room complications. *Anaesth Intens Care* 1987;15:168–74.

161 Bowman WC. Non-relaxant properties of neuromuscular blocking drugs. *Br J Anaesth* 1982;54:147–60.

162 Basta SJ. Modulation of histamine release by neuromuscular blocking drugs. *Curr Opin Anaesthesiol* 1992;5:572–6.

163 Levy JH, Davis GK, Duggan J, Szlam F. Determination of the hemodynamics and histamine release of rocuronium (Org 9426) when administered in increased doses under N_2O/O_2-sufentanil anesthesia. *Anesth Analg* 1994;78:318–21.

164 Matteo RS, Liebermann IG, Salnitre E, McDaniel DD, Diaz J. Distribution, elimination, and action of d-tubocurarine in neonates, infants, children, and adults. *Anesth Analg* 1984;63:799–804.

165 Fisher DM, O'Keefe C, Stanski DR, Cronnelly R, Miller RD, Gregory GA. Pharmacokinetics and pharmacodynamics of d-tubocurarine in infants, children, and adults. *Anesthesiology* 1982;57:203–8.

166 Brandom BW, Stiller RL, Cook DR, Woelfel SK, Chakravorti S, Lai A. Pharmacokinetics of atracurium in anesthetized infants and children. *Br J Anaesth* 1986;58:1210–13.

167 Fisher DM, Canfell PC, Spellman MJ, Miller RD. Pharmacokinetics and pharmaco-dynamics of atracurium in infants and children. *Anesthesiology* 1990;73:33–7.

168 Kitts JB, Fisher DM, Canfell PC, *et al*. Pharmacokinetics and pharmacodynamics of atracurium in the elderly. *Anesthesiology* 1990;72:272–5.

169 Goudsouzian NG, Alifimoff JK, Liu LMP, Foster VJ, McNulty BF, Savarese JJ. Neuromuscular and cardiovascular effects of doxacurium in children anaesthetized with halothane. *Br J Anaesth* 1989;**62**:263–8.

170 Sarner JB, Brandom BW, Cook DR, *et al.* Clinical pharmacology of doxacurium chloride (BW 938U) in children. *Anesth Analg* 1988;**67**:303–6.

171 Goudsouzian NG, Alifirmoff JK, Eberly C, *et al.* Cardiovascular effects of mivacurium in children. *Anesthesiology* 1989;**70**:237–42.

172 Meistelman C, Agoston S, Kersten UW, Saint-Maurice C, Bencini AF, Loose JP. Pharmacokinetics and pharmacodynamics of vecuronium and pancuronium in anesthetized children. *Anesth Analg* 1986;**65**:1319–23.

173 Pittet JF, Taasonyi E, Morel DR, Gemperle G, Rouge JC. Neuromuscular effect of pipecuronium bromide in infants and children during nitrous oxide–alfentanil anesthesia. *Anesthesiology* 1909;**72**:432–5.

174 Vuksanaj D, Fisher DM. Pharmacokinetics of rocuronium in children aged 4–11 years. *Anesthesiology* 1995;**82**:1104–10.

175 Rupp SM, Fisher DM, Miller RD, Catagnoli K. Pharmacokinetics and pharmacodynamics of vecuronium in the elderly. *Anesthesiology* 1983;**59**:A270.

176 Matteo RS, Backus WW, McDaniel DD, Brotherton WP, Abraham R, Diaz J. Pharmacokinetics and pharmacodynamics of d-tubocurarine and metocurine in the elderly. *Anesth Analg* 1985;**64**:23–9.

177 Stephens ID, Ho PC, Holloway AW, Bourne DWA, Triggs EJ. Pharmacokinetics of alcuronium in elderly patients undergoing total hip replacements or aortic reconstructive surgery. *Br J Anaesth* 1984;**56**:465–71.

178 Dresner DL, Basta SJ, Ali HH, *et al.* Pharmacokinetics and pharmacodynamics of doxacurium in young and elderly patients during isoflurane anesthesia. *Anesth Analg* 1990;**71**:498–502.

179 Duvaldestin P, Saada J, Berger JL, D'Hollander A, Desmonts JM. Pharmacokinetics, pharmacodynamics and dose–response relationships of pancuronium in control and elderly subjects. *Anesthesiology* 1982;**56**:36–40.

180 Lien CA, Matteo RS, Ornstein E. Distribution, elimination, and action of vecuronium in the elderly. *Anesth Analg* 1991;**73**:39–42.

181 McLeod K, Hull CJ, Watson MJ. Effect of ageing on the pharmacokinetics of pancuronium. *Br J Anaesth* 1979;**51**:435–8.

182 Bell PF, Mirakhur RK, Clarke RSJ. Dose–response studies of atracurium, vecuronium and pancuronium in the elderly. *Anaesthesia* 1989;**44**:925–7.

183 Koscielniak-Nielsen ZJ, Law-Min JC, Donati F, Bevan DR, Clement P, Wise R. Dose–response relations of doxacurium and its reversal with neostigmine in young adults and healthy elderly patients. *Anesth Analg* 1992;**74**:845–50.

184 Parker CJP, Hunter JM, Snowdon SL. Effect of age, gender and anaesthetic technique on the pharmacodynamics of atracurium. *Br J Anaesth* 1993;**70**:38–42.

185 Duvaldestin P, Saada J, Berger JL, D'Hollander A, Desmonts JM. Pharmacokinetics, pharmacodynamics and dose–response relationships of pancuronium in control and elderly subjects. *Anesthesiology* 1982;**56**:36–40.

186 Cronnelly R, Fisher SM, Miller RD, Gencarelli P, Nguyen-Gruneke L, Castagnoli N Jr. Pharmacokinetics and pharmacodynamics of vecuronium (Org NC45) and pancuronium in anesthetized humans. *Anesthesiology* 1983;**58**:405–8.

187 Ornstein E, Matteo RS, Schwartz AE, Jamdar SC, Diaz J. Pharmacokinetics and pharmacodynamics of pipecuronium bromide (Arduan) in elderly surgical patients. *Anesth Analg* 1992;**74**:841–4.

188 Matteo RS, Ornstein E, Schwartz AE, Ostapkovich N, Stone JG. Pharmacokinetics and pharmacodynamics of rocuronium (Org 9426) in elderly surgical patients. *Anesth Analg* 1993;**77**:1193–7.

189 Fiset P, Balendram P, Bevan DR. Onset, duration, and recovery from Org 9426 in the elderly. *Anesthesiology* 1990;**73**:A881.

190 Matteo RS, Ornstein E, Schwartz AE, *et al.* Pharmacokinetics and pharmacodynamics of Org 9426 in elderly surgical patients. *Anesthesiology* 1991;**75**:A1065.

191 Kent AP, Parker CJR, Hunter JM. Pharmacokinetics of atracurium and laudanosine in the elderly. *Br J Anaesth* 1989;**63**:661–6.

192 Slavov V, Khalil M, Merle JC, Agostini MM, Ruggier R, Duvaldestin P. Comparison of duration of neuromuscular blocking effect of atracurium and vecuronium in young and elderly patients. *Br J Anaesth* 1995;**74**:709–11.

193 Gariepy LP, Varin F, Donati F, Salib Y, Bevan DR. Influence of aging on the pharmacokinetics and pharmacodynamics of doxacurium. *Clin Pharmacol Ther* 1993; **53**:340–7.

194 Schmith VD, Lai A, Dresner DL. Pharmacodynamic modeling of doxacurium in young adult and elderly patients [Abstract]. *Pharmacol Res* 1991;**8**:S275.

195 Matteo RS, Schwartz AE, Ornstein E, et al. Pharmacokinetics and pharmacodynamics of pipecuronium in elderly surgical patients. *Anesth Analg* 1991;**72**:S172.

196 Diefenbach C, Mellinghof H, Buzello W. Variability of pipecuronium neuromuscular blockade. *Acta Anaesthesiol Scand* 1993;**37**:189–91.

197 Meistelman C, Agoston S, Kersten UW, Saint Maurice C, Bencini AF, Loose JP. Pharmacokinetics and pharmacodynamics of vecuronium and pancuronium in anesthetized children. *Anesth Analg* 1986;**65**:1319–23.

198 Caldwell JE, Castagnoli KP, Canfell PC, et al. Pipecuronium and pancuronium: comparison of pharmacokinetics and duration of action. *Br J Anaesth* 1988;**61**:693–7.

199 Duvaldestin P, Demetriou M, Henzel D, Desmonts JM. The placental transfer of pancuronium and its pharmacokinetics during caesarian section. *Acta Anaesthesiol Scand* 1978;**22**:327–33.

200 Dailey PA, Fisher DM, Shnider SM, et al. Pharmacokinetics, placental transfer, and neonatal effects of vecuronium and pancuronium administered during Caesarean section. *Anesthesiology* 1984;**60**:569–74.

201 Flynn PJ, Frank M, Hughes R. Use of atracurium in caesarean section. *Br J Anaesth* 1984;**56**:599–605.

202 Abouleish E, Wingard Jr, S, De La Vega S, Uy N. Pancuronium in Caesarean section and its placental transfer. *Br J Anaesth* 1980;**52**:531–6.

203 Ho PC, Stephens ID, Triggs EJ. Caesarean section and placental transfer of alcuronium. *Anaesth Intens Care* 1981;**9**:113–18.

204 Hogue CW, Jr, Ward JM, Itani MS, Martyn JAJ. Tolerance and upregulation of acetylcholine receptors follow chronic infusion of d-tubocurarine. *J Appl Physiol* 1992;**72**:1326–31.

205 Segredo V, Matthay MA, Sharma ML, Gruenke LD, Caldwell JE, Miller RD. Prolonged neuromuscular blockade after long term administration of vecuronium in two critically ill patients. *Anesthesiology* 1990;**72**:566–70.

206 Patridge BL, Abrams JH, Bazemore C, Rubin R. Prolonged neuromuscular blockade after long term infusion of vecuronium bromide in the intensive care unit. *Crit Care Med* 1990;**18**:1177–9.

207 Gooch JL, Suchtya MR, Balbierz JM, Petajan JH, Clemmer TP. Prolonged paralysis after treatment with neuromuscular junction blocking agents. *Crit Care Med* 1991; **19**:1125–31.

208 Heckmatt JZ, Pitt MC, Kirkham F. Peripheral neuropathy and neuromuscular blockade presenting as prolonged respiratory paralysis following critical illness. *Neuropediatrics* 1993;**24**:123–5.

209 Kupfer Y, Namba T, Kaldawi E, Tessler S. Prolonged weakness after long-term infusion of vecuronium bromide. *Ann Intern Med* 1992;**117**:484–6.

210 Zochodne DW, Bolton CF, Wells GA, et al. Critical illness polyneuropathy—a complication of sepsis and multiorgan failure. *Brain* 1987;**110**:819–42.

211 Witt NJ, Zochodne DW, Bolton CF, et al. Peripheral nerve function in sepsis and multiple organ failure. *Chest* 1991;**99**:176–84.

212 Bolton CF, Young GB, Zochodne DW. The neurological complications of sepsis. *Ann Neurol* 1993;**33**:94–100.

213 Helliwell TR, Coakley JH, Wagenmakers AJM, et al. Necrotizing myopathy in critically-ill patients. *J Pathol* 1991;**164**:307–14.

214 Zochodne DW, Ramsay DA, Saly V, Shelley S, Moffatt S. Acute necrotizing myopathy of intensive care: electrophysiological studies. *Muscle Nerve* 1994;**17**:285–92.

215 Segredo V, Caldwell JE, Matthay MA, Sharma ML, Gruenke LD, Miller RD. Persistent paralysis in critically ill patients after long-term administration of vecuronium. *N Engl J Med* 1992;**327**:524–8.

216 Brun-Buisson C, Gheraldi R. Hydrocortisone and pancuronium bromide: acute myopathy during status asthmaticus (letter to the editor). *Crit Care Med* 1988;**16**:731–2.

217 Barohn RJ, Jackson CE, Rogers SJ, Ridings LW, McVey AL. Prolonged paralysis due to nondepolarising neuromuscular blocking agents and corticosteroids. *Muscle Nerve* 1994;**17**:647–54.

218 Op de Coul AAW, Lambregts PCLA, Koeman J, van Puyenbroek MJE, Ter Laak HJ, Gabreëls-Festen AAWM. Neuromuscular complications in patients given Pavulon (pancuronium bromide) during artificial ventilation. *Clin Neurol Neurosurg* 1985; **887**:17–22.

219 Griffin D, Fairman N, Coursin DB, Rawsthorne L, Grossman JE. Acute myopathy during treatment of status asthmaticus with corticosteroids and steroidal relaxants. *Chest* 1992;**102**:510–14.

220 Meyer KC, Prielipp RC, Grossman JE, Coursin DB. Prolonged weakness after infusion of atracurium in two intensive care unit patients. *Anesth Analg* 1994;**78**:772–4.

221 Gwinnutt CL, Eddleston JM, Edwards D, Pollard BJ. Concentrations of atracurium and laudanosine in cerebrospinal fluid and plasma in three intensive care patients. *Br J Anaesth* 1990;**65**:829–32.

222 Parker CJR, Jones JE, Hunter JM. Disposition of infusions of atracurium and its metabolite, laudanosine, in patients with renal and respiratory failure in an ITU. *Br J Anaesth* 1988;**61**:531–40.

223 Nigrovic V, Klaunig JE, Smith SL, Schulz NE, Wajskol A. Comparative toxicity of atracurium and metocurine in isolated rat hepatocytes. *Anesth Analg* 1986;**65**:1107–11.

224 Callanan DL. Development of resistance to pancuronium in adult respiratory distress syndrome. *Anesth Analg* 1985;**64**:1126–8.

225 Coursin DB, Klasek G, Goelzer SL. Increased requirements for continuous infused vecuronium in critically ill patients. *Anesth Analg* 1989;**69**:518–21.

226 Yate PM, Flynn PJ, Arnold RW, Weatherly BC, Simmonds RJ, Dobson T. Clinical experience and plasma laudanosine concentrations during infusion of atracurium in the intensive therapy unit. *Br J Anaesth* 1987;**59**:211–17.

227 Mesry S, Baradaran J. Accidental intrathecal injection of gallamine triethiodide. *Anaesthesia* 1974;**29**:301–4.

228 Peduto VA, Gungii P, Di Martino MR, Napoleone M. Accidental subarachnoid injection of pancuronium. *Anesth Analg* 1989;**69**:516–17.

229 Matteo RS, Pua EK, Khambotta KJ, Spector S. Cerebrospinal fluid levels of d-tubocurarine in man. *Anesthesiology* 1977;**46**:396–400.

7: Muscle relaxants and concurrent diseases

LEO HDJ BOOIJ

Muscle relaxants nowadays are indispensable tools for anaesthetists. The effects of neuromuscular blocking agents in patients is characterised by a wide variability, in both the intensity and the time course of action.[1] Apart from anatomical and physiological factors, such as interindividual variability in body size and composition, muscular maturity (age), gender, and variability in plasma cholinesterase activity, many other factors are important. These factors include interactions of relaxants with concurrent medication and the physical status of the patient. A variety of diseases such as hepatic and renal failure, acid–base imbalance, electrolyte shift, and neuromuscular disturbances do cause pharmacodynamic or pharmacokinetic change in the properties of the relaxant administered.

Muscle relaxants themselves have effects on the normal functioning of the body. Such side effects may interfere with concurrent diseases and administered drugs. Especially in cases where altered effects of relaxants can be expected, or where the side effects of the relaxants are causing an increased risk for the patients, close monitoring of neuromuscular function throughout the case is desirable. Furthermore, good clinical practice demands the administration of the smallest dose necessary to achieve adequate relaxation in the individual patient.

Effect of concurrent diseases on the pharmacological effect of muscle relaxants

Many diseases can interfere with either the pharmacodynamics or the pharmacokinetics of muscle relaxants. Both result in an increased or decreased sensitivity to the relaxant (degree of neuromuscular blockade), and a change in the time course of action (onset, duration, and recovery rate).

There are various reasons why diseases interact with the pharmacodynamics of a muscle relaxant. Some diseases interfere with the generation and conductance of stimuli in the central or peripheral motor nervous system. This will lead to a change in acetylcholine release at the neuromuscular junction. Other diseases directly interfere with the neuro-muscular junction, through interference either with the amount of acetylcholine synthesised, mobilised, released, or metabolised, or with the number of postjunctional acetylcholine receptors (upregulation and down-regulation) available. The resulting change in the margin of safety of neuromuscular transmission leads to an altered effect of the relaxants. Yet other diseases interfere with the contractility of the muscles themselves, and appear to lead to a change in the pharmacodynamics of the relaxants.

All such interactions may not only be a direct result of the disease itself, but may also be related to the drugs that are administered for the treatment of that disease.[2] Drug interactions with muscle relaxants are discussed in chapter 4.

Muscle relaxation is caused by occupation of acetylcholine receptors by depolarising or non-depolarising relaxants (see chapter 2). A relationship exists between the plasma concentration of the relaxant and the receptor occupancy. The plasma concentration of the relaxant is determined by the pharmacokinetic behaviour of the drug. Pharmacokinetic interactions with relaxants may thus be mediated by interference of the disease with their volume of distribution, protein binding, metabolism, and excretion. Change in the haemodynamics may, for example, change the distribution of a relaxant over the body, and its extraction and metabolism in the liver or kidney. Another example is that increase in blood volume will lead to an increased initial volume of distribution, resulting in a slower onset and possibly a lesser degree of neuromuscular block. Again, drugs that are administered for the treatment of a concurrent disease may interfere with the pharmacokinetic behaviour of the muscle relaxant, for example, via protein binding or drug metabolism.

Both pharmacodynamic and pharmacokinetic alterations of drug effects will be visible as a change in the time course of action of the relaxants. Here we discuss some of the diseases that do interfere with the effect of the relaxants.

Effect of renal disease

Most muscle relaxants are water soluble, ionised, quaternary ammonium compounds, and thus depend on glomerular filtration, tubular excretion, and tubular reabsorption for their rate of body clearance (table 7.1).[3]

Gallamine is completely dependent, and pancuronium, tubocurarine, and metocurine are largely dependent on renal excretion. Only sux-amethonium (succinylcholine), atracurium, mivacurium, and to some extent vecuronium and rocuronium are more or less independent of renal excretion.

When renal function is diminished, a higher plasma concentration of relaxant is maintained for a longer period of time unless other routes of elimination exist. Also there is a decrease in elimination of endogenous substances which may now bind to non-specific relaxant binding sites. This will affect plasma clearance of the relaxant by a decrease in distribution

Table 7.1 Percentage and route of elimination of currently used relaxants over 24 hours

Drug	Renal elimination (%)	Biliary elimination (%)	Metabolism
Suxamethonium	0	0	100% pseudocholinesterase
Tubocurarine	45–60	10–40	0% metabolism
Metocurine	60–90	<10	0% metabolism
Atracurium	6–10	0	90% Hofmann elimination/carboxylesterase
Doxacurium	25–50		
Mivacurium	<10		100% pseudocholinesterase
Alcuronium	80–90	10	0% metabolism
Gallamine	95–98	2–5	0% metabolism
Fazadinium	25–60		
Pancuronium	60–90	20–30	35% metabolism
Pipecuronium	30–40	20–30	20% metabolism
Vecuronium	20–30	50–60	35% metabolism
Rocuronium	20–30		

Data randomly chosen from the literature.

across compartments. In renal disease other factors also often play a role, such as altered fluid status, metabolic imbalance, electrolyte shift, acid–base imbalance, and concurrent administration of drugs. For all these reasons abnormal response to the administration of muscle relaxants can be expected in patients with renal diseases. Some of the muscle relaxants may be removed from the body by haemofiltration.

Depolarising muscle relaxants

The effect of suxamethonium depends on the plasma cholinesterase activity, which is independent of renal function. Thus the effect of suxamethonium is principally not altered in patients with isolated renal disease. However, in these patients suxamethonium can lead to a more pronounced potassium release leading to dangerous serum potassium concentrations (see later). In fact renal failure is frequently accompanied by hepatic disturbances, and these can decrease plasma cholinesterase activity. If alkalosis exists the effect of suxamethonium may be prolonged in renal patients, whereas in acidosis the effect can be shorter.

Following renal transplantation, cyclosporin (cyclosporine) is frequently administered for immunosuppression. A case in which cyclosporin prolonged the effect of pancuronium has been reported,[4] and such an effect has been confirmed in animal experiments. Furthermore, plasma cholinesterase activity is decreased for about two weeks after renal transplantations; the decrease is so small, however, that it is unlikely that suxamethonium will have a longer effect by this mechanism.[5]

Non-depolarising relaxants

With all non-depolarising agents, a greater variability in effect exists in patients with renal failure than in patients with normal renal function. It has been demonstrated that these alterations are the result of changed pharmacokinetic behaviour of the drugs.

Table 7.2   Pharmacokinetic data on muscle relaxants in patients with renal failure as found in the literature

	VD_{ss} (l/kg)		Cl_p (ml/kg per min)		Elimination half life (min)	
	Normal	Renal	Normal	Renal	Normal	Renal
Atracurium	0·18	0·22	6·1	6·7	21	24
Doxacurium	0·22	0·27	2·66	1·16	99	221
Fazadinium	0·21	0·31	2·1	1·6	96	140
Gallamine	0·21	0·28	1·2	0·24	131	752
Metocurine	0·15	0·24	1·3	0·38	360	684
Mivacurium	0·11	0·15	70·3	76·5	18	34
Pancuronium	0·15	0·24	1·0	0·3	100	489
Pipecuronium	0·31	0·44	2·3	1·66	137	263
Rocuronium	0·21	0·21	3·7	2·5	97	104
Tubocurarine	0·25	0·25	2·4	1·5	84	132
Vecuronium	0·20	0·24	5·3	3·1	53	83

As the data are illustrative, the figures are rounded, and references are not given.
VD_{ss}, volume of distribution into central and prejunctional components; Cl_p, plasma clearance.

The initial volume of distribution (central compartment) of relaxants does not differ in patients with renal failure, but the elimination half life does with most relaxants (table 7.2). The reason for this is that there is a larger volume of distribution and a reduced plasma clearance. Protein binding only makes a minimal contribution because relaxants are not highly protein bound (40–50%). α_1-Globulin binding is the major component in binding.[6]

As a result of a decrease in clearance, administration of incremental doses or continuous infusion of relaxants will cause prolonged neuromuscular blockade.

In renal failure the time course of action is altered with most relaxants. The elimination of gallamine is most affected in renal failure because it is not metabolised, but is almost entirely dependent on renal excretion (>95%). An increase in the duration of action is observed, especially when larger or repeated doses are administered.[7] The effect of tubocurarine, 25–60% of which is excreted via the kidneys, is known to be prolonged in renal failure—the elimination half life is increased.[8] Also alcuronium and metocurine (60–90% renal excretion) have a prolonged effect through decreased clearance.[9] Pancuronium is 60–90% excreted by the kidneys, although 25–40% is first metabolised in the liver; in renal failure the plasma clearance is decreased.[10 11] All these drugs thus have a prolonged duration of action in renal failure.

The plasma clearance of vecuronium and atracurium is said to be minimally affected by renal failure. Atracurium is dependent on the Hofmann elimination (temperature and pH determined) and non-specific hydrolysis in plasma by carboxylesterase,[12 13] so its effect is not affected by renal failure.[14 15] Vecuronium is mainly excreted in the bile; nevertheless it does show some accumulation in patients with renal failure.[16]

This will lead to a prolonged effect, especially after repeated administration or continuous infusion.[17 18] After prolonged administration it has been proved that, in renal failure, a higher plasma concentration of 3-desacetylvecuronium is present.[17] This compound has a neuromuscular blocking effect that is about half that of vecuronium. In patients receiving isoflurane anaesthesia, vecuronium has a decreased plasma clearance and a prolonged elimination half life as compared with that in patients with normal renal function.[19]

Fazadinium is excreted largely unchanged by the kidneys (25–60%) and is only metabolised in the liver to a minor extent. The effect of fazadinium is, however, not prolonged in renal failure.[20] About 40% of pipecuronium is excreted unchanged via the kidneys; more is excreted by the kidneys after metabolism in the liver. The elimination half life is prolonged in renal failure, but the duration of the effect is not prolonged.[21]

In one paper,[22] renal failure does not seem to have influenced the time course of action of rocuronium. In another paper, however, the duration of action is prolonged, although unlike other agents the onset of action of rocuronium is not affected.[23]

As a large part of doxacurium is excreted unchanged via the kidneys, the duration of action is prolonged in patients with renal failure.[24] It has in fact been demonstrated that a greater variability effect exists in doxacurium.[25]

Mivacurium is metabolised by plasma cholinesterase at a rate that is 70–90% that of suxamethonium;[25] the experimental drugs BW 985U, BW 785U, and BW 444U[26-28] are also all hydrolysed by plasma cholinesterase, and so all are expected to be independent of renal function. In a study on continuous infusion of mivacurium in renal failure, however, a lower infusion rate was needed to maintain a certain degree of blockade, and recovery lasted longer compared with in patients with normal renal function.[29] A case was recently reported in which a single dose of mivacurium lasted a long time in a patient with renal failure.[30]

Some patients in renal failure are resistant to atracurium or vecuronium, and no explanation has been found for this.[31] It might, however, be that an increased volume of distribution is present in these patients. In patients with renal failure a higher plasma concentration of the major metabolite of atracurium—laudanosine—is present.[32] This, however, has never been reported as a cause of problems.

In another study,[15] it was found that the duration of action of atracurium in patients in renal failure is reduced compared with that in patients with normal renal function; with repeated administration the authors were unable to demonstrate a prolongation in the effect. In the same study, the effect of pancuronium in patients in renal failure was found to be longer, and an increase in duration after repeated administration was also observed.[15]

In addition to the prolonged effect that most muscle relaxants exhibit in patients with renal failure, anticholinesterases also have a longer duration of action. This makes the prospect of recurarisation after their administration almost impossible (see chapter 8).

The effect of hepatic diseases on muscle relaxants

As muscle relaxants are water soluble, the liver only plays a minor role in the excretion of these compounds (see table 7.1). The liver is, however, important in the metabolism of some of them, especially the steroidal relaxants. As drug metabolism is, most of the time, only affected in the later stages of cirrhosis, this disease will not in general have an influence on the duration of neuromuscular blockade. In cholestasis, however, uptake in the liver is decreased, which decreases plasma clearance and leads to a prolonged effect.[33] Hepatic elimination of relaxants is dependent on hepatic blood perfusion, hepatic drug extraction, and drug binding to proteins.[34] Changes in these factors will result in different pharmacokinetics and hence in altered pharmacodynamics.[35]

Depolarising relaxants

Plasma cholinesterase, on which the metabolism of suxamethonium, the non-depolarising relaxant mivacurium,[25] and the experimental drugs BW 985U, BW 785U, and BW 444U[26-28] is dependent, is produced in the liver. Thus in patients with liver diseases that result in altered plasma cholinesterase activity, an enhanced effect of these relaxants is to be expected.

Non-depolarising relaxants

The liver only plays a secondary role in the excretion of most non-depolarising muscle relaxants. Nevertheless, in patients with liver diseases, their effects are often prolonged. The liver is not involved in the elimination of atracurium and gallamine, and is of minimal importance in the elimination of metocurine. Only about 10% of alcuronium, pancuronium, vecuronium, and tubocurarine is excreted in the bile. This amount may be increased when there is renal failure. The liver is, however, important in the metabolism of, for example, pancuronium (25–40%) and vecuronium (20–35%), which are mainly excreted in the urine after such metabolism. Hepatic diseases interfere with this metabolism and thus alter the pharmacokinetic profile of the drugs involved (table 7.3).

Alterations in the pharmacokinetic profile may lead to alterations in the pharmacodynamic profile.

Patients with chronic liver disease are resistant to a number of muscle relaxants that also have a slower onset of action. In cirrhotic patients this is the result of an increase in the volume of distribution, leading to a lower plasma concentration when the same dose is administered. This phenomenon can be observed with pancuronium, tubocurarine, and atracurium, but not with gallamine. The larger volume of distribution will also result in an increased terminal half life and, thus, prolong the duration of action. There is no resistance to vecuronium in cirrhotic patients, but the duration of

Table 7.3 Pharmacokinetic data on muscle relaxants in patients with cirrhotic liver disease as found in the literature

	VD_{ss} (l/kg)		Cl_p (ml/kg min)		Elimination half life (min)	
	Normal	Cirrhosis	Normal	Cirrhosis	Normal	Cirrhosis
Alcuronium						
Atracurium	0·20	0·28	6·6	8·0	21	25
Doxacurium	0·22	0·29	2·66	2·33	99	115
Fazadinium	0·23	0·45	2·1	1·9	76	140
Gallamine	0·20	0·25	1·0	1·21	125	160
Metocurine						
Mivacurium	0·11	0·12	70·3	33·16	18	34
Pancuronium	0·28	0·42	1·9	1·5	114	208
Pipecuronium	0·35	0·45	2·96	2·61	111	143
Rocuronium	0·18	0·24	2·8	2·4	87	96
Tubocurarine						
Vecuronium	0·30	0·35	4·3	2·7	58	84

As the data are only illustrative, the figures are rounded, and references are not given.
VD_{ss}, volume of distribution into central and peripheral components; Cl_p, plasma clearance.

action of this drug is prolonged. The pharmacokinetics and duration of action of vecuronium at a dose of 0·1 mg/kg were shown in one study to be no different from those in normal patients.[36] An unexplainable slower onset of action was, however, present. The distribution and elimination half lives of pancuronium are prolonged in cirrhosis.[37] Mivacurium has a prolonged duration of action, which correlates with a decrease in plasma cholinesterase activity.[38]

In patients with primary biliary cirrhosis immunoglobulin IgG and IgM class antibodies against acetylcholine receptors are present, and consequently myasthenia gravis, like muscle weakness, has been demonstrated,[39 40] although these antibodies are different from those found in myasthenia gravis.[41] Whether these antibodies contribute to an increased sensitivity for relaxants in such patients remains to be determined.

The plasma clearance of rocuronium is mainly through liver uptake and biliary excretion.[42] The duration of action is prolonged in patients with hepatic dysfunction,[43] but the onset and recovery rate are slower. The initial volume of distribution in this situation is higher, as is the mean residence time (MRT). The other pharmacokinetic parameters are similar to those in normal patients.[44]

Hepatic diseases appear to have no influence on the effect of doxacurium.[45] In hepatic disease (cirrhosis) there is accumulation of laudanosine after administration of atracurium (see later).[46] In patients with liver cirrhosis there is no change in the pharmacokinetics of pipecuronium as compared with that in normal patients. Nevertheless the onset of action is delayed.[47]

In cholestatic patients the decrease in plasma elimination results in a prolonged half life time in the elimination phase, and hence a prolonged duration of action with tubocurarine, pancuronium, and vecuronium, and, to a lesser degree, also with gallamine.[48 49] The increased plasma concentration of bile salts in these patients reduces the liver uptake of vecuronium and pancuronium.[50]

In hepatitis, there is a decrease in plasma clearance, resulting in a longer duration of action.

The effect of acid–base imbalance on muscle relaxants

Acid–base imbalance interferes with muscle relaxation through various mechanisms such as alteration in protein binding, and changes in electrolyte distribution and acetylcholine release, etc. It is clear currently that the interactions are more complicated than originally thought.

Depolarising relaxants

It is generally accepted that, on the one hand, respiratory or metabolic acidosis antagonises the effect of suxamethonium; on the other, respiratory or metabolic alkalosis potentiates the effect of suxamethonium.

Non-depolarising relaxants

In older studies it was demonstrated that the effect of gallamine is decreased in respiratory acidosis and enhanced in respiratory alkalosis. On the contrary, tubocurarine, pancuronium, and vecuronium are potentiated by respiratory acidosis and antagonised by respiratory alkalosis. Acidosis slightly increases and alkalosis slightly decreases the effect of atracurium. Alcuronium and metocurine are barely influenced by changes in acid–base balance.

Recently, using a rat hemidiaphragm preparation, it was demonstrated that respiratory acidosis potentiated the effects of tubocurarine and vecuronium, but antagonised the effect of metocurine, pancuronium, and alcuronium.[51] In respiratory alkalosis tubocurarine and vecuronium were found to be antagonised and metocurine, pancuronium, and alcuronium to be potentiated. These results conflict partly with the previous studies, and may be an expression of the many factors involved in acid–base imbalance, such as electrolyte shift, changes in ionisation of relaxants, changes in protein binding, and so forth. The same group, using the same model, later demonstrated that there is no difference between respiratory or metabolic origin of the pH change: decrease in pH potentiated monoquaternary relaxants (tubocurarine and vecuronium), but antagonised bisquaternary relaxants (metocurine and pancuronium).[52] Rocuronium acts in this regard in a similar way to vecuronium, and pipecuronium to pancuronium.[53]

Respiratory acidosis and metabolic alkalosis do decrease the blockade reversing effect of the anticholinesterases (see chapter 8).

The effect of burn trauma on muscle relaxants

A number of altered effects have been described in patients with burns involving a larger part of the body.

Depolarising relaxants

After burn trauma, patients are more sensitive to suxamethonium;[54] when administered to these patients it can increase the serum potassium concentration to levels that induce cardiac arrest.[55 57] This will occur from the first few days after up to months afterwards. The more extensive the burn trauma, the more pronounced the potassium release. It is speculated to be caused by an increase in the number of acetylcholine receptors and their spread over the entire (extrajunctional) muscle membrane.[57]

Non-depolarising relaxants

In patients with burns in excess of 30% of their total body surface area (TBSA), resistance to non-depolarising muscle relaxants has been demonstrated. It starts about one week after the accident and lasts for more than one year. The relaxant plasma concentration at which a particular neuromuscular blockade occurs is increased. The origin of this effect is probably the multiplication and spread of acetylcholine receptors over the muscle membrane. Such an effect has been described for atracurium,[58] metocurine,[59] pancuronium,[60] and tubocurarine.[61] In 31 paediatric cases with burns, the potency of atracurium during the first week after the burn was found to be the same as in another control group of children.[62] After the first week, however, there was a decrease in the potency of atracurium. In thermally injured rats a maximal resistance at 40 days after the burn injury was demonstrated.[63] Higher plasma concentrations were needed to cause the same degree of blockade, indicating a lower sensitivity/affinity of the acetylcholine receptor. In rat experiments using muscles distant from the burn sites, an increase in the number of acetylcholine receptors was found in these muscles.[64]

The increased requirement for tubocurarine and atracurium cannot be explained by pharmacokinetic change.[65 66] With other relaxants such studies have not been done.

The effect of neural and neuromuscular diseases on muscle relaxants

Neural and neuromuscular diseases present a number of implications with respect to the administration of anaesthesia.[67] In many such patients, autonomic nervous system dysregulation is present. In addition, in many neuromuscular diseases, the myocardium is also involved, and, in general, there is a higher sensitivity to muscle relaxants than in normal patients. After administration for a long period muscle relaxants can reach considerable concentrations in the brain and interfere with the cerebral acetylcholine receptors. This is especially a possibility for consideration in patients with disturbed blood–brain barriers (either from disease or the administration of mannitol and other hyperosmolar fluids). It is well known that non-depolarising relaxants do have an excitatory central nervous system effect.[68 69]

132

Depolarising relaxants

In many neural and neuromuscular diseases the administration of suxamethonium is accompanied by massive potassium release, resulting in hyperkalaemia.[56] Such hyperkalaemia has been seen in hemiplegia,[70] paraplegia,[71] encephalitis,[72] diffuse intracranial lesions,[73] ruptured cerebral aneurysm,[74] peripheral neuropathy,[75] and peripheral denervation.[76] The potassium release is most probably the result of extension of the muscular junctions (and acetylcholine receptors) beyond the original motor endplate and is called "extrajunctional chemosensitivity." It is seen in all muscle denervation lesions, starting as early as one week and as late as six months after the accident; it has an unknown duration.

Non-depolarising relaxants

Many neural and neuromuscular diseases cause a change in the pharmacodynamic behaviour of the non-depolarising relaxants, that is, increased sensitivity and a prolonged duration of action are seen. Most of these patients are also extremely sensitive to the cardiovascular effects of the relaxants.

Effect of relaxants in specific neural diseases

Motoneuron lesions—Central motoneuron lesions (cerebral location, that is, hemiplegia) have been associated with resistance to non-depolarising muscle relaxants at the afflicted side, and with hyperkalaemia following administration of suxamethonium.[56 77–79] The changes occur two days after the start of the hemiplegia, and are probably caused by sprouting of remaining axons, with spread of the increased number of acetylcholine receptors (extrajunctional chemosensitivity). In addition, in patients with diffuse intracranial lesions, ruptured cerebral aneurysm, and closed head injury, there is increased potassium release on suxamethonium administration and resistance to non-depolarising relaxant has been observed.[80] This may lead to inadvertent mortality.

In lower motoneuron lesions (spinal cord location, that is, paraplegia, quadriplegia), however, increased response to non-depolarising relaxants is observed at the afflicted side.[81] There is supersensitivity to suxamethonium, which can also in this situation lead to hyperkalaemia.[82 83] The origin of the effects in lower motoneuron lesions is a sprouting of acetylcholine receptors.[84] It has even been reported after transient paraplegia.[85] Muscular contractures may occur spontaneously or following suxamethonium administration in denervated muscles.[76] In amyotrophic lateral sclerosis suxamethonium may induce a myotonia like contracture.[86]

One to two weeks after peripheral muscular denervation (peripheral nerve damage), extrajunctional chemosensitivity and decrease in plasma cholinesterase activity develop. Thus an increased response to suxamethonium will occur; even myotonic contractures may be seen. There is normal response to non-depolarising relaxants in denervation disorders.[87] Reinnervation restores both the number of acetylcholine receptors and their function, whereas induced muscle activity only restores their function. This normalises the sensitivity for suxamethonium.

In multiple sclerosis[88] contractures and rhabdomyolysis may occur after administration of suxamethonium.

Myotonia—In the three groups of myotonia (dystrophic, congenita, and paramyotonia), suxamethonium may induce myotonic crisis with hyperkalaemia and inability to intubate the trachea.[89 90] Also rhabdomyolysis may occur. The effect of non-depolarising relaxants is normal in some patients and enhanced in others.[91] Reversal with neostigmine or use of a nerve stimulator may also result in sustained muscle contraction.[92–94]

Muscular dystrophy—In Duchenne muscular dystrophy the administration of suxamethonium may lead to rhabdomyolysis.[95] Also acidosis and hyperkalaemia occur and may even lead to death of the patient.[96] Patients are easily paralysed by non-depolarising relaxants, thus their titration with monitoring of neuromuscular transmission is advocated.[97] Suxamethonium can induce hyperkalaemia in apparently healthy children and adolescents who were subsequently found to have myopathies.[98] In 50% of the cases it caused death. Administration of suxamethonium in patients with mitochondrial myopathy may induce malignant hyperthermia.[99]

Peripheral polyneuropathy—Patients with peripheral polyneuropathy from all kinds of origin (diabetes, alcoholism, vascular insufficiency, vitamin deficiencies, tumours, heavy metal poisoning, etc) are extremely sensitive to non-depolarising muscle relaxants and resistant to suxamethonium. In Guillain–Barré syndrome suxamethonium can induce hyperkalaemia.[100]

Myasthenic syndromes—In myasthenia gravis an autoimmune process causes reduction of functional acetylcholine receptors at the neuromuscular junction. The quantal acetylcholine content is unchanged. Patients have an increased sensitivity for non-depolarising relaxants.[101 102] The increased sensitivity is strongly related to individual anti-acetylcholine/receptor antibody titres. Patients with "cured myasthenia gravis" remain more sensitive.[103] Resistance to suxamethonium is seen in myasthenia. With repeated doses of suxamethonium a progressive prolongation of blockade occurs and phase II block easily develops.[104–107] When, however, patients receive anticholinesterase treatment, a decrease in plasma cholinesterase may occur. Then increased sensitivity to suxamethonium can be expected.[108] Myasthenic patients are more sensitive to non-depolarising relaxants than normal patients. When, however, equipotent dosages are given, the duration of blockade is no different.[109] Patients are also more sensitive to mivacurium, although this drug is dependent on plasma cholinesterase activity.[110] When acetylcholinesterase inhibitors are administered to reverse a non-depolarising blockade in myasthenic patients, a depolarising blockade may occur.[111] Thus reversal of blockade should be done very carefully, and only if absolutely indicated. In myasthenic patients a number of other drugs, including some antibiotics, can cause paralysis. This is an expression of the decreased margin of safety in neuromuscular transmission in such patients.

In myasthenic syndrome (Lambert–Eaton syndrome) the number of receptors is not affected, but the amount of acetylcholine released is diminished. This is the result of production of autoantibodies against neuronal voltage operated calcium channels. There is also some change in the morphology and function of the acetylcholine receptors. The patients have an exaggerated response to both suxamethonium and non-depolarising relaxants.[112]

AIDS—In a study in patients with AIDS the onset time and duration of action of vecuronium were longer than in normal patients.[113] A number of factors, such as the associated peripheral neuropathy, the associated myopathy, or the administration of antiviral drugs, may be involved.

Effect of decreased plasma cholinesterase activity on muscle relaxants

Plasma cholinesterase (acetylcholine acetylhydrolase) is involved in the metabolism of a number of relaxants, and so a change in its activity may change the effect of the relaxant (see chapter 5). Plasma cholinesterase activity is not only low in patients with inherited atypical cholinesterase,[114] but also in patients with liver disease,[115] in pregnancy,[116 117] during cardiopulmonary bypass,[118] and with use of cytotoxic drugs and anticholinesterases. It has been demonstrated that cardiopulmonary bypass does decrease plasma cholinesterase activity by 60%, independently of whether this was run under normothermic or hypothermic conditions.[119] After about six weeks the activity is back to normal. Furthermore the plasma cholinesterase activity from birth to about six months of age is 50% that of adults. Between the ages of three and six years it is 30% higher than in adults.[120] In elderly people (>70 years), the plasma cholinesterase activity is about 25% lower than in younger adults.[121]

Depolarising relaxants

It has been demonstrated that suxamethonium has a large interindividual variability in its effect. The duration of action is inversely correlated with the plasma cholinesterase activity of the patient, even in patients with genotypically normal enzyme.[122] In a recent study it was demonstrated that this is also true for the potency (degree of blockade) of suxamethonium.[123] The interindividual difference in plasma cholinesterase activity is thus one of the major factors involved in the variability in response to suxamethonium. As plasma cholinesterase activity is, as mentioned above, decreased in a variety of situations, it is unlikely that variability in effect can ever be prevented. Another point is that, as a result of a fast hydrolysis by plasma cholinesterase, only a small part of the suxamethonium injected reaches the neuromuscular junction. Such a small amount is effective because only 25–30% of the acetylcholine receptors need to be occupied.

Decreased cholinesterase activity with an increased sensitivity to and prolonged effect of suxamethonium has been demonstrated in patients with the Churg–Strauss syndrome (allergic angiitis with granulomatosis) who have been treated with immunosuppressive agents.[124] Drugs which are broken down by plasma cholinesterase (procaine, procainamide, ecothiopate, etc) also interfere with suxamethonium.

Non-depolarising relaxants

Mivacurium is metabolised by plasma cholinesterase at a rate 70–90% that of suxamethonium.[25] The metabolites are inactive. There is an inverse relationship between the plasma cholinesterase activity and the duration of action of mivacurium,[125] so that there is prolonged effect in patients with atypical or decreased pseudocholinesterase.[126] Also, in elderly people, mivacurium is longer lasting.[127] It is known that elderly people do have a lower plasma cholinesterase activity, but whether this is the cause remains to be proved. It has been speculated that prolonged mivacurium blockade may be reversed with neostigmine.[128]

The experimental neuromuscular blocking drugs, BW 985U, BW 785U, and BW 444U,[26–28] are all also hydrolysed by plasma cholinesterase into inactive derivatives.

Atracurium is 40–50% spontaneously metabolised by Hofmann degradation (pH and temperature dependent) and ester hydrolysis.[13 129] In patients with decreased plasma cholinesterase activity, a prolonged effect of atracurium has not been described because atracurium metabolism involves carboxylesterase and not plasma cholinesterase.[130]

The effect of tumours on muscle relaxants

In children with abdominal, bone, or cerebral tumours, it was demonstrated that a delayed onset of action and decreased sensitivity occur after administration of tubocurarine and alcuronium.[131] Upon successful treatment (surgery or chemotherapy) the sensitivity reverted to normal. An explanation for this discrepancy is not yet available. Also in children with liver tumours there is decreased sensitivity to tubocurarine and alcuronium.[132]

In patients with various types of tumours a so called myasthenic syndrome (Lambert–Eaton syndrome) may develop. These patients have increased sensitivity for muscle relaxants.

The effect of temperature on muscle relaxants

Hypothermia decreases the contraction force of the adductor pollicis muscle even without the presence of muscle relaxants when measured with mechanomyography but an increase is seen when measured with electromyography (EMG).[133] Hypothermia during anaesthesia can occur spontaneously or may be induced, as is the case in cardiopulmonary bypass. In cardiopulmonary bypass it was demonstrated that cooling caused an increase in potency and a prolongation in the duration of pancuronium and vecuronium, via an effect at the neuromuscular junction rather than a change in pharmacokinetics.[134] This is in agreement with the increased sensitivity at the cat neuromuscular junction found in the past.[135] The effect of hypothermia is reversed upon rewarming. Similar data in cardiopulmonary bypass have been found with d-tubocurarine and alcuronium.[136] In addition, the atracurium effect is enhanced in hypothermia.[17 137] Studies without the use of cardiopulmonary bypass demonstrated that the twitch contraction of the adductor pollicis muscle remains unchanged above 35·2°C and below this it then decreased linearly with the temperature.[138] There was a difference between patients with active and those with passive cooling. In a subsequent study it was demonstrated that the effect of local surface cooling on muscle contraction was less than that of central core cooling.[139] Maintaining central temperature is therefore of primary importance. Cooling does not affect the train-of-four ratio. In mild intraoperative hypothermia, a significantly increased duration of action and significantly decreased recovery rate were observed for vecuronium.[140] Higher sensitivity during hypothermia has also been demonstrated for continuous infusion of vecuronium.[141]

Chronic administration of relaxants: effects of muscle relaxants in intensive care patients

Chronic administration of non-depolarising relaxants has been demonstrated in rats to cause upregulation (increase in number) of acetylcholine receptors and hence to decrease sensitivity for competitive antagonistic relaxants.[142] Theoretically this could also lead to increased potassium release when suxamethonium is administered. From other animal studies it has also been suggested that prolonged pharmacological denervation (neuromuscular block) can lead to morphological injury of the motor endplate.[143]

Muscle relaxants were originally developed and tested for relatively short duration administration. Currently, relaxants are even used for up to several weeks in the intensive care unit. Recently muscle areflexia, atrophy, and sensory impairment in patients with multiorgan failure have been attributed to the prolonged administration of muscle relaxants.[144–147] Muscle weakness may delay weaning from artificial ventilation. In one study 50% of the patients in the intensive care unit developed polyneuropathy upon administration of vecuronium for a long period.[148]

Signs of polyneuropathy are, however, also observed in other critically ill patients who have not received muscle relaxants (critical illness neuropathy).[149] In one study up to 70% of the intensive care patients with sepsis and multiple organ failure had symptoms of this syndrome.[150 151] In 50% of the patients with the syndrome, muscle fibre necrosis has been demonstrated and thus myopathy also exists.[152] In addition to motor function deficits, sensory deficits are also present. EMG readings in patients with critical illness neuropathy do not demonstrate neuromuscular transmission disorders.[153] It must therefore be concluded that this entity has more characteristics of a myopathy than of a neuropathy.

The neuropathy resulting from administration of relaxants in intensive care patients is a different entity. It is usually symmetrical and most of the time it does not involve the sensory system; in addition the neuromuscular transmission is affected. EMG readings frequently resemble those seen in Guillain–Barré syndrome or myonecrosis, but they also resemble readings resulting from residual neuromuscular blockade. Furthermore, it was demonstrated that about 50% of the patients receiving vecuronium over a long period of time developed prolonged paralysis. All these patients had renal insufficiency, and about half also had hepatic dysfunction. Most patients developing prolonged paralysis were women who had metabolic acidosis. All had a higher plasma concentration of 3-desacetylvecuronium compared with the patients not experiencing prolonged paralysis.[154] This compound does have a significant neuromuscular blocking effect which could have contributed to the blockade in these patients. Residual paralysis after prolonged administration of relaxants may be the reason for the polyneuropathy or myopathy seen on EMG readings in intensive care patients. It is also possible for other drugs, for example, aminoglycosides, polypeptides, and lincosamines, which are usually administered to this type of patient, to lead to neuromuscular and muscular abnormalities. Another example is seen with long term administration of corticosteroids.[155] The muscle weakness usually resolves slowly over weeks to months, after stopping administration of the relaxants. Although these results were confirmed by others,[156] further studies are needed to evaluate these neuropathic and myopathic effects.

It is mainly the steroidal relaxants that seem to cause the prolonged muscle weakness that is mentioned, especially in patients with renal failure or those who receive simultaneous administration of large doses of corticosteroids.[157 158] It must be realised, however, that steroids are used far more frequently in the intensive care unit than benzylisoquinolines.

After administration of atracurium prolonged muscle weakness has also been observed.[159] In intensive care patients, laudanosine, the major metabolite of atracurium, may also accumulate both in plasma and in cerebrospinal fluid.[160] This metabolite is also seen at higher concentrations in patients with renal and hepatic disease. In animal experiments laudanosine causes seizures, although this seems to be of minimal risk in patients.[161] In in vitro studies in isolated rat hepatocytes it was demonstrated furthermore that another metabolite of atracurium, a monoacrylate, results from alkylation of endogenous nucleophiles in cell damage.[162] This effect can also be neglected in humans. Thus it is unlikely that the metabolism of atracurium will, during short or long term clinical administration, lead to problems related to its metabolic products.

Contrary to cases of prolonged weakness, cases have been reported with development of resistance to pancuronium,[163] vecuronium,[164] and atracurium[165] over their long period of administration. This may be related to increased extrajunctional sensitivity to acetylcholine and/or receptor upregulation as a result of neuromuscular blockade.

There is a possibility that muscle relaxants, after administration for a long period, can reach high concentrations in the brain, and interfere with cerebral acetylcholine receptors.

This should be considered especially in patients with disturbed blood–brain barriers (from either disease or the administration of mannitol and other hypersomolar fluids). It is well known that non-depolarising relaxants do have an excitatory central nervous system effect with myotonia, convulsions, and autonomic changes.[166 167] Presence of relaxants in cerebrospinal fluid has been demonstrated after administration of large doses.[168]

Effect of muscle relaxants on concurrent diseases

The effect of muscle relaxants is not only affected by diseases; muscle relaxants can also exert potentially deleterious effects on the normal functioning of the body. They may thereby enhance or induce symptoms or diseases. It is known that the depolarising relaxants can cause cardiac dysrhythmias, hyperkalaemia, myalgia, myoglobinuria, increased intraocular pressure, increased intracranial pressure, and sustained skeletal muscle contraction.

The effect of muscle relaxants on intraocular and intracranial pressure

Increase in intraocular and intracranial pressure can cause severe damage, and must therefore be avoided. Such an increase can be mediated by an increase in blood flow or a direct pharmacological effect.

Depolarising relaxants

Both the administration of suxamethonium and tracheal intubation are known to increase the intraocular and intracranial pressures. In a recent study in children, suxamethonium 1 mg/kg increased the intraocular pressure by 84%, and endotracheal intubation added another 5% to this value.[169] The increase in pressure was maintained for a significant period of time and could not be prevented by prior intravenous administration of lignocaine (lidocaine) 2 mg/kg. Suxamethonium therefore has at least a relative contraindication in patients with open eye injury or in patients with increased intraocular pressure (glaucoma).

Suxamethonium increases intraocular pressure for 7–10 minutes,[170] which may be deleterious in glaucoma and in patients with open eye injury. A series of patients with such injury has, however, received suxamethonium without extrusion of the global contents.[171] In a recent study it was also demonstrated that suxamethonium causes a significant increase in intraocular pressure, mainly through a cycloplegic effect of the drug and not through fasciculations of the extraocular muscles.[172]

Increases in intracranial pressure (ICP) must be prevented in patients with a high ICP (that is, head trauma, brain tumours). In addition, intragastric pressure increases after administration of suxamethonium, and may therefore raise the risk for regurgitation and aspiration of stomach contents.

Although it has been demonstrated, in animals, that suxamethonium increases intracranial pressure, presumably by an increase in cerebral blood flow, this could not be confirmed in patients with neurological injury.[173] Suxamethonium is theoretically suspected of increasing intracranial pressure by various mechanisms, and should not presumably be used in patients with high ICPs.[174 175]

Suxamethonium also increases intragastric pressure via fasciculation of skeletal muscles. In patients with a patent oesophagus sphincter the increase in intragastric pressure should not exceed the "barrier pressure."[176] The increase in intragastric pressure, may, however, be a disadvantage in patients with impaired lower oesophageal sphincter pressure.

Non-depolarising relaxants

Atracurium,[177] alcuronium,[178] fazadinium,[179] pancuronium,[180] and vecuronium[181] are free from effects on intraocular pressure. In addition, rocuronium has no effect on intraocular pressure.[182] It should be realised, however, that in clinical anaesthesia laryngoscopy and intubation result in increased intracranial pressure. This effect cannot be prevented by administration of relaxants, but deep anaesthesia and some particular opioids or anaesthetics do attenuate the response.[183]

Tubocurarine markedly increases the intracranial pressure;[184] atracurium has no effect. If, however, histamine release occurs the intracranial perfusion pressure may decrease, and put the brain at risk.[185] Pancuronium,[186] vecuronium,[187] and atracurium[188] do not increase intracranial pressure.

Effect of muscle relaxants on serum electrolyte concentrations

The most well known effect of muscle relaxants on serum electrolyte concentrations is that on potassium. In normal patients a clinical dose of suxamethonium will lead to an increase in potassium level of 0·5–1·0 mmol/l. The potassium release caused by this has been reported to be larger in a number of diseases and nervous system disorders, including tetanus, burns, massive muscle trauma, uraemia, head and spinal cord injury, and cerebrovascular accidents.[189] The resulting hyperkalaemia can lead to cardiac arrhythmias and arrest.[56] The potassium release can be exaggerated by acid–base balance disturbances.[190 191] It has been confirmed in animal experiments that severe acidosis and haemorrhage can lead to hyperkalaemia after suxamethonium administration.[192] These authors demonstrated, in rabbits, that the potassium release in acidosis and haemorrhage probably takes place in the liver and gut.[193] In patients with severe intra-abdominal infections, hyperkalaemia can also occur after administration of suxamethonium.[194] It has been suggested that pre-treatment with non-depolarising relaxants would prevent potassium release. This has, however, never been proved in all situations, and is also the case for myalgia induced by suxamethonium.

Recently deaths were reported in children after administration of suxamethonium in combination with halothane. All had massive rhabdo-myolysis and most had hyperkalaemia and acidosis. Eleven similar cases were reported from Germany in the same study. There is evidence that all deaths were caused by hyperkalaemia,[195] and it appeared that all patients had neuromuscular disorders (that is, myotonia and dystrophia); this had not, however, been diagnosed because of the absence of symptoms. The report prompted the US Food and Drug Administration (FDA) and the Northern American manufacturers to change the package insert, and they recommended that suxamethonium should not be used routinely in children and adolescents except for emergency intubation. This instigated lengthy discussions.[196–198] The FDA brought up, in the discussion, the 14 cases of sudden hyperkalaemic cardiac arrest after suxamethonium that had occurred in the United States of America from 1990 to 1992; of these seven were fatal.[199] In addition one of the manufacturers brought up the 20 cases that occurred in 1990–2 with a mortality rate of 55%,[200] plus the fact that another 36 cases can be found in the literature in which the children and adolescents were apparently healthy. Again, in all cases myopathies were subsequently demonstrated, primarily Duchenne muscular dystrophy.

Effect of muscle relaxants on the cardiovascular system

Most muscle relaxants are known to exert cardiovascular responses on administration.[201] A variety of mechanisms (vagolytic effect, ganglion blockade, block of noradrenaline (norepinephrine) reuptake, histamine

Table 7.4   Autonomic nervous system effects of muscle relaxants

Drug	Autonomic ganglia	Cardiac muscarinic receptors	Histamine release	Neuromuscular block: vagal ratio
Suxamethonium	Stimulation	Stimulation	Slight	
d-Tubocurarine	Block	None	Strong	1–2
Metocurine	Weak block	None	Slight	17
Atracurium	None	None	Moderate	25
Doxacurium	None	None	Slight	300
Mivacurium	None	None	Mild	100
Alcuronium	None	None	Slight	5
Gallamine	None	Strong block	None	3–5
Pancuronium	None	Weak block	None	3
Pipecuronium	None	None	None	25
Vecuronium	None	None	None	50
Rocuronium	None	None	None	5

release) is responsible for such effects, and these have been demonstrated both in animal experiments and in human studies (table 7.4).

Depolarising relaxants

Suxamethonium can release histamine,[202] but the resulting hypotensive effects are masked most of the time by the stimulating effect on the autonomic ganglia (muscarinic) and the cardiac muscarinic receptors. Overall bradycardia and peripheral vasoconstriction are observed.

Bradycardia is seen particularly when suxamethonium is used in combination with higher doses of fentanyl or its analogues.[203] At higher dosages ganglionic (muscarinic) and postganglionic (nicotinic) sympathetic effects can also occur, resulting in increased catecholamine levels, and tachycardia and hypertension.[204] Recently it has been confirmed that suxamethonium increases plasma levels of catecholamines (predominantly noradrenaline) and is inhibited by pre-treatment with non-depolarising relaxants.[205] The use of suxamethonium is accompanied by many and varied dysrhythmias (sinus bradycardia, nodal rhythm, ventricular ectopic beats) from stimulation of all cholinergic (nicotinic and muscarinic) receptors;[206] probably it is also accompanied by increased release of catecholamines when halothane anaesthesia is administered.[207] These dysrhythmias can have haemodynamic consequences.[208]

The suxamethonium metabolites succinylmonocholine and choline may play a role in the cardiovascular side effects.[209 210] In a study including 7306 patients of whom 266 (3·6%) had intraoperative cardiovascular complications, eight (0·11%) had a cardiac arrest, with three after administration of suxamethonium.[211]

Non-depolarising relaxants

The benzylisoquinolines tubocurarine[212] and, to a lesser degree, metocurine,[213] atracurium, and mivacurium[214] cause tachycardia and hypotension mainly by histamine release. Doxacurium does not cause histamine release in clinical dosages. In the case of tubocurarine and, to a lesser extent, of metocurine the symptoms are intensified by blockade of autonomic ganglia. Benzylisoquinolines do not have vagolytic properties. If histamine release is absent, atracurium, mivacurium, and doxacurium do not cause clinically relevant cardiovascular effects.

Histamine release is rare with alcuronium, but this compound has a weak vagolytic and ganglionic blocking activity, which can lead to hypotension and tachycardia. Gallamine does not have ganglionic blocking properties, but blocks cardiac muscarinic receptors, resulting in tachycardia.

The steroidal relaxants pancuronium, pipecuronium, vecuronium, and rocuronium do not cause histamine release. Pancuronium and gallamine cause tachycardia and hypertension through blockade of cardiac muscarinic receptors and blockade of myocardial noradrenaline (type II) reuptake. These drugs should therefore be avoided in, for example, heroin addicts. Cardiac muscarinic M_2 receptors are affected by all steroidal relaxants with the following rank order: pancuronium > vecuronium > pipecuronium >

rocuronium. Only pancuronium, however, with an acetylcholine moiety in the A ring, causes cardiac effects via this mechanism in clinical dosages.[215] Fazadinium and alcuronium also block cardiac muscarinic receptors. The cardiovascular effects from pancuronium are dangerous in patients with aortic stenosis,[216] and may be harmful when there is myocardial ischaemia. In many instances, however, the effects of pancuronium are masked by other drugs used during anaesthesia, that is, opioid analgesics.

Sympathetic effects of pancuronium may also result in pulmonary vasoconstriction and in ventilation–perfusion mismatch. This has, for example, been noted during intensive care treatment in neonates.[217]

Vecuronium, pipecuronium, and doxacurium appear to have no cardio-vascular effects at all, and so the bradycardic effects of other drugs, that is, opioids, or other vagal stimulation will be seen.[218-222] Vecuronium does not cause cardiovascular effects even at very high doses, therefore high doses can be used to speed the onset of action.[223] This is the opposite of atracurium, which, at high doses, will cause hypotension via histamine release. In patients undergoing coronary artery bypass grafting (CABG) neither vecuronium nor pipecuronium causes changes in the haemo-dynamics.[224] With mivacurium, some patients undergoing CABG showed haemodynamic changes.[225] Doxacurium has no haemodynamic effects in such patients.[226] In patients with aortic or mitral valvular heart disease, especially with aortic stenosis, maintenance of afterload is extremely important. It has been proved that atracurium and vecuronium, or a combination of pancuronium and metocurine, is favourable in patients with aortic stenosis, but in patients with mitral stenosis vecuronium seems to be the best choice.[227] Also pipecuronium and doxacurium, even at large doses, have no haemodynamic effects in patients with valvular disease and pulmonary hypertension.[228]

Recently it has been reported that rocuronium causes a slight increase in heart rate and a significant rise in blood pressure, presumably through a sympathomimetic mechanism.[229 230]

In in vitro studies in the guinea pig heart, it was demonstrated that laudanosine exhibits a strong noradrenaline releasing action.[231] This may contribute to the tachycardia exhibited following administration of atra-curium and may increase the hypertension in patients with phaeo-chromocytoma. The hypertension occurring when atracurium is admin-istered in patients with phaeochromocytoma has been described in a number of cases.[232] Also suxamethonium, tubocurarine, pancuronium, and metocurine cause cardiovascular instability in patients with phaeochromo-cytoma.[233] Vecuronium is more cardiovascularly stable in such patients.[234]

It has been proved in one study that cardiac arrhythmias after laryngoscopy and intubation occur more frequently when muscle relaxation is obtained by suxamethonium, atracurium, pancuronium, or vecuronium than when tubocurarine or alcuronium is used.[235] This seems to be the result of sympathetic stimulation caused by these drugs.

It is difficult to prove that the cardiovascular effects of the muscle relaxants are of importance in the outcome of anaesthesia. At least theoretically, drugs that cause increased myocardial oxygen consumption (tachycardia) should not, however, be used in patients with myocardial ischaemia.

Effect of muscle relaxants on the pulmonary system

Muscle relaxants can influence airway tone through two different mechanisms. The first is histamine release[236–238] which may potentially cause constriction of the airways, and the second is action on muscarinic receptors in the smooth airway muscles.[239]

Depolarising relaxants

Suxamethonium can release histamine in humans and can therefore cause bronchoconstriction and anaphylactoid reactions.[240]

Non-depolarising relaxants

The relaxants that release histamine can, at least theoretically, induce bronchospasm. It has been demonstrated that d-tubocurarine[241] and altracurium[242] significantly increase airway muscle tone. Others were unable to demonstrate such effects.[243 244] Bronchospasm after pancuronium is rare, but has been described in the literature in a few cases;[245 246] this also is true for vecuronium.[247] Anaphylactoid reactions have also been described after administration of gallamine[248] and alcuronium.[249]

Another possible effect of muscle relaxants is on the hypoxic ventilatory response. It has been demonstrated that, in partial vecuronium induced neuromuscular blockade, inhibition of the carotid body hypoxic chemo-sensitivity occurs.[250] It is still unclear whether other relaxants also have this effect and what the clinical implications are.

Effect of muscle relaxants on hepatic function

Atracurium is metabolised through the Hofmann degradation and hydrolysis by carboxylesterase into a quaternary acid, a quaternary alcohol, laudanosine, and a quaternary monoacrylate. In vitro these products exert considerable hepatotoxicity, expressed as massive lactate dehydrogenase leakage from rat hepatocytes.[251 252] In an isolated perfused rat liver model this could not be substantiated.[253] Others found that atracurium, admin-istered in rats, may lead to inhibition of hepatic drug metabolism by decrease in hepatic cytochrome P450 content.[254]

Effect of muscle relaxants on allergic patients: histamine release

Of all the anaphylactoid reactions that occur during anaesthesia 80% are caused by relaxants.[255] Allergic reactions resulting from muscle relaxants are mainly caused by their potential to release histamine. Such histamine release can be caused by three mechanisms:

1 Antigen mediated release, causing immediate and delayed cardiovascular

responses. In most cases an earlier exposure to the relaxant has taken place. It involves IgE antibodies related to substituted ammonium ions.

2 Complement activation by combination of relaxant with IgG or IgM antibodies on the mast cell surface. Previous exposure is not required.

3 Direct chemical action of the relaxant on the mast cell. This mainly causes local reactions such as weals and flares, and in some situations vasodilatation and bronchoconstriction. This is the most frequent cause of histamine release in the use of relaxants.

Intradermal injection of histamine releasing drugs, including some relaxants, in humans causes the production of weals and flares.[213 256] In animal studies the ratio between the neuromuscular blocking potency (ED_{90}) and the histamine releasing potency (ED_{50}) of most relaxants has been determined.

Depolarising relaxants

About 50% of patients, with a history of generalised allergic reactions during anaesthesia, have a positive skin test to suxamethonium. Determination of antibodies with a suxamethonium–RAST test was, however, always negative (RAST, radioallergosorbent test).[257] This indicates that the mechanism is a direct histamine releasing effect.

Non-depolarising relaxants

Tubocurarine is the strongest histamine releaser, followed by atracurium, metocurine, and mivacurium.[258 259] After administration of clinical dosages of mivacurium, 15% of the patients show skin flushing, lasting for 3–5 minutes. Suxamethonium and alcuronium are also known to release histamine. The steroidal relaxants pancuronium, pipecuronium, vecuronium, and rocuronium[260] do not cause histamine release.

It should be advised that histamine releasing compounds are not used in allergic and asthmatic patients.

Anticholinesterases may provoke histamine release, but these compounds also have direct muscarinic effects causing bronchoconstriction.

Histamine release can not only cause anaphylactoid reactions in allergic and normal patients, but it may also lead to cerebral vasodilatation and increased cerebral blood flow in patients with a disrupted blood–brain barrier. This will lead to an increase in intracranial pressure. Histamine releasing relaxants should thus be avoided in situations where the blood–brain barrier is impaired or where intracranial pressure is elevated.[261] The histamine induced hypotension itself may also result in decrease in cerebral perfusion.[262]

Effect of muscle relaxants on muscles, other than relaxation

Sustained muscle contraction after administration of suxamethonium occurs in patients with myotonia. Increase in masseter muscle baseline tension is a rather common response, not only in children, but also in adults.[263] In children this may be noticed by anaesthetists as masseter muscle spasm. Such spasm is, according to some studies, not necessarily followed by the hypermetabolic activity connected to malignant hyperthermia.[264] It has been demonstrated that the halothane–caffeine test in muscle biopsies of patients with masseter muscle spasm is, however, positive in 59% of the cases, indicating susceptibility for malignant hyperthermia. Of the patients 7% developed malignant hyperthermia after masseter spasm.[265]

In patients susceptible to malignant hyperthermia suxamethonium can induce its onset. Atracurium has been administered to susceptible patients without untoward effects. In a prospective study in 44 patients undergoing muscle biopsy, of whom 20 were susceptible to malignant hyperthermia, five were equivocal and 19 were non-susceptible, demonstrating the safety of vecuronium.

Suxamethonium results in a high incidence of postoperative myalgia, especially after early mobilisation of the patient.[267] It is speculated that the myalgia is the result of incoordinated muscle contractions from the agonistic effect of suxamethonium. There is a relationship between the dose of suxamethonium and the incidence of myalgia.[268] It has, however, been demonstrated that, in short procedures in outpatients, the incidence of myalgia after administration of intermediate duration non-depolarising relaxants is not different.[269] This would indicate that other factors such as the position of the patient on the table and the use of wound retractors, etc are more important. In clinical patients pre-treatment with a variety of drugs,[270] including non-depolarising relaxants,[271] analgesics,[272] benzodiazepines,[273] antiepileptics,[274] and local anaesthetics[275] has been used for the prevention of suxamethonium induced myalgia. A variety of other drugs such as aspirin, vitamin C, dantrolene, lignocaine, fentanyl, and calcium gluconate has also been used for this purpose. Only the non-depolarising relaxants were to some extent able to prevent/decrease myalgia. Pre-treatment with these drugs can, however, lead to respiratory depression and can certainly result in prolonged neuromuscular blockade.[276] The results are therefore equivocal and contradictory, so other factors may be involved.[277]

The occurrence of myoglobinaemia after administration of suxamethonium suggests that it can cause muscle damage.[278] It seems to occur particularly in paediatric patients and if halothane is used.[279]

Muscle relaxants and drug interactions

More than 250 drugs have an effect on neuromuscular transmission and hence interfere pharmacodynamically with muscle relaxants.[2] Other drugs may interfere with the metabolism or excretion of the relaxants, and thus interact pharmacokinetically.

The effect of suxamethonium is enhanced and prolonged when drugs that decrease plasma cholinesterase activity (ecothiopate, monoamine oxidase inhibitors, lignocaine, procaine, etc) are administered.

Inhalational anaesthetics increase the potency of and prolong the neuromuscular blockade of most non-depolarising relaxants. Enflurane has the strongest effect, then isoflurane, followed by halothane; the new inhalants, sevoflurane and desflurane,[280 281] also potentiate the effect of the relaxants. Such effects are dependent on the concentration[282] and the duration of administration. The effect is more pronounced with the longer acting relaxants than with the shorter acting ones. In addition, some intravenous anaesthetics have a potentiating effect (that is, benzodiazepines, ketamine), although this is rarely of clinical relevance.

Antibiotics of the aminoglycoside, lincosamide, polypeptide, and tetracycline series are other examples of drugs showing interactions with muscle relaxants. These compounds can cause curarisation when administered up to 4–6 hours after complete recovery of the neuromuscular blockade, even when antagonised with neostigmine or pyridostigmine (Booij, unpublished data). The polymyxins have a local anaesthetic effect in that they block acetylcholine receptor ion channels;[283] this effect is not reversed by anticholinesterases and only partly by 4-aminopyridine.[284] Aminoglycosides decrease acetylcholine release and lower the postjunctional sensitivity for acetylcholine.[285] Again neostigmine has little reversing effect on such a blockade. Tetracyclines interfere with calcium, which is involved in acetylcholine release;[286] neostigmine has no effect. Lincomycin and clindamycin block ion channels and depress muscle contractility.[287] Both neostigmine and 4-aminopyridine are partially effective in antagonising the blockade.[288] It should be remembered that, in patients with myasthenia gravis, muscle paralysis can develop when the aminoglycoside, lincosamide, or polypeptide type of antibiotics is administered without concomitant administration of relaxants. This is also the case when procainamide, quinine, or quinidine is given for the treatment of cardiac arrhythmias.[289]

Local anaesthetics, quinidine, and calcium channel blockers interfere with neuromuscular transmission via blockade of open acetylcholine receptor operated ion channels.[290] The blockade from calcium channel blockers (nifedipine, diltiazem) remains reversible by anticholinesterases.[291]

Phosphodiesterase inhibitors (aminophylline, theophylline) potentiate the effect of suxamethonium and antagonise the non-depolarising relaxants.[292] The mechanism is probably via an increase in acetylcholine release from a phosphodiesterase inhibition leading to increased prejunctional cyclic AMP.

Magnesium sulphate, frequently used in (pre-)eclampsia, prolongs the effect of the non-depolarising relaxants in a dose related manner. It inhibits the effect of suxamethonium.[293]

Cyclosporin, used to prevent rejection after organ transplantation, has been reported to prolong the effect of pancuronium.[294]

Patients with epilepsy are chronically treated with anticonvulsants. In the past a resistance towards non-depolarising relaxants, that is, pancuronium, vecuronium, and metocurine, has been described in patients receiving carbamazepine or phenytoin.[295] There seems to be no effect on atracurium. In a prospective study, however, resistance to atracurium was also found in 23 patients chronically treated with phenytoin.

It is clear that, on the one hand, many diseases do have an effect on the pharmacokinetics and pharmacodynamics of muscle relaxants; on the other hand muscle relaxants have an influence on vital functions. Many drugs also interfere with the effect of the muscle relaxants. Muscle relaxants should therefore be administered with care and neuromuscular transmission should be monitored while doing so.

1 Katz RL. Neuromuscular effects of d-tubocurarine, edrophonium and neostigmine in man. *Anesthesiology* 1967;**28**:327–36.
2 Argov Z, Mastaglia FL. Disorders of neuromuscular transmission caused by drugs. *N Engl J Med* 1979;**301**:409–13.
3 Garrett ER. Pharmacokinetics and clearances related to renal processes. *Int J Clin Pharmacol Biopharm* 1978;**16**:155–72.
4 Crosby E, Robblee JA. Cyclosporine-pancuronium interaction in a patient with a renal allograft. *Can J Anaesth* 1988;**35**:300–2.
5 Ryan DW. Postoperative serum cholinesterase activity following successful renal transplanatation. *Br J Anaesth* 1979;**51**:881–4.
6 Hunter JM. Resistance to non-depolarising neuromuscular blocking agents. *Br J Anaesth* 1991;**67**:511–14.
7 Agoston S, Vermeer GA, Kersten UW. A preliminary investigation of the renal and hepatic elimination of gallamine triethiodide in man. *Br J Anaesth* 1978;**50**:345–51.
8 Miller RD, Matteo RD, Benet LZ, Sohn YJ. The pharmacokinetics of d-tubocurarine in man with and without renal failure. *J Pharmacol Expl Ther* 1977;**12**:23–9.
9 Smith CL, Hunter JM, Jones RS. Prolonged paralysis following an infusion of alcuronium in a patient with renal dysfunction. *Anaesthesia* 1987;**42**:522–25.
10 McLeod K, Watson MJ, Rawlins MD. Pharmacokinetics of pancuronium in patients with normal and impaired renal function. *Br J Anaesth* 1976;**48**:341–5.
11 Somogyi AA, Shanks CA, Triggs EJ. The effect of renal failure on the disposition and neuromuscular blocking action of pancuronium bromide. *Eur J Clin Pharmacol* 1977; **12**:23–9.
12 Hughes R, Chapple DJ. The pharmacology of atracurium: a new competitive neuromuscular blocking agent. *Br J Anaesth* 1981;**53**:31–44.
13 Nigrovic V, Auen M, Wajskol A. Emzymatic hydrolysis of atracurium in vivo. *Anesthesiology* 1985;**62**:606–9.
14 Hunter JM, Jones RS, Utting JE. Use of atracurium in patients with no renal function. *Br J Anaesth* 1982;**54**:1251–8.
15 Berntman L, Rosberg B, Schweikh I, Yousef H. Atracurium and pancuronium in renal insufficiency. *Acta Anaesthesiol Scand* 1989;**33**:48–52.
16 Bevan DR, Donati F, Gyasi H. Vecuronium in renal failure. *Can Anaesth Soc J* 1984;**31**:491–6.
17 Segredo V, Matthay MA, Sharma ML, Gruenke LD, Caldwell JE, Miller RD. Prolonged neuromuscular blockade after long-term administration of vecuronium in two critically ill patients. *Anesthesiology* 1990;**72**:566–70.
18 Slater RM, Pollard BJ, Doran BRH. Prolonged neuromuscular blockade with vecuronium in renal failure. *Anaesthesia* 1988;**43**:250–1.
19 Lynam DP, Cronnelly R, Castagnoli KP, *et al.* The pharmacodynamics and pharmacokinetics of vecuronium in patients anesthetized with isoflurane with normal function or with renal failure. *Anesthesiology* 1988;**69**:227–31.
20 Camu F, D'Hollander A. Neuromuscular blockade of fazadinium bromide (AH8165) in renal failure patients. *Acta Anaesthesiol Scand* 1978;**22**:221–6.
21 Caldwell JE, Canfell PC, Castagnoli KP, *et al.* The influence of renal failure on the pharmacokinetics and duration of action of pipecuronium bromide, in patients anesthetized with halothane and nitrous oxide. *Anesthesiology* 1989;**70**:7–12.

22 Szenohradszky J, Segredo V, Caldwell JE, Sharma M, Gruenke LD, Miller RD. Pharmacokinetics, onset and duration of action of Org 9426 in humans: Normal vs. absent renal function. *Anesth Analg* 1991;72:S290.

23 Cooper RA, Maddineni VR, Mirakhur RK, Wierda JMKH, Brady M, Fitzpatrick KTJ. Time course of neuromuscular effects and pharmacokinetics of rocuronium bromide (Org 9426) during isoflurane anaesthesia in patients with and without renal failure. *Br J Anaesth* 1993;71:222–6.

24 Cashman JN, Luke JJ, Jones RM. Neuromuscular block with doxacurium (BW A938U) in patients with normal or absent renal function. *Br J Anaesth* 1990;64:186–92.

25 Cook DR, Freeman JA, Gai AA, *et al.* Pharmacokinetics and pharmacodynamics of doxacurium in normal patients and in those with hepatic or renal failure. *Anesth Analg* 1991;72:145–50.

26 Savarese JJ, Wastila WB. Pharmacology of BW985U: A short acting nondepolarizing neuromuscular blocking agent. *Anesthesiology* 1979;51:S277.

27 Savarese JJ, Wastila WB. BW444U: an intermediate-duration nondepolarizing blocking agent with significant lack of cardiovascular and autonomic effect. *Anesthesiology* 1979;51:S279.

28 Wastila WB, Savarese JJ. Antonomic/neuromuscular dose-ratios and hemodynamic effects of BW785U, a short-acting nondepolarizing ester neuromuscular blocking agent. *Anesthesiology* 1979;51:S278.

29 Phillips BJ, Hunter JM. Use of mivacurium chloride by constant infusion in the anephric patient. *Br J Anaesth* 1992;68:492–8.

30 Mangar D, Kirchhoff GT, Rose PL, Castellano FC. Prolonged neuromuscular block after mivacurium in a patient with end-stage renal disease. *Anesth Analg* 1993;76:866–7.

31 Hunter JM, Jones RS, Utting JE. Comparison of vecuronium, atracurium and tubocurarine in normal patients and in patients with no renal function. *Br J Anaesth* 1984;56:941–51.

31 Fahey MR, Rupp SM, Canfell C, *et al.* Effect of renal failure on laudanosine excretion in man. *Br J Anaesth* 1985;57:1049–51.

33 Westra P, Keulemans GTP, Houwertjes MC, Hardonk MJ, Meijer DKF. Mechanisms underlying the prolonged duration of action of muscle relaxants caused by extrahepatic cholestasis. *Br J Anaesth* 1981;53:217–27.

34 Wilkinson GR, Shand DG. A physiological approach to hepatic drug clearance. *Clin Pharmacol Ther* 1975;18:377–90.

35 Williams RL, Mamelok RD. Hepatic diseases and drug pharmacokinetics. *Clin Pharmacokinet* 1980;5:528–47.

36 Arden JR, Lynam DP, Castagnoli KP, Canfell PC, Cannon JC, Miller RD. Vecuronium in alcoholic liver disease: A pharmacokinetic and pharmacodynamic analysis. *Anesthesiology* 1988;68:771–6.

37 Duvaldestin P, Agoston S, Henzel D, Kersten UW, Desmonts JM. Pancuronium pharmacokinetics in patients with liver cirrhosis. *Br J Anaesth* 1978;50:1131–6.

38 Devlin JC, Head-Rapson AG, Parker VJR, Hunter JM. Pharmacodynamics of mivacurium chloride in patients with hepatic cirrhosis. *Br J Anaesth* 1993;7:227–31.

39 Culp KS, Fleming CR, Duffy J, Baldus WP, Dickson ER. Autoimmune associations in primary biliary cirrhosis. *Mayo Clin Proc* 1982;57:365–70.

40 Sundewall AC, Lefvert AK, Olsson R. Antiacetylcholine receptor antibodies in primary biliary cirrhosis. *Acta Med Scand* 1985;217:519–25.

41 Sundewall AC, Lefvert AK. Acetylcholine receptor antibodies in primary biliary cirrhosis: characterization of antigen and idiotypic specificity. *Scand J Immunol* 1990;31:477–84.

42 Khuenl-Brady K, Castagnoli KP, Canfell C, Caldwell JE, Agoston S, Miller RD. The neuromuscular blocking effect and pharmacokinetics of Org 9426 and Org 9616 in the cat. *Anesthesiology* 1990;72:669–74.

43 Magorian T, Wood P, Caldewell JE, *et al.* Pharmacokinetics, onset, and duration of action of rocuronium in humans: normal vs hepatic dysfunction. *Anesthesiology* 1991;75:A1069.

44 Khalil M, D'Honneur G, Duvaldestin P, Slavov V, De Hyus C, Gomeni R. Pharmacokinetics and pharmacodynamics of rocuronium in patients with cirrhosis. *Anesthesiology* 1994;80:1241–7.

45 Cook DR, Freeman JA, Lai AA, *et al.* Pharmacokinetics and pharmacodynamics of doxacurium in normal patients and those with hepatic or renal failure. *Anesth Analg* 1991;72:145–50.

46 Parker CRJ, Hunter JM. Pharmacokinetics of atracurium and laudanosine in patients with hepatic cirrhosis. *Br J Anaesth* 1989;**62**:177–83.
47 D'Honneur G, Khalil M, Dominique C, Harberer JP, Kleef UW, Duvaldestin P. Pharmacokinetics and pharmacodynamics of pipecuronium in patients with cirrhosis. *Anesth Analg* 1993;**77**:1203–6.
48 Lebrault G, Duvaldestin P, Henzel D, Chauvin M, Guesnon P. Pharmacokinetics and pharmacodynamics of vecuronium in patients with cholestasis. *Br J Anaesth* 1986; **58**:983–7.
49 Somogyi AA, Shanks CA, Triggs EJ. Disposition kinetics of pancuronium bromide in patients with total biliary obstruction. *Br J Anaesth* 1977;**49**:1103–8.
50 Westra P, Houwertjes MC, Wesseling H, Meyer DKF. Bile salts and neuromuscular blocking agents. *Br J Anaesth* 1981;**53**:407–15.
51 Ono K, Ohta Y, Morita K, Kosaka F. The influence of respiratory-induced acid–base changes on the action of non-depolarizing muscle relaxants in rats. *Anesthesiology* 1988;**68**:357–62.
52 Ono K, Nagano O, Ohta Y, Kosaka F. Neuromuscular effects of respiratory and metabolic acid–base changes in vitro with and without non-depolarizing muscle relaxants. *Anesthesiology* 1990;**73**:710–16.
53 Aziz L, Ono K, Ohta Y, Morita K, Hirakawa M. The effect of CO_2-induced acid-base changes on the potencies of muscle relaxants and antagonism of neuromuscular block by neostigmine in rat in vitro. *Anesth Analg* 1994;**78**:322–7.
54 Brown TCK, Bell B. Electromyographic responses to small doses of suxamethonium in children after burns. *Br J Anaesth* 1987;**59**:1017–21.
55 Viby-Mogensen J, Hanel HK, Hansen E, Sorensen B, Graae J. Serum cholinesterase activity in burned patients. I. Biochemical findings. *Acta Anaesthesiol Scand* 1975; **19**:159–79.
56 Gronert GA, Theye RA. Pathophysiology of hyperkalemia produced by succinylcholine. *Anesthesiology* 1975;**43**:89–99.
57 Martyn J, Goldhill DR, Goudsouzian NG. Clinical pharmacology of muscle relaxants in patients with burns. *J Clin Pharmacol* 1986;**26**:680–5.
58 Dwersteg JF, Pavlin EG, Heimbach DM. Patients with burns are resistant to atracurium. *Anesthesiology* 1986;**65**:517–20.
59 Martyn JAJ, Goudsouzian NG, Matteo RS, Liu MP, Szyfelbein SK, Kaplan RF. Metocurine requirements in burned pediatric patients: relaxation of plasma concentration to neuromuscular blockade. *Br J Anaesth* 1983;**55**:263–8.
60 Martyn JAJ, Liu MP, Szyfelbein SK, Ambalavanar ES, Goudsouzian NG. The neuromuscular effects of pancuronium in burned children. *Anesthesiology* 1983; **59**:561–4.
61 Martyn JAJ, Szyfelbein SK, Ali HH, Matteo RS, Savarese JJ. Increased d-tubocurarine requirement following major thermal injury. *Anesthesiology* 1980;**52**:352–5.
62 Mills AK, Martyn JAJ. Evaluation of atracurium neuromuscular blockade in paediatric patients with burn injury. *Br J Anaesth* 1988;**60**:450–5.
63 Pavlin EG, Haschke RH, Marathe P, Slattery JT, Howard ML, Butler SH. Resistance to atracurium in thermally injured rats. *Anesthesiology* 1988;**69**:696–701.
64 Kim C, Fuke N, Martyn JAJ. Burn injury to rat increases nicotinic acetylcholine receptors in the diaphragm. *Anesthesiology* 1988;**68**:401–6.
65 Martyn JAJ, Matteo RS, Greenblatt DJ, Lebowitz PW, Savarese JJ. Pharmacokinetics of d-Tubocurarine in patients with thermal injury. *Anesth Analg* 1982;**61**:241–6.
66 Marathe PH, Dwersteg JF, Pavlin EG, Haschke RH, Heimbach DM, Slattery JT. Effect of thermal injury on the pharmacokinetics and pharmacodynamics of atracurium in humans. *Anesthesiology* 1989;**70**:752–5.
67 Choi WW, Sokoll MD. Anaesthesia and neuromuscular disease. *Anesthesiol Rev* 1988;**15**(6):13–22.
68 Mesry S, Baradaran J. Accidental intrathecal injection of gallamine triethiodide. *Anaesthesia* 1974;**29**:301–4.
69 Peduto VA, Gungii P, Di Martino MR, Napoleone M. Accidental subarachnoid injection of pancuronium. *Anesth Analg* 1989;**69**:516–17.
70 Smith RB, Grenvik A. Cardiac arrest following succinylcholine in patients with central nervous system injuries. *Anesthesiology* 1970;**33**:558-60.
71 Cooperman LH, Strobel GE Jr, Kennell EM. Massive hyperkalemia after administration of succinylcholine. *Anesthesiology* 1979;**32**:161–4.

72 Cowgill DB, Mostello LA, Shapiro HM. Encephalitis and a hyperkalemic response to succinylcholine. *Anesthesiology* 1974;**40**:409–11.

73 Stevenson PH, Birch AA. Succinylcholine-induced hyperkalemia in a patient with a closed head injury. *Anesthesiology* 1979;**51**:89–90.

74 Iwatsuki N, Kuroda N, Amaha K, Iwatsuki K. Succinylcholine induced hyperkalemia in patients with ruptured cerebral aneurysm. *Anesthesiology* 1980;**53**:64–7.

75 Feldman JM. Cardiac arrest after succinylcholine administration in a pregnant patient recovering from Guillain–Barré syndrome. *Anesthesiology* 1990;**72**:942–4.

76 Gronert GA, Lambert EH, Theye RA. The response of denervated skeletal muscle to succinylcholine. *Anesthesiology* 1973;**39**:113–22.

77 Moorthy SS, Hilgenberg JC. Resistance to non-depolarizing muscle relaxants in paretic upper extremities of patients with residual hemiplegia. *Anesth Analg* 1980;**59**:624–7.

78 Shayevitz JR, Matteo RS. Decreased sensitivity to metocurine in patients with upper motoneuron disease. *Anesth Analg* 1985;**64**:767–72.

79 Gronert GA, Theye RA. Effect of succinylcholine on skeletal muscle with immobilization atrophy. *Anesthesiology* 1974;**40**:268–71.

80 Fiacchino F, Gemma M, Bricchi M, Giombini S, Regi B. Sensitivity to curare in patients with upper and lower motor neurone dysfunction. *Anaesthesia* 1991;**46**:980–2.

81 Rosenbaum KJ, Neigh JL, Strobel GE. Sensitivity to non-depolarizing muscle relaxants in amyotrophic lateral sclerosis: report of two cases. *Anesthesiology* 1971;**35**:638–41.

82 Stone WA, Beach TP, Hamelberg W. Succinylcholine-danger in the spinal-cord-injured patient. *Anesthesiology* 1970;**32**:168–9.

83 Tobey RE. Paraplegia, succinylcholine and cardiac arrest. *Anesthesiology* 1970;**32**: 359–64.

84 Hogue Jr CW, Itani MS, Martyn JAJ. Resistance to d-tubocurarine in lower motor neuron injury is related to increased acetylcholine receptors at the neuromuscular junction. *Anesthesiology* 1990;**73**:703–9.

85 Greenawalt III JW. Succinylcholine-induced hyperkalemia 8 weeks after a brief paraplegic episode. *Anesth Analg* 1992;**75**:294–5.

86 Orndahl G, Sternberg K. Myotonic human musculature: stimulation with depolarizing agents. Mechanical registration of the effect of succinylcholine, succinylmonocholine, and decamethonium. *Acta Med Scand* 1962;**172**(3)(suppl 389):2–29.

87 Azar I. The response of patients with neuromuscular disorders to muscle relaxants: a review. *Anesthesiology* 1984;**61**:173–87.

88 Weintraub MI, Megahed MS, Smith BH. Myotonic-like syndrome in multiple sclerosis. *NY State J Med* 1970;**70**:677–9.

89 Peterson IS. Generalized myotonia following suxamethonium. *Br J Anaesth* 1962; **34**:340–2.

90 Crody JR. Muscle rigidity following administration of succinylcholine. *Anesthesiology* 1968;**29**:159–62.

91 Nightingale P, Healy TEJ, McGuinness K. Dystrophia myotonica and atracurium. A case report. *Br J Anaesth* 1985;**57**:1131–5.

92 Muller J, Suppan P. Case report. Anaesthesia in myotonic dystrophy. *Anaesth Intens Care* 1977;**5**:70–3.

93 Mitchell MM, Ali HH, Savarese JJ. Myotonica and neuromuscular blocking agents. *Anesthesiology* 1978;**49**:44–8.

94 Boheimer N, Harris JW, Ward S. Neuromuscular blockade in dystrophia myotonica with atracurium besylate. *Anaesthesia* 1985;**40**:872–4.

95 Boltshauser E, Steinman B, Meyer A, Jerusalem F. Anaesthesia induced rhabomyolysis in Duchenne muscular dystrophy. *Br J Anaesth* 1980;**52**:559.

96 Seay AR, Ziter FA, Thompson JA. Cardiac arrest during induction of anesthesia in Duchenne muscular dystrophy. *J Pediatr* 1978;**93**:88–90.

97 Buzello W, Huttarsch H. Muscle relaxation in patients with Duchenne's muscular dystrophy. *Br J Anaesth* 1988;**60**:228–31.

98 Kent RS. Revised label regarding use of succinylcholine in children and adolescents. *Anesthesiology* 1994;**80**:244–5.

99 Ohtani Y, Miike T, Ishitsu T, Matsuda I, Tamari H. A case of malignant hyperthermia with mitochondrial dysfunction. *Brain and Development* 1985;**7**:249.

100 Reilly M, Hutchinson M. Suxamethonium is contraindicated in the Guillain–Barré syndrome. *J Neurol Neurosurg Psychiatry* 1991;**54**:1018–19.

151

101 Ward S, Wright DJ. Neuromuscular blockade in myasthenia gravis with atracurium besylate. *Anaesthesia* 1984;**39**:51–3.

102 Ramsey FM, Smith GD. Clinical use of atracurium in myasthenia gravis: a case report. *Can Anaesth Soc J* 1985;**32**:642–5.

103 Lumb AB, Calder I. 'Cured' myasthenia gravis and neuromuscular blockade. *Anaesthesia* 1989;**44**:828–30.

104 Baraka A, Baroody M, Yazbeck V. Repeated doses of suxamethonium in the myasthenic patient. *Anaesthesia* 1993;**48**:782–4.

105 Eisenkraft JB, Book WJ, Mann SM, Papatestas AE, Hubbard M. Resistance to succinylcholine in myasthenia gravis: a dose response study. *Anesthesiology* 1988; **69**:760–3.

106 Wainwright AP, Brodrick PM. Suxamethonium in myasthenia gravis. *Anaesthesia* 1987;**42**:950–7.

107 Vanlinthout LEH, Robertson EN, Booij LHDJ. Response to suxamethonium during propofol–fentanyl–N_2O/O_2 anaesthesia in a patient with active myasthenia gravis receiving chronic anticholinesterase therapy. *Anaesthesia* 1994;**49**:509–11.

108 Baraka A. Suxamethonium block in the myasthenic patient. Correlation with plasma cholinesterase. *Anaesthesia* 1992;**47**:217–19.

109 Nilsson E, Meretoja OA. Vecuronium dose-response and maintenance requirements in patients with myasthenia gravis. *Anesthesiology* 1990;**73**:28–32.

110 Seigne RD, Scott RPF. Mivacurium chloride and myasthenia gravis. *Br J Anaesth* 1994;**72**:468–9.

111 Kim JM, Mangold J. Sensitivity to both vecuronium and neostigmine in a sero-negative myasthenic patient. *Br J Anaesth* 1989;**63**:497–500.

112 Wise RP. A myasthenic syndrome complication in bronchial carcinoma. *Br J Anaesth* 1962;**17**:488.

113 Fassoulaki A, Desmonts JM. Prolonged neuromuscular blockade after a single bolus dose of vecuronium in patients with acquired immunodeficiency syndrome. *Anesthesiology* 1994;**80**:457–9.

114 Whittaker M, Britten JJ. Phenotyping of individuals sensitive to suxamethonium. *Br J Anaesth* 1987;**59**:1052–5.

115 Robertson GS. Serum cholinesterase deficiency I. Disease and inheritance. *Br J Anaesth* 1966;**38**:355–60.

116 Robertson GS. Serum cholinesterase deficiency II pregnancy. *Br J Anaesth* 1966; **38**:361–4.

117 Robson N, Robertson I, Whittaker M. Plasma cholinesterase changes in the puerperium. *Anaesthesia* 1986;**41**:243–9.

118 Matsuki A, Oyama T. Effects of extracorporeal circulation on plasma cholinesterase activity in man. *Agressologie* 1981;**22**:79–81.

119 Shearer ES, Russell GN. The effect of cardiopulmonary bypass on cholinesterase activity. *Anaesthesia* 1993;**48**:293–6.

120 Whittaker M. Plasma cholinesterase variants and the anaesthetist. *Anaesthesia* 1980; **35**:174–97.

121 Maddineni VR, Mirakhur RK, McCoy EP. Plasma cholinesterase activity in elderly and young patients. *Br J Anaesth* 1994;**72**:497.

122 Ritter DM, Rettke SR, Ilstrup DM, Burritt MF. Effect of plasma cholinesterase activity on the duration of action of succinylcholine in patients with genotypically normal enzyme. *Anesth Analg* 1988;**67**:1123–6.

123 VanLinthout LEC, VanEgmond J, De Boo T, Lerou JGC, Wevers R, Booij LHDJ. Factors affecting magnitude and time course of neuromuscular block produced by suxamethonium. *Br J Anaesth* 1992;**69**:21–7.

124 Taylor BL, Whittaker M, van Heerden V, Britten J. Cholinesterase deficiency and the Churg–Strauss syndrome. *Anaesthesia* 1990;**45**:649–52.

125 Ostergaard D, Jensen FS, Jensen E, Viby-Morgensen J. Influence of plasma cholinesterase activity on recovery from mivacurium-induced neuromuscular blockade. *Acta Anaesthesiol Scand* 1989;**33**(suppl 191):A164.

126 Cook DR, Freeman ASA, Lai AA, *et al.* Pharmacokinetics of mivacurium in normal patients and in those with hepatic or renal failure. *Br J Anaesth* 1992;**69**:580–5.

127 Maddineni VR, McCoy EP, Mirakhur RK, Stanley JC, Lyons SM. Mivacurium in the elderly: comparison of neuromuscular and hemodynamic effects with adults. *Anesthesiology* 1993;**79**:A964.

128 Goudsouzian NG, d'Hollander AA, Viby-Mogensen J. Prolonged neuromuscular block from mivacurium in two patients with cholinesterase deficiency. *Anesth Analg* 1993;77:183–5.

129 Fisher DM, Canfell PC, Fahey MR, *et al.* Elimination of atracurium in humans: contribution of Hofmann elimination and ester hydrolysis versus organ-based elmination. *Anesthesiology* 1986;65:6–12.

130 Merrett RA, Thompson CW, Webb FW. In vitro degradation of atracurium in human plasma. *Br J Anaesth* 1983;55:61–6.

131 Brown TCK, Gregory M, Bell B, Clare D. Response to nondepolarizing muscle relaxants in children with tumours. *Anaesth Intens Care* 1990;18:460–5.

132 Brown TCK, Gregory N, Bell B, Campbell PC. Liver tumours and muscle relaxants. *Anaesthesia* 1987;42:1284–6.

133 Buzello W, Pollmaecher T, Schluermann D, Urbanyi B. The influence of hypothermic cardiopulmonary bypass on neuromuscular transmission in the absence of muscle relaxants. *Anesthesiology* 1986;64:279–81.

134 Buzello W, Schluerman D, Schindler M, Spillner G. Hypothermic cardiopulmonary bypass and neuromuscular blockade by pancuronium and vecuronium. *Anesthesiology* 1985;62:201–4.

135 Miller RD, Agoston S, van der Pol F, Booij LHDJ, Crul JF, Ham J. Hypothermia and the pharmacokinetics and pharmacodynamics of pancuronium in the cat. *J Pharmacol Expl Ther* 1978;207:532–8.

136 Buzello W, Schluermann D, Pollmaecher T, Spillner G. Unequal effects of cardiopulmonary bypass-induced hypothermia on neuromuscular blockade from constant infusion of alcuronium, d-tubocurarine, pancuronium, and vecuronium. *Anesthesiology* 1987;66:842–6.

137 Denny NM, Kneeshaw JD. Vecuronium and atracurium infusions during hypothermic cardiopulmonary bypass. *Anaesthesia* 1986;41:919–22.

138 Heier T, Caldwell JE, Sessler DI, Kitts JB, Miller RD. The relationship between adductor pollicis twitch tension and core, skin, and muscle temperature during nitrous oxide isoflurane anaesthesia in humans. *Anesthesiology* 1989;71:381–4.

139 Heier T, Caldwell JE, Sessler DI, Miller RD. The effect of local surface and central cooling on adductor pollicis twitch tension during nitrous oxide/isoflurane and nitrous oxide/fentanyl anesthesia in humans. *Anesthesiology* 1990;72:807–11.

140 Heier T, Caldwell JE, Sessler DI, Miller RD. Mild hypothermia increaes duration of action and spontaneous recovery of vecuronium blockade during nitrous oxide–isoflurane anesthesia in humans. *Anesthesiology* 1991;74:815–19.

141 Heier T, Caldwell JE, Eriksson LI, Sessler DI, Miller RD. The effect of hypothermia on adductor pollicis twitch tension during continuous infusion of vecuronium in isoflurane-anesthetized humans. *Anesth Analg* 1994;78:312–17.

142 Hogue CW Jr, Ward JM, Itani MS, Martyn JAJ. Tolerance and upregulation of acetylcholine receptors follow chronic infusion of d-tubocurarine. *J Appl Physiol* 1992;72:1326–31.

143 Wernig A, Pécot-Dechavassine M, Stövner H. Sprouting and regression of the nerve at the frog neuromuscular junction in normal conditions and after prolonged paralysis with curare. *J Neurocytol* 1980;9:277–303.

144 Segredo V, Matthay MA, Sharma ML, Gruenke LD, Caldwell JE, Miller RD. Prolonged neuromuscular blockade after long term administration of vecuronium in two critically ill patients. *Anesthesiology* 1990;72:566–70.

145 Patridge BL, Abrams JH, Bazemore C, Rubin R. Prolonged neuromuscular blockade after long term infusion of vecuronium bromide in the intensive care unit. *Crit Care Med* 1990;18:1177–9.

146 Gooch JL, Suchyta MR, Balbierz JM, Petajan JH, Clemmer TP. Prolonged paralysis after treatment with neuromuscular junction blocking agents. *Crit Care Med* 1991;19:1125–31.

147 Heckmatt JZ, Pitt MC, Kirkham F. Peripheral neuropathy and neuromuscular blockade presenting as prolonged respiratory paralysis following critical illness. *Neuropediatrics* 1993;24:123–5.

148 Kupfer Y, Namba T, Kaldawi E, Tessler S. Prolonged weakness after long-term infusion of vecuronium bromide. *Ann Intern Med* 1992;117:484–6.

149 Zochodne DW, Bolton CF, Wells GA, *et al.* Critical illness polyneuropathy—a complication of sepsis and multiorgan failure. *Brain* 1987;110:819–42.

150 Witt NJ, Zochodne DW, Bolton CF, et al. Peripheral nerve function in sepsis and multiple organ failure. Chest 1991;99:176–84.

151 Bolton CF, Young GB, Zochodne DW. The neurological complications of sepsis. Ann Neurol 1993;33:94–100.

152 Helliwell TR, Coakley JH, Wagenmakers AJM, et al. Necrotizing myopathy in critically-ill patients. J Pathol 1991;164:307–14.

153 Zochodne DW, Ramsay DA, Saly V, Shelley S, Moffatt S. Acute necrotizing myopathy of intensive care: electrophysiological studies. Muscle Nerve 1994;17:285–92.

154 Segredo V, Caldwell JE, Matthay MA, Sharma ML, Gruenke LD, Miller RD. Persistent paralysis in critically ill patients after long-term administration of vecuronium. N Engl J Med 1992;327:524–8.

155 Brun-Buisson C, Gherardi R. Hydrocortisone and pancuronium bromide: acute myopathy during status asthmaticus (letter to the editor). Crit Care Med 1988;731–2.

156 Barohn RJ, Jackson CE, Rogers SJ, Ridings LW, McVey AL. Prolonged paralysis due to nondepolarizing neuromuscular blocking agents and corticosteroids. Muscle Nerve 1994;17:647–54.

157 Op de Coul AAW, Lambregts PCLA, Koeman J, van Puyenbroek MJE, Ter Laak JH, Gabreëls-Festen AAWM. Neuromuscular complications in patients given Pavulon (pancuronium bromide) during artificial ventilation. Clin Neurol Neurosurg 1985; 887:17–22.

158 Griffin D, Fairman N, Coursin DB, Rawsthorne L, Grossman JE. Acute myopathy during treatment of status asthmaticus with corticosteroids and steroidal relaxants. Chest 1992;102:510–14.

159 Meyer KC, Prielipp RC, Grossman JE, Coursin DB. Prolonged weakness after infusion of atracurium in two intensive care unit patients. Anesth Analg 1994;78:772–4.

160 Gwinnutt CL, Eddleston JM, Edwards D, Pollard BJ. Concentrations of atracurium and laudanosine in cerebrospinal fluid and plasma in three intensive care patients. Br J Anaesth 1990;65:829–32.

161 Parker CJR, Jones JE, Hunter JM. Disposition of infusions of atracurium and its metabolite, laudanosine, in patients with renal and respiratory failure in an ITU. Br J Anaesth 1988;61:531–40.

162 Nigrovic V, Klaunig JE, Smith SL, Schulz NE, Wajskol A. Comparative toxicity of atracurium and metocurine in isolated rat hepatocytes. Anesth Analg 1986;65:1107–11.

163 Callanan DL. Development of resistance to pancuronium in adult respiratory distress syndrome. Anesth Analg 1985;64:1126–8.

164 Coursin DB, Klasek G, Goelzer SL. Increased requirements for continuous infused vecuronium in critically ill patients. Anesth Analg 1989;69:518–21.

165 Yate PM, Flynn PJ, Arnold RW, Weatherly BC, Simmonds RJ, Dobson T. Clinical experience and plasma laudanosine concentrations during infusion of atracurium in the intensive therapy unit. Br J Anaesth 1987;59:211–17.

166 Mesry S, Baradaran J. Accidental intrathecal injection of gallamine triethiodide. Anaesthesia 1974;29:301–4.

167 Peduto VA, Gungii P, Di Martino MR, Napoleone M. Accidental subarachnoid injection of pancuronium. Anesth Analg 1989;69:516–17.

168 Matteo RS, Pua EK, Khambotta KJ, Spector S. Cerebrospinal fluid levels of d-tubocurarine in man. Anesthesiology 1977;46:396–400.

169 Warner LO, Brener DL, Davidson PJ, Rogers GL, Beach TP. Effects of lidocaine, succinylcholine, and tracheal intubation on intraocular pressure in children anaesthetized with halothane–nitrous oxide. Anesth Analg 1989;69:687–90.

170 Warner LO, Brener DL, Davidson PJ, Rogers GL, Beach TP. Effects of lidocaine, succinylcholine, and tracheal intubation on intraocular pressure in children anesthetized with halothane–nitrous oxide. Anesth Analg 1989;69:687–90.

171 Libonati MM, Leahy JJ, Ellison N. The use of succinylcholine in open eye surgery. Anesthesiology 1985;62:637–40.

172 Kelly RE, Dinner M, Turner LS, Haik B, Abramson DH, Daines P. Succinylcholine increased intraocular pressure in the human eye with the extraocular muscles detached. Anesthesiology 1993;79:948–52.

173 Kovarik WD, Mayberg TS, Lam AL, Mathisen TL, Winn HR. Succinylcholine does not change intracranial pressure, cerebral blood flow velocity or the electroencephalogram in patients with neurologic injury. Anesth Analg 1994;78:469–73.

174 Artru AA. Muscle relaxation with succinylcholine or vecuronium does not alter the rate of CFS production or resistance to reabsorption of CSF in dogs. *Anesthesiology* 1988;**68**:392–6.

175 Thiagarajah S, Sophie S, Lear E, Azar I, Frost EAM. Effect of suxamethonium on the ICP of cats with and without thiopentone pretreatment. *Br J Anaesth* 1988;**60**:157–60.

176 Smith G, Dalling R, Williams TIR. Gastro-oesophageal pressure gradient changes produced by induction of anaesthesia and suxamethonium. *Br J Anaesth* 1978; **50**:1137–43.

177 Lavery GG, McGalliard JN, Mirakhur RK, Shepherd WFI. The effects of atracurium on intraocular pressure during steady state anaesthesia and rapid sequence induction: a comparison with succinylcholine. *Can Anaesth Soc J* 1986;**33**:437–42.

178 George R, Nursingh A, Downing JW, Welsh NH. Non-depolarizing neuromuscular blockers and the eye: a study of intraocular pressure. *Br J Anaesth* 1979;**51**:779–92.

179 Couch JA, Eltringham RJ, Magauran DM. The effect of thiopentone and fazadinium on intraocular pressure. *Anaesthesia* 1979;**34**:586–90.

180 Litwiller RW, Difazio CA, Ruslian EL. Pancuronium and intraocular pressure. *Anesthesiology* 1975;**42**:750–2.

181 Mirakhur RK, Shepherd WFI, Lavery GG, Elliott P. The effects of vecuronium on intra-ocular pressure. *Anaesthesia* 1987;**42**:944–9.

182 Robertson EN, Hull JM, Verbeek AM, Booij LHDJ. A comparison of rocuronium and vecuronium: the pharmacodynamic, cardiovascular and intra-ocular effects. *Eur J Anaesthesiol* 1994;**11**(suppl 9):116–21.

183 Mirakhur RK, Shepherd WFI, Elliott P. Intraocular pressure changes during rapid sequence induction of anaesthesia: comparison of propofol and thiopentone in combination with vecuronium. *Br J Anaesth* 1988;**60**:379–83.

184 Tarkkanen L, Laitinen L, Johanssen G. Effects of d-tubocurarine on intracranial pressure and thalamic electrical impedance. *Anesthesiology* 1974;**40**:247–51.

185 Rosa G, Orfei P, Sanfilippo M, Vilardi V, Gasparetto A. The effects of atracurium besylate (Tracrium) on intracranial pressure and cerebral perfusion pressure. *Anesth Analg* 1986;**65**:381–4.

186 McLeskey CH, Cullen BF, Kennedy RD, Galindo A. Control of cerebral perfusion pressure during induction of anesthesia in high-risk neurosurgical patients. *Anesth Analg* 1974;**53**:985–92.

187 Stirt JA, Maggio W, Haworth C, Minton MD, Bedford RF. Vecuronium: effect on intracranial pressure and hemodynamics in neurosurgical patients. *Anesthesiology* 1987;**67**:570–3.

188 Stirt JA, Chiu GJ. Intraocular pressure during rapid sequence induction: use of moderate-dose sufentanil or fentanyl and vecuronium or atracurium. *Anaesth Intens Care* 1990;**18**:390–4.

189 Yentis SM. Suxamethonium and hyperkalaemia. *Anaesth Intens Care* 1990;**18**:92–101.

190 Koller ME, Breivik H, Grieder P, Jones DJ, Smith RB. Synergistic effect of acidosis and succinyl-induced hyperkalemia in spinal cord transected rats. *Acta Anaesthesiol Scand* 1984;**28**:87–90.

191 Schwartz DE, Kelly B, Caldwell JE, Carlisle AS, Cohen NH. Succinylcholine-induced hyperkalemic arrest in a patient with severe metabolic acidosis and exsanguinating hemorrhage. *Anesth Analg* 1992;**75**:291–3.

192 Antognini JF, Gronert GA. Succinylcholine causes profound hyperkalemia in hemorrhagic, acidotic rabbits. *Anesth Analg* 1993;**77**:585–8.

193 Antognini JF. Splanchnic release of potassium after hemorrhage and succinylcholine in rabbits. *Anesth Analg* 1994;**78**:697–90.

194 Kohlschütter B, Bauer H, Roth F. Suxamethonium-induced hyperkalaemia in patients with severe intra-abdominal infections. *Br J Anaesth* 1976;**48**:557–62.

195 Rosenberg H, Gronert GA. Intractable cardiac arrest in children given succinylcholine. *Anesthesiology* 1992;**77**:1054.

196 Marell RC, Berman JM, Royster RI, Petrozza PH, Kelly JS, Colonna DM. Revised label regarding use of succinylcholine in children and adolescents: I. *Anesthesiology* 1994;**80**:242.

197 Badgwell JM, Hall SC, Lockhart C. Revised label regarding use of succinylcholine in children and adolescents: II. *Anesthesiology* 1994;**80**:243.

198 Lerman J, Berdock SE, Bissonnett B, *et al.* Succinylcholine warning. *Can J Anaesth* 1993;**41**:165.

199 Katz L, Wright C, Harter J, Zung M, Scally D, Spyker D. In reply. *Anesthesiology* 1994;**80**:243-4.
200 Kent RS. In reply. *Anesthesiology* 1994;**80**:244-5.
201 Booij LHDJ, Edwards RP, Sohn YJ, Miller RD. Cardiovascular and neuromuscular effects of Org NC 45, pancuronium, metocurine and d-tubocurarine in dogs. *Anesth Analg* 1980;**59**:26-30.
202 Vervloet D, Arnaud A, Senft M, *et al.* Leucocyte histamine release to suxamethonium in patients with adverse reactions to muscle relaxants. *J Allergy Clin Immunol* 1985; **75**:338-42.
203 Inoue K, Reichelt W. Asystole and bradycardia in adults after a single dose of suxamethonium. *Acta Anaesthesiol Scand* 1986;**30**:571-3.
204 Nigrovic V, McCullough LS, Wajskol A, Levin JA, Martin JT. Succinylcholine-induced increases in plasma catecholamine levels in man. *Anesth Analg* 1983;**62**:627-32.
205 Oshita S, Denda S, Fujiwara Y, Takeshida H, Kosaka F. Pretreatment with d-tubocurarine, vecuronium, and pancuronium attenuates succinylcholine-induced increases in plasma norepinephrine concentrations in humans. *Anesth Analg* 1991; **72**:84-8.
206 Yasuda I, Hirano T, Amaha K, Fudeta H, Obara S. Chronotropic effects of succinylcholine and succinylmonocholine on sinoatrial node. *Anesthesiology* 1982; **57**:289-92.
207 Leiman BC, Katz J, Butler BD. Mechanisms of succinylcholine-induced arrhythmias in hypoxic or hypoxic-hypercarbic dogs. *Anesth Anal* 1987;**66**:1292-7.
208 Elia ST, Lebowitz PW. Succinylcholine induced idioventricular rhythm. *Anesth Analg* 1988;**67**:588-9.
209 Williams CH, Deutsch S, Linde HW. Effects of intravenously administered succinylcholine on cardiac rate, rhythm, and arterial blood pressure in anesthetized man. *Anesthesiology* 1961;**22**:947-54.
210 Ohmura A, Wong KC, Shaw L. Cardiac effects of succinylcholine and succinylmonocholine. *Can Anaesth Soc J* 1976;**23**:567-73.
211 Pedersen T, Eliasen K, Henriksen E. A prospective study of risk factors and cardiopulmonary complications associated with anaesthesia and surgery: risk indicators of cardiopulmonary morbidity. *Acta Anaesthesiol Scand* 1990;**34**:144-55.
212 Moss J, Rosow CE, Savarse JJ, Philbin DM, Kniffen KJ. Role of histamine in the hypotensive action of d-tubocurarine in humans. *Anesthesiology* 1981;**55**:19-25.
213 Booij LHDJ, Krieg NN, Crul JF. Intradermal histamine releasing effect caused by Org-NC 45. A comparison with pancuronium, metocurine and d-tubocurarine. *Acta Anaesthesiol Scand* 1980;**24**:393-4.
214 Savarese JJ, Ali HH, Basta SJ, *et al.* The cardiovascular effects of mivacurium chloride (BW B1090U) in patients receiving nitrous oxide-opiate-barbiturate anesthesia. *Anesthesiology* 1989;**70**:386-94.
215 Appadu BL, Lambert DG. Studies on the interaction of steroidal neuromuscular blocking drugs with cardiac muscarinic receptors. *Br J Anaesth* 1994;**72**:86-8.
216 Sethna DH, Starr NJ, Estafanous FG. Cardiovascular effects of non-depolarizing neuromuscular blockers in patients with aortic valve disease. *Can J Anaesth* 1987;**34**:582-8.
217 Bergin AM, Clarke TA, Matthews TG. Problems with pancuronium in the neonatal intensive care unit. *Irish Med J* 1988;**81**:39-40.
218 Clayton D. Asystole associated with vecuronium. *Br J Anaesth* 1986;**58**:937-8.
219 Starr MH, Sethna DH, Estafanous FG. Bradycardia and asystole following the rapid administration of sufentanil with vecuronium. *Anesthesiology* 1986;**64**:521-3.
220 Cozanitis DA, Erkola O. A clinical study into the possible intrinsic bradycardiac activity of vecuronium. *Anaesthesia* 1989;**44**:648-50.
221 Wierda JMKH, Maestrone E, Bencini AF, *et al.* Haemodynamic effects of vecuronium. *Br J Anaesth* 1989;**62**:194-8.
222 Morton CPJ, Drummond GB. Bradycardia and vecuronium: comparison with alcuronium during cholecystectomy. *Br J Anaesth* 1992;**68**:619-20.
223 Tullock WC, Diana P, Cook DR, *et al.* Neuromuscular and cardiovascular effects of high-dose vecuronium. *Anesth Analg* 1990;**70**:86-90.
224 Starr NJ, Kraenzler EJ, Wong D, Koehler LS, Estafanous FG. Comparison of cardiovascular effects of pipecuronium versus vecuronium in patients receiving sufentanil anesthesia for mycoardial revascularization. *J Cardiothorac Vasc Anesth* 1991;**5**:116-19.

225 Stoops CM, Curtis CA, Kovach DA, et al. Hemodynamic effects of mivacurium chloride administered to patients during oxygen-sufentanil anesthesia for coronary artery bypass grafting or valve replacement. Anesth Analg 1989;68:333–9.

226 Emmott RS, Bracey BJ, Goldhill DR, Yate PM, Flynn PJ. Cardiovascular effects of doxacurium, pancuronium and vecuronium in anaesthetized patients presenting for coronary artery bypass surgery. Br J Anaesth 1990;65:480–6.

227 Larach DR, Hensley Jr, FA, Martin DE, High KM, Rung GW, Skeehan TM. Hemodynamic effects of muscle relaxant drugs during anesthetic induction in patients with mitral or aortic valvular heart disease. J Cardiothorac Vasc Anesth 1991;5:126–31.

228 Simons LB, Wyble SS, Hirsch LJ, Rooney MW. Comparison of hemodynamic response to pipecuronium and doxacurium in patients undergoing valvular surgery while anesthetized with fentanyl. J Cardiothor Vasc Anesth 1994;8:297–301.

229 Robertson EN, Hull JM, Verbeek AM, Booij LHDJ. A comparison of rocuronium and vecuronium: the pharmacodynamic, cardiovascular and intra-ocular effects. Eur J Anaesthesiol 1994;11(suppl 9):116–21.

230 McCoy EP, Maddineni VR, Elliot P, Mirakhur RK, Caroon IW, Cooper RA. Haemodynamic effects of rocuronium during fentanyl anaesthesia: comparison with vecuronium. Can J Anaesth 1993;408:703–8.

231 Kinjo M, Nagashima H, Vizi ES. Effect of atracurium and laudanosine on the release of ³H-noradrenaline. Br J Anaesth 1989;62:683–90.

232 Amaranath L, Zanettin GG, Bravo EL, Barnes A, Estafanous FG. Atracurium and pheochromocytoma: a report of three cases. Anesth Analg 1988;67:1127–30.

233 Stirt JA, Brown Jr RE, Ross Jr WT, Althaus JS. Atracurium in a patient with pheochromacytoma. Anesth Analg 1985;64:547–50.

234 Gencarelli PJ, Roizen MF, Miller RD, Joyce J, Hunt TK, Tyrrell JB. Org NC45 (Norcuron) and pheochromocytoma: a report of three cases. Anesthesiology 1981;55:690–3.

235 Saarnivaara L, Klemora UM, Lindgren L. QT interval of the ECG, heart rate and arterial pressure using five non-depolarizing muscle relaxants for intubation. Acta Anaesthesiol Scand 1988;32:623–8.

236 Stellato C, dePaulis A, Cirillo R, Mastronardi P, Mazzarella B, Marone G. Heterogeneity of human mast cells and basophils in response to muscle relaxants. Anesthesiology 1991;74:1078–86.

237 North FC, Kettelkamp N, Hirshman CA. Comparison of cutaneous and in vitro histamine release by muscle relaxants. Anesthesiology 1987;66:543–6.

238 Robertson EN, Fragen RJ, Booij LHDJ, Crul JF. Intradermal histamine release by 3 muscle relaxants. Acta Anaesthesiol Scand 1983;27:203–5.

239 Vetterman J, Beck KC, Lindahl SHE, Brichant JF, Rehder K. Actions of enflurane, isoflurane, vecuronium, atracurium and pancuronium on pulmonary resistance in dogs. Anesthesiology 1988;69:688–95.

240 Assem ESK, Frost PG, Levis RD. Anaphylactic-like reaction to suxamethonium. Anaesthesia 1981;36:405–10.

241 Crago RR, Bryan AC, Laws AK, Winestock AE. Respiratory flow resistance after curare and pancuronium measured by forced oscillations. Can Anaesth Soc J 1972;19:607–14.

242 Mehr EH, Hirshman CA, Lindeman KS. Mechanism of action of atracurium on airways. Anesthesiology 1992;76:448–54.

243 Gerbershagen HU, Bergmann HA. The effect of d-tubocurarine on respiratory resistance in anesthetized man. Anesthesiology 1967;28:981–4.

244 Simpson DA, Wright DJ, Hammond JE. Influence of tubocurarine, pancuronium and atracurium on bronchomotor tone. Br J Anaesth 1985;57:753–7.

245 Brauer FS, Ananthanarayan CR. Histamine release by pancuronim. Anesthesiology 1978;49:434–5.

246 Buckland RW, Avery AF. Histamine release following pancuronium. Br J Anaesth 1973;45:518–21.

247 O'Callaghan AC, Scadding G, Watkins J. Bronchospasm following the use of vecuronium. Anaesthesia 1986;41:940–2.

248 Evans PJD, Mckinnon I. An anaphylactoid reaction to gallamine triethiodide. Anaesth Intens Care 1977;5:539–43.

249 Fisher M McD, Hallowes RC, Wilson RM. Anaphylaxis to alcuronium. Anaesth Intens Care 1978,6:125–8.

250 Eriksson LI, Sato M, Severinghaus JW. Effect of a vecuronium-induced partial neuromuscular block on hypoxic ventilatory response. *Anesthesiology* 1993;78:693–9.

251 Nigrovic V, Klaunig JE, Smith SL, Schultz NE. Potentiation of atracurium toxicity in isolated rat hepatocytes by inhibition of its hydrolytic degradation pathway. *Anesth Analg* 1987;66:512–16.

252 Nigrovic V, Klaunig JE, Smith SL, Schultz NE, Wajskol A. Comparative toxicity of atracurium and metocurine in isolated rat hepatocytes. *Anesth Analg* 1986;65:1107–11.

253 Sperlich M, Reckendorfer H, Burgmann H, *et al.* Altered hepatic function by atracurium or its breakdown products. *Transpl Proc* 1993;25:1851–2.

254 Böhrer H, Schmidt H, Bach A, *et al.* Inhibition of hepatic microsomal drug metabolism by atracurium administration in the rat. *Pharmacol Toxicol* 1993;73:137–41.

255 Laxenaire MC, Moneret-Vautrin DA, Widmer S, Mouton C, Guéant JL. Anaesthetic drugs responsible for anaphylactic shock. French multi-center study. *Ann Franc d'Anaesth Reanim* 1990;9:501–6.

256 Levy JH, Adelson D, Walker B. Wheal and flare responses to muscle relaxants in humans. *Agents Actions* 1991;34:302–8.

257 Binkley K, Cheema A, Sussman G, *et al.* Generalized allergic reactions during anesthesia. *J Allergy Clin Immunol* 1992;89:768–74.

258 Basta SJ, Savarese JJ, Ali HH, Moss J, Gionfriddo M. Histamine-releasing properties of atracurium, dimethyl tubocurarine and tubocurarine. *Br J Anaesth* 1983;55:105S–6S.

259 Brandom BW, Woelfel SK, Cook DR, Weber S, Powers DM, Weakly JN. Comparison of mivacurium and suxamethonium administered by bolus and infusion. *Br J Anaesth* 1989;62:488–93.

260 Levy JH, Davis GK, Duggan J, Szlam F. Determination of the hemodynamics and histamine release of rocuronium (Org 9426) when administered in increased doses under N_2O/O_2-sufentanil anesthesia. *Anesth Analg* 1994;78:318–21.

261 Vesely R, Hoffman WE, Gil KSL, Albrecht RF, Miletich DJ. The cerebrovascular effects of curare and histamine in the rat. *Anesthesiology* 1987;66:519–23.

262 Sokoloff L. The action of drugs on the cerebral circulation. *Pharmacol Rev* 1959;11:1–85.

263 Smith CE, Donati F, Bevan DR. Effects of succinylcholine at the masseter and adductor pollicis muscles in adults. *Anesth Anal* 1989;69:158–62.

264 VanderSpek AFL, Reynolda PI, Fang WB, Ashton-Miller JA, Stohler CS, Schork MA. Changes in resistance to mouth opening induced by depolarizing and non-depolarizing neuromuscular relaxants. *Br J Anaesth* 1990;64:21–7.

265 O'Flynn RP, Shutack JG, Rosenberg H, Fletcher JE. Masseter muscle rigidity and malignant hyperthermia susceptibility in pediatric patients. *Anesthesiology* 1994;80:1228–33.

266 Ording H, Fonsmark L. Use of vecuronium and doxapram in patients susceptible to malignant hyperthermia. *Br J Anaesth* 1988;60:445–9.

267 Trépanier CA, Brousseau C, Lacerte L. Myalgia in outpatient surgery: comparison of atracurium and succinylcholine. *Can J Anaesth* 1988;35:255–9.

268 Stewart KG, Hopkins PM, Dean SG. Comparison of high and low doses of suxamethonium. *Anaesthesia* 1991;46:833–6.

269 Zahl K, Apfelbaum JL. Muscle pain occurs after outpatient laparoscopy despite the substitution of vecuronium for succinylcholine. *Anesthesiology* 1989;70:408–11.

270 Laurence AS. Myalgia and biochemical changes following intermittent suxamethonium administration. Effects of alcuronium, lignocaine, midazolam and suxamethonium pretreatments on serum myoglobin, creatinine kinase and myalgia. *Anaesthesia* 1987;42:503–10.

271 Sosis M, Broad T, Larijani CE, Marr AT. Comparison of atracurium and d-tubocurarine for prevention of succinylcholine myalgia. *Anesth Analg* 1987;66:657–9.

272 Kahraman S, Ercan SA, Aypar U, Erdem K. Effects of preoperative i.m. administration of diclofenac on suxamethonium induced myalgia. *Br J Anaesth* 1993;71:238–41.

273 Verma RS. Diazepam and suxamethonium muscle pain (a dose–response study). *Anaesthesia* 1982;37:668–90.

274 Hatta V, Saxena A, Kaul HL. Phenytoin reduces suxamethonium induced myalgia. *Anaesthesia* 1992;47:664–7.

275 Fassaulaki A, Kaniaris P. Use of lignocaine throat spray to reduce suxamethonium muscle pains. *Br J Anaesth* 1981;53:1087–9.

276 Houghton IT, Aun CST, Gin T, Lau JFT, Oh TE. Suxamethonium myalgia: an ethnic comparison with and without pancuronium pretreatment. *Anaesthesia* 1993;**48**:377–81.

277 Bennets FE, Khalil KI. Reduction of post-suxamethonium pain by pretreatment with four non-depolarizing agents. *Br J Anaesth* 1981;**53**:531–6.

278 Ryan JF, Kagen LJ, Hyman AI. Myoglobinemia after a single dose of succinylcholine. *N Engl J Med* 1971;**285**:824–7.

279 Laurence AS. Serum myoglobin release following suxamethonium administration to children. *Eur J Anaesthesiol* 1988;**5**:31–8.

280 Caldwell JE, Magorian T, Lynam DP, Segredo V, Eger II EI, Miller RD. Desflurane versus isoflurane: dose–response relationships of pancuronium and succinylcholine. *Anesthesiology* 1990;**73**:A860.

281 Witkowski TA, Azad SS, Bartkowski RR, Epstein RH, Marr A, Lessin J. Desflurane (I-653) potentiation of pancuronium bromide: a comparison with isoflurane. *Anesthesiology* 1990;**73**:A903.

282 Smiley RM, Ornstein E, Mathews D, Matteo RS. A comparison of the effects of desflurane and isoflurane on the action of atracurium in man. *Anesthesiology* 1990;**73**:A882.

283 Fiekers JF. Neuromuscular block produced by polymyxin B—interaction with endplate ion channels. *Eur J Pharmacol* 1981;**70**:77–81.

284 Singh YN, Marshall IG, Harvey AL. Depression of transmitter release and postjunctional sensitivity during neuromuscular block produced by antibiotics. *Br J Anaesth* 1979; **51**:1027–33.

285 Singh YN, Marshall IG, Harvey AL. Some effects of the aminoglycoside antibiotic amikacin on neuromuscular and autonomic transmission. *Br J Anaesth* 1978;**50**:109–17.

286 Wright JM, Collier B. The site of the neuromuscular block produced by polymyxin B and rolitetracycline. *Can J Physiol Pharmacol* 1976;**54**:926–36.

287 Wright JM, Collier B. Characterization of the neuromuscular block produced by clindamycin and lincomycin. *Can J Physiol Pharmacol* 1976;**56**:937–44.

288 Booij LHDJ, Miller RD, Crul JF. Neostigmine and 4-aminopyridine antagonism of lincomycin-pancuronium neuromuscular blockade in man. *Anesth Analg* 1978;**57**: 316–21.

289 Kornfeld P, Horowitz SH, Genkins G, Papatestas AE. Myasthenia gravis unmasked by antiarrhythmic agents. *Mount Sinai J Med* 1976;**43**:10–14.

290 Lambert JJ, Durant NN, Handerson EG. Drug-induced modification of ionic conductance at the neuromuscular junction. *Annu Rev Pharmacol Toxicol* 1983;**23**:505–39.

291 Wali FA. Interactions of nifedipine and diltiazem with muscle relaxants and reversal of neuromuscular blockade with edrophonium and neostigmine. *J Pharmacol (Paris)* 1986;**17**:244–53.

292 Doll DC, Rosenberg H. Antagonism of neuromuscular blockage by theophylline. *Anesth Analg* 1979;**58**:139–40.

293 Ramanathan J, Sibai BM, Pillai R, Angel JJ. Neuromuscular transmission studies in preeclamptic women receiving magnesium sulfate. *Am J Obstet Gynecol* 1988;**158**:40–6.

294 Crosby E, Robblee JA. Cyclosporine–pancuronium interaction in a patient with a renal allograft. *Can J Anaesth* 1988;**35**:300–2.

295 Hickey DR, Sangwan S, Bevan JC. Phenytoin-induced resistance to pancuronium. *Anaesthesia* 1988;**43**:757–9.

159

8: Active reversal and monitoring of neuromuscular blockade

Closed loop infusion of non-depolarising relaxants

LEO HDJ BOOIJ

Ever since the introduction of muscle relaxants into routine clinical practice problems have occurred with the prediction of their duration of action, and the estimate of their degree of effect. Partial paralysis has always played a major role in the morbidity and mortality of anaesthesia. Therefore methods were developed to measure the degree of muscle paralysis. They are, however, for indistinct reasons not routinely practised in clinical anaesthesia in most clinics.

In cases of residual curarisation at the end of surgery, the ability to reverse such a paralysis is a basic requirement. At present the anti-cholinesterases neostigmine, pyridostigmine, and edrophonium are used clinically for this purpose. In many practices, for unjustifiable legal reasons, reversing agents are routinely administered if muscle relaxants had been used during anaesthesia. In such cases, deep non-reversible blockade or complete recovery may exist when reversing agents are administered. Such administration of anticholinesterases without previous determination of the degree of blockade is potentially dangerous. Deep blockade with most relaxants cannot be reversed, and the administration of anticholinesterases can cause paralysis. Furthermore, routine administration of anticholin-esterases provides the anaesthetist with an unjustified feeling of safety.

Reversing agents do, in fact, increase the acetylcholine concentration at all cholinergic receptors (nicotinic and muscarinic), and so exert many side effects, which are frequently more pronounced than the side effects of the muscle relaxants. There is no reason for the choice of a clean, but expensive, relaxant, and then to reverse its effects with a "dirty" compound, that is, a compound having many adverse effects. As with all drugs, compounds

160

reversing neuromuscular blockade should also be administered only on indication, and for this monitoring of the neuromuscular transmission is essential.

Monitoring neuromuscular transmission

Why should neuromuscular transmission by monitored routinely?

Shortly after their introduction in routine clinical practice, it was noticed that muscle relaxants could cause severe complications and even death, with the consequence that, particularly in patients with concurrent diseases, the relaxant must be administered with extreme caution.[1] It is currently recognised that muscle relaxants are responsible for about 50% of the adverse reactions during and immediately after anaesthesia.[2] The most common of such reactions are prolonged paralysis, hyperkalaemia, muscle rigidity, and drug interactions, although others do occur, especially when prolonged total or partial paralysis exists. Severe respiratory complications can occur, leading to permanent damage and even mortality.

All muscle relaxants have the inherent potential risk of interference with respiratory function because they all paralyse skeletal muscles. This is not a problem during anaesthesia itself when the patient is artificially ventilated and under the continuous attention of the anaesthetist, but it may be of importance during the recovery phase when the patient is breathing spontaneously, and is no longer continuously attended by the anaesthetist. Residual curarisation contributes heavily to such postoperative respiratory depression.[3] There is no difference in the outcome of residual curarisation with regard to the type (depolarising or non-depolarising, benzylisoquinoline, or steroid) of relaxant. Shorter acting relaxants are, however, less likely to cause residual curarisation than longer acting ones.[4-6] In one study the incidence of complications after pancuronium was 45% and after vecuronium 8%.[7] The long acting ones tend to cumulate, especially on repeated administration.

Postoperative residual curarisation is a real problem, and this has been confirmed in a study where it was demonstrated that, in a recovery room, 55% of the patients had mild hypoxia and 13% had severe hypoxia.[8] This was the case in 55% of the patients, although they received supplemental oxygen. The hypoxia was not recognised by the staff in 95% of the cases, and was present on arrival in the recovery room in 32%. Many anaesthetists have stated that residual curarisation is related to the experience of the anaesthetists, with less experienced ones having more problems. It has been proved repeatedly that this experience is not, however, an important factor in the prevention of residual curarisation.[9] In 72 patients, anaesthetised by experienced anaesthetists the neuromuscular function was assessed upon arrival in the recovery room using train-of-four stimulation, and clinical evaluation made of ability to cough, protrude the tongue, open the eyes, and sustain a head lift for five seconds.[10] Although 67 patients had received neostigmine on clinical indication and, although in all patients the recovery of the blockade was considered adequate, in 16 patients (22%) the observed train-of-four ratio was less than 0·60, and in 30 (42%) less than 0·70. Of these patients, 24% could not sustain a head lift for five seconds. In 1984 a similar study was conducted, and the results indicated that 25% of the patients still had a train-of-four ratio of less than 0·7, some of whom could not lift their heads.[11] In another study, about 10 years later in the same hospital, in a group of 7306 patients, 33 (0·4%) had severe clinical signs of respiratory insufficiency immediately upon arrival in the recovery room. Eight of them responded to neostigmine administration.[12] In this study it was also demonstrated that use of muscle relaxants was connected with a significantly increased risk of pulmonary complications when compared with patients not receiving relaxants.

Residual paralysis not only carries the risk of respiratory depression, but it also decreases the ability to cough or sigh, and to transport mucus. Thus the development of atelectasis and pulmonary infections is more likely to occur.

The interindividual variability in the response to muscle relaxants is large. Such variability was demonstrated in a study in which tubocurarine 0·1 mg/kg caused no depression of the contraction force at all in 6% of the patients, complete blockade in 7% of the patients, and other varying degrees of blockade in 87% of the patients.[13] Such studies have later been repeated with other relaxants, and with similar results. The duration of action of the relaxants also varies from patient to patient. The interindividual variability in response is caused by a number of factors. Although statistically there is good correlation between the plasma relaxant concentration and the degree of paralysis, in reality there is a large scatter in concentration for the same degree of blockade.[14] This points in the direction of a pharmacodynamic origin of the variability.

Other reasons for the large interindividual variability among patients are differences in body size and composition, differences in renal or hepatic function, the presence of concurrent diseases, and possible interactions with chronically or simultaneously administered drugs (see chapter 7). More than 250 drugs do have an effect on neuromuscular transmission, and many of these are given to patients in the perioperative period. Some examples are the antibiotics of the aminoglycoside, polypeptide, tetracycline, or lincosamide type.[15 16] Curarisation from antibiotics can even occur if the previous blockade has been adequately reversed with anticholinesterase (Booij, unpublished results).

It must therefore be concluded that not only a large variability in neuromuscular blockade and its recovery exists when the same dose of relaxant is administered, but also clinical judgment of such a blockade is totally unreliable. Many more examples that prove that monitoring of neuromuscular transmission is demanded for the sake of the patient's safety are to be found in the literature.[17] More quantitative monitoring of the blockade is therefore needed. Monitoring neuromuscular transmission can serve the following goals:

- Determination of the magnitude of neuromuscular blockade
- Determination of the type of relaxant administered
- Estimation of the need for additional administration
- Measurement of the degree of spontaneous recovery
- Evaluation of the efficiency of anticholinesterases
- Recognition of the interaction with other drugs or diseases
- Differential diagnosis in apnoea
- Instruction on the use of relaxants and antagonists during training.

Methods of evaluation of neuromuscular transmission

Patency of neuromuscular transmission can be evaluated either sub-jectively by clinical signs, or more objectively by measurement of the response upon nerve stimulation. If a patient can sustain head lift for five seconds, then it is unlikely that adequate airway protection is present. This seems to be the most sensitive clinical sign of adequate recovery of paralysis.[18] Sustainment of voluntary hand grip strength and elevation of the stretched arm are also sensitive measures.[19] They all, however, depend heavily on the cooperation of the patient, and are not an absolute guarantee for continuous adequate respiration and maintenance of a clear airway. Measurement of ventilatory parameters such as tidal volume, vital capacity, minute ventilation, and inspiratory force are other possible tools, but they also require the cooperation of the patient, and are cumbersome to measure in the operating and recovery rooms.

A more reliable method, which does not need the cooperation of the patient, is the evaluation of the response to nerve stimulation. Such an evaluation can either be qualitative or quantitative. Qualitative evaluation uses visual or tactile judgment of the response and is again unreliable. Although it seems easy to estimate the response in this way, both methods tend to underestimate the neuromuscular blockade.[20 21] More quantitative methods should therefore be used.

It is generally accepted that, when the response to train-of-four stimulation is 0·75 or higher, there is adequate recovery of neuromuscular blockade.[22] The single twitch response is about 90% of the control. During very profound blockade a tactile or visual judgment can be made accurately because there is no response to stimulation at all. With a lesser degree of blockade the count for train-of-four responses is accurate. With even more superficial block, however, accurate subjective determination of the degree of depression in twitch response or train-of-four ratio is impossible, and so objective quantification is necessary. Visual or tactile evaluation of the response to train-of-four stimulation is also unreliable as compared with objective quantification.[20 21 23] Misinterpretations seem to be less severe, however, when tactile judgment is used. Tactile judgment of the response to double burst stimulation is more accurate than that to train-of-four stimulation, but it remains questionable during recovery.[24] Visual or tactile judgment of fading in response to tetanic stimulation has an acceptable accuracy; as this is a painful stimulus, however, this method cannot be applied to awakening patients during the recovery phase. Frequent application of tetanic stimulation in fact interferes with the neuromuscular blockade in the stimulated muscles, although not in the other muscles.

Quantitative measurement of neuromuscular blockade uses electromyography, mechanomyography, or acceleromyography. In electromyography either the amplitude or the surface area under the curve of the biphasic electrical muscle action potential is quantified, and used as an expression of the degree of transmission. There is no difference in outcome between surface area and amplitude.[25] In this method a measurement time gate is used, which must be meticulously chosen and depend on the distance between the place of stimulation and the place of quantification of the response. Another problem with electromyography is that, in time, there is usually a drift towards a 20% decrease in response; preload seems to be a determining factor in this.[26]

Both mechanomyography and acceleromyography use the contractile force of the muscle. They measure the whole transmission process, including the contractility of the muscle, which is physiologically of clinical importance. In all three methods the nerve can be stimulated in various patterns, which determine the pattern of response. As the methods measure different things, there is a difference in outcome between the methods of quantification for the individual stimulation patterns.[27 28] With non-depolarising relaxants, the mechanomyogram is more depressed than the electromyogram; with suxamethonium, the opposite is seen.[29 30] In addition, with electromyography the train-of-four ratio tends to be 10–15% greater than the same ratio with mechanomyography. This means that the ratio should be above 0·8 for electromyography compared with 0·7 for mechanomyography, so as to ensure the patient's safety.[31]

Mechanomyography is critically dependent on maintenance of a constant preload, so fixation of the arm and thumb is requested. This is not necessary with acceleromyography. In acceleromyography the acceleration of movement consequent upon muscle contraction is measured with a special transducer. A linear relationship exists between contraction force and acceleration. With acceleromyography, in contrast to mechanomyography, there is an underestimation during onset of block and an overestimation during recovery.[32] Both electromyography and mechanomyography are influenced by temperature.[33] Tetanic responses cannot be evaluated with acceleromyography, because movement is requested with this method.

The stimulator and the stimulation patterns for monitoring neuromuscular transmission

The nerve stimulator and the stimulation electrodes

The stimulator should provide monophasic square wave stimuli at constant current output. If the stimulus is biphasic, bursts of action may occur. The constant current is needed because in time variations in skin impedance occur, which will then lead to change in stimulation force on the nerve, and inconsistency in response.[34][35] The stimulus must be supramaximal to guarantee recruitment of all muscle fibres.[35] Such stimulus does exist when it is at 2·5–3 times the threshold stimulation current. This demands that, in almost all circumstances, the maximal output of the stimulator should be at least 60 mA, but preferably 80–100 mA, at all stimulation frequencies.[35] In most patients the output needed for supramaximal stimulation will be 20–30 mA. In some patients (obese, oedematous), a higher output current is needed. It must be remembered that supramaximal stimulation with tetanus, train-of-four, and double burst is painful.[36] For reasons explained later the stimulator must be able to provide single twitch, train-of-four, tetanic stimulation at 50 Hz, and double burst stimulation, both single and repeatedly, applied at the proper intervals. It is an advantage if the apparatus is programmable, so that, for example, post-tetanic potentiation and post-tetanic count can be automatically chosen after administration of a tetanic stimulation. The duration of each individual stimulus must be between 0·1 and 0·2 ms, and the negative electrode should be placed distally from the positive one.

Stimuli can be applied to the patient via surface electrodes placed over the nerve to be stimulated.[37] For the transfer of the stimulus the impedance is of importance, and is mainly determined by electrode contact with the skin. In the past needle electrodes have been used, but they are invasive, with all potential risks related to this. The results with proper surface electrodes are as good as those with needle electrodes. For routine clinical measurement the use of surface electrodes with a silver/silver chloride jelly is advocated. The contact surface of the electrodes must be not too large, because otherwise dispersion of the current will occur. If the surface is too small, the density of the current may be too high, and this could cause damage to skin, nerve, or other tissues. This could also be the case when needle electrodes are used in the wrong way. Needle electrodes carry a greater risk of direct muscle stimulation than surface electrodes. High quality children's ECG electrodes are used for clinical evaluation of neuromuscular transmission; they should be placed over the nerve that mediates contraction of the muscle being evaluated. With surface electrodes the skin should be carefully prepared, that is, shaven, degreased, and part of the cornefied layer removed to decrease and to stabilise skin impedance. In obese or oedematous patients needle electrodes do give more reliable supramaximal stimulation than surface electrodes.

The stimulation patterns

A number of stimulation patterns and resulting parameters are nowadays used for monitoring the neuromuscular transmission, that is, single twitch, train-of-four, double burst, tetanus. Other parameters derived from such stimulation are train-of-four count, post-tetanic potentiation, and post-tetanic count. All stimuli should be administered at a supramaximal voltage and a constant current.[38][39] Supramaximal stimulation ensures that all muscle fibres are contracting upon each stimulation. This results in more consistent responses. It has, however, been demonstrated that, in the postoperative period, submaximal stimulation results in adequate responses to evaluate recovery.[40]

Single twitch stimulation—This is a square wave supramaximal stimulus of 0·1 ms duration at a frequency of 0·1–0·15 Hz. The duration of the single twitch stimulus should not exceed 0·2 ms to avoid repetitive nerve firing.

Muscle relaxants decrease the response to single twitch stimulation. The response starts to decrease when 75–80% of the acetylcholine receptors are occupied with a non-depolarising relaxant. When more than 90–95% of the receptors are occupied, there is complete neuromuscular blockade.[41] In the case of suxamethonium (depolarising) this is 25% and 90% respectively of the receptors. This means that for non-depolarising relaxants 70% of the receptors are still occupied when the response to twitch stimulation has fully recovered. With increase in stimulation frequency, the number of receptors which are still occupied when the response shows complete recovery decreases, and the decrease in response to twitch stimulation as a percentage of the control height (amplitude) expresses the degree of neuromuscular blockade. Before the relaxant is administered, a baseline response must be obtained to quantify the effect. Full single twitch response does not guarantee complete recovery of muscle contraction because normal muscle activity is generated by a physiological tetanic stimulation pattern at 30–50 Hz, which already fades when fewer receptors are occupied.

The response to single twitch stimulation is usually used to describe the pharmacodynamics of relaxants, that is, potency (degree of block), delay to first effect, onset, clinical and total duration, and recovery. At a 75% depression of the response, good surgical relaxation starts to occur.

Train-of-four stimulation—This consists of train-of-four stimuli at a frequency of 2 Hz; each individual stimulus lasts 0·1 ms. The train is repeated at 10–12 second intervals.

When the stimulation frequency is above 1·5 Hz, fading in response will be observed upon administration of repeated stimuli in the presence of non-depolarising muscle relaxants. This is the result of a decrease in acetylcholine release. Fade after tetanic or train-of-four stimulation is essentially a prejunctional effect; suppression of the single twitch response is primarily a postjunctional effect.[42] At 2 Hz, maximum fading is reached at the fourth stimulus. Poststimulation potentiation is not seen in this situation, so the 2 Hz frequency was chosen for the train-of-four stimulation. The interval between the individual train-of-four stimulations is important. The shorter the interval, the higher the degree of blockade and the faster the onset.[43] Thus to compare data from various studies the same stimulation rate at intervals of 0·1–0·12 s should be used.

The ratio of the height of the first and the fourth response is called the *train-of-four ratio*; a baseline control value is not needed. The response to train-of-four stimulation is believed to be the clinically most suitable method of evaluation of neuromuscular blockade.[39] There is a relaxant independent relationship between the train-of-four ratio and the degree of depression of muscle contraction upon single twitch stimulation.[44] This is best seen when one or more of the four responses is disappearing, that is, in the *train-of-four count*. Disappearance of the fourth, third, and second responses to train-of-four stimulation relates to 60–70%, 70–80%, and 80–90% decrease in response to single twitch stimulation respectively.[44] At a train-of-four ratio of 0·70 at the adductor pollicis muscle, all patients can sustain eye opening, tongue protrusion, and hand grip during recovery, whereas most can sustain head lift for only five seconds.[45] Sustained response to tetanic stimulation (50 Hz for five seconds) of the adductor pollicis muscle is also present. This counts when the evoked responses are quantified with mechanomyography. If there is quantification with electromyography, a train-of-four ratio of 0·9 at the adductor pollicis muscle is required.[46] As it has been demonstrated that, under enflurane anaesthesia, the train-of-four response reappears at a deeper degree of single twitch depression, the actual relationship might depend on the type of anaesthetic administered.[47] Fade, especially during onset of blockade, is also dependent on the relaxant used, being more pronounced with tubocurarine and atracurium than with pancuronium and vecuronium. Fading is more apparent during recovery than during onset of blockade.[48]

Double burst stimulation—With double burst stimulation two bursts of three stimuli at a frequency of 50 Hz are administered with a 0·75 s interval. They result in two short duration contractions, which are equal in strength in non-paralysed patients.[49] With non-depolarising relaxants the second response is weaker than the first. This is a more reliable measure than the train-of-four responses.[50] Double burst stimulation is, however, more painful than train-of-four and cannot therefore be recommended during the recovery room period. The interval between two double burst stimuli should be at least 12 s.

Tetanic stimulation, post-tetanic potentiation, and post-tetanic count—When a train of supramaximal stimuli at a frequency of 50 Hz is administered for five seconds, the individual responses will converge into one sustained muscle contraction which lasts as long as the stimulus is applied.

At stimulation frequencies above 5 Hz, there is a fusion of the individual responses, that is, tetanisation. When non-depolarising muscle relaxants are administered, the peak tetanic contraction is not maintained and fading occurs. Stimulation frequencies above 50 Hz may also result in spontaneous fade in response (fatigue), even in the absence of muscle relaxants.[51]

If, immediately after a five second duration tetanic stimulation, a 1 Hz single twitch stimulation is applied, a potentiation (facilitation) in the response will be seen for 90–120 seconds (post-tetanic potentiation). This results from increased mobilisation and release of acetylcholine (see chapter 1). The deeper the degree of blockade, the less likely it is that such post-tetanic responses are seen, and thus their appearance is an indication of recovery of blockade.[52] Such recovery is correlated with the number of potentiated single twitch responses observed after tetanic stimulation (post-tetanic count). Other characteristics of post-tetanic potentiation are a decrease in the fade in response to train-of-four and double burst stimulation, and a decrease in the latency period from the beginning of an muscle action potential to the rise in muscle tension. The mechanism of post-tetanic potentiation and post-tetanic count is an increase in acetylcholine release, with liberation of postjunctional receptors from relaxant, and increased muscle contractility.

The time relationship between the first appearance of a post-tetanic response, and a response to normal single twitch stimulation without previous application of a tetanus, proved to be the following in children:

- vecuronium   5·8   (0·3 SD) min
- atracurium   7·8   (0·5 SD) min
- pancuronium   19·8   (3·0 SD) min
- alcuronium   29·3   (3·3 SD) min
- tubocurarine   33·3   (3·3 SD) min.

The post-tetanic count, in relation to the appearance of the first response in the train-of-four in children, was the following in the same study:

- vecuronium   7·3   (0·8 SD) twitches
- atracurium   7·2   (0·4 SD) twitches
- pancuronium   7·2   (0·5 SD) twitches
- alcuronium   6·3   (0·4 SD) twitches
- tubocurarine   5·7   (0·4 SD) twitches.

Post-tetanic count should not be applied more than once every 5–6 minutes because tetanic stimulation will speed up recovery of blockade in the stimulated muscles.[54 55] Post-tetanic facilitation is a prejunctional phenomenon, and hence depends on the relaxant administered. Vecuronium, for example, has less prejunctional effect than atracurium, so that during onset its fading is less marked. Studies with vecuronium have suggested that the post-tetanic count remains unchanged at the same degree of blockade after repeated administration of relaxant.[56] Another method for monitoring deep blockade is stimulation of the orbicularis oculi muscle. This method is, however, less sensitive than post-tetanic count.[57] Of course the post-tetanic count, that is, the time interval of reappearance of single twitch responses after a tetanic stimulation, depends on the type of relaxant used. Although the duration of action of muscle relaxants depends on the type of anaesthetic administered, there is, however, no effect on the time delay in post-tetanic count.[58]

Post-tetanic potentiation is not seen at a frequency of 2 Hz; therefore this frequency was chosen for the train-of-four stimulation.

After a 50 Hz stimulation, the fade in response to train-of-four and double burst stimulation is decreased for a period of about 2 minutes.

There is a relationship between the responses to the various stimulation

Table 8.1   Relationships between response to stimulation and receptor occupancy

Receptor occupancy (%)	Twitch response (%)	Train-of-four ratio response	Train-of-four count	Tetanus fade at frequency
0	100	1	4	None
30	100	1	4	Fade at 200 Hz
50	100	1	4	Fade at 100 Hz
75	99	0·75–1·0	4	Fade at 50 Hz
80	95	0·7–0·75	4	More fade
	80–90	0·6–0·7	4	More fade
	25	0	3	Fade at 30 Hz
90	20	0	2	
	10	0	1	
95–100	0	0	0	

patterns and the number of receptors occupied by non-depolarising relaxants (table 8.1).

At which muscle should neuromuscular transmission be monitored?

All superficial nerves can be used for stimulation; the responses of the muscles innervated by them have not, however, been correlated with either surgical relaxation or respiratory function.

In evaluation of a neuromuscular blockade, stimulation of the ulnar or median nerve near the wrist is particularly appropriate. These nerves are not only easily accessible for stimulation most of the time, but there is also a good correlation between the response of the innervated muscles and the ability of the patient to breathe spontaneously. Only minor, clinically irrelevant differences are evident in the sensitivity of the various hand muscles, if measured by the same method.[30] There are major differences, however, between the muscles in the hand and those in other body areas.[60]

As anaesthetists also have easy access to the head of the patients most of the time, stimulation and evaluation of the response in facial muscles have been used clinically. This muscle is, however, much more resistant to relaxants than the adductor pollicis, so underestimation of relaxation of the respiratory muscles is likely to occur.[61] Accordingly it has been proved that these muscles have made a complete recovery before the adductor pollicis or the respiratory muscles, which leads to underestimation of the neuromuscular blockade.[61] Other sites that may be evaluated include the peroneal and posterior tibial nerves. All muscle groups, however, have different responses in potency, delay of effect, onset, duration, and recovery of relaxants.[61-64]

It has been recognised for a long time that there is respiratory sparing effect of non-depolarising relaxants.[65] Respiration is unaffected when the muscles in the hand are completely paralysed.[66] The potency of pancuronium on the diaphragm is half that on the adductor pollicis muscle,[67] and intercostal and abdominal muscles have a greater sensitivity to pancuronium than the diaphragm.[68] In fact the onset of action of relaxants is faster in the diaphragm than in the adductor pollicis muscle.[69] These facts may explain the good correlation between surgical relaxation, as judged by the surgeon, and the relaxation of the adductor pollicis muscle. It can also be concluded that monitoring of the adductor pollicis muscle is a valuable method of guaranteeing either sufficient surgical muscle paralysis or adequate recovery of the respiratory muscles.

The adductor muscles of the larynx have a similar resistance to relaxants as the diaphragm and show a faster onset and recovery.[70] Recently, a model was described which showed that the faster onset is caused by an earlier peak concentration of the relaxant in the respiratory muscles, probably because of greater perfusion.[71] This explains why there are adequate intubation conditions even when blockade in the adductor pollicis muscle is only 80–90%.

For adequate relaxation during abdominal surgery, 80% reduction in adductor pollicis single twitch contraction, or the presence of only one or two responses in the train-of-four count, is usually sufficient. Further suppression is superfluous and may put the anaesthetist in a difficult position if reversal of blockade is suddenly needed.

There can be variability in response in muscles affected by diseases, so such areas should be avoided when monitoring neuromuscular transmission (see chapter 7).

If, after administration of a muscle relaxant, the response of the adductor pollicis muscle to single twitch stimulation has decreased to 5–10% of control, then conditions are suitable for laryngoscopy and endotracheal intubation. The abdominal musculature shows adequate relaxation for abdominal surgery when the response is less than 25% of control. A sustained head lift is possible when the response is more than 90% of control. Suitable abdominal wall relaxation exists at a train-of-four count of less than three responses. The conditions for laryngoscopy and intubation are good when the train-of-four count is one. Head lift starts to come back at a train-of-four ratio of more than 0·4; at a ratio of more than 0·75 the patient can open the eyes, protrude the tongue, and cough. At a ratio of 0·8 or more the vital capacity and inspiratory force are normal. Reversal of neuromuscular blockade by administration of cholinesterase inhibitors should not be started before there is a reaction to single twitch stimulation.

Thus optimal surgical conditions exist at a single twitch response of between 25% and 5% of control, or a train-of-four count of 2:1. Under these conditions reversal can always be guaranteed.

Factors affecting neuromuscular monitoring

It has been demonstrated that hypothermia affects the contraction of the adductor pollicis muscle, which must be taken into consideration when neuromuscular blockade is monitored. The decrease in contraction force in the absence of muscle relaxants is more than 10% per °C decrease in core temperature.[72] In hypothermia the pharmacokinetic and/or pharmacodynamic behaviour of most relaxants is also changed, which will lead to deeper and more prolonged neuromuscular blockade (see chapter 7).

Hemiplegia and quadriplegia should be taken into consideration while monitoring neuromuscular transmission (see chapter 7).

The approach of maintaining a particular level of relaxation with the aid of a transmission monitor can be used for closed loop administration of muscle relaxants.[73] In such situations it must be realised that a decrease in temperature influences the response, so the temperature of the arm should be kept above 32°C.[74]

Reversal of neuromuscular blockade

If necessary, at the end of surgery, the effect of the non-depolarising neuromuscular blockers can be reversed. Two principles are important in the reversal process; first neuromuscular blockade is obtained by competitive occupancy of acetylcholine receptors by non-depolarising relaxants and, second, spontaneous recovery of non-depolarising relaxants is attained by lowering their concentration in the biophase. This second principle is achieved by relaxant plasma clearance (redistribution, metabolism, or excretion). It is also important in reversal to shift the competition for receptor occupancy in the direction of acetylcholine, which can be reached theoretically through two mechanisms: increase in the amount of acetylcholine available or active decrease in the amount of relaxant present.

Drugs that can reverse neuromuscular blockade

Active decrease in the amount of relaxant

At present it is clinically impossible to achieve an active decrease in the amount of relaxant present. Theoretically, the plasma concentration of atracurium could be decreased more rapidly by enhancing the Hofmann degradation through induction of acidosis; this is not, however, acceptable in practice. The metabolism of suxamethonium and mivacurium may be enhanced by administration of pseudocholinesterase, which leads to serious side effects. Theoretically, haemodialysis, using a membrane permeable to relaxants, could decrease the amount of relaxant, but again this method is clinically not feasible.

Increase in the amount of acetylcholine available

The amount of acetylcholine available for competition with non-depolarising relaxants at the postjunctional acetylcholine receptor can be increased by either decreasing its breakdown or by increasing its prejunctional release. Increase in acetylcholine is feasible with the administration of 4-aminopyridine or one of its analogues. Decrease in metabolism can be reached with one of the quaternary anticholinesterases neostigmine, pyridostigmine, or edrophonium.

Anticholinesterases—The antagonistic effect of physostigmine on curare

171

induced neuromuscular blockade was demonstrated at the turn of this century.[75] Its chemical structure was discovered in 1925, after which neostigmine was synthesised.[76] As physostigmine passes the blood–brain barrier, and thus causes central nervous system effects, it is no longer used for the reversal of neuromuscular blockade.

The anticholinesterases bind to acetylcholinesterase, thereby inhibiting the hydrolytic breakdown of acetylcholine at both the nicotinic and the muscarinic receptor sites. Acetylcholinesterase is produced in the myotubules, and transported to the muscle cell surface, where, under the influence of neural activity, it accumulates in the basal lamina of the membrane, especially in the secondary folds of the neuromuscular junction.[77] There is more acetylcholinesterase activity in fast contracting muscles (more acetylcholine release) than in slow contracting muscles.[78] The products of hydrolysis are taken up again in the nerve terminal for resynthesis of acetylcholine. Only 50% of the acetylcholine molecules liberated from the nerve terminal reach the postjunctional receptors, the rest being hydrolysed before that (see chapters 1 and 2). Acetylcholinesterase has two action sites: an anionic and an ester site. Neostigmine and pyridostigmine are themselves hydrolysed by acetylcholinesterase (acid transferring anticholinesterases, which bind to both the anionic and the ester sites), whereas edrophonium is not (prosthetic anticholinesterase that binds to the anionic site).[79] This last compound rapidly dissociates, however, from the enzyme, although it can reassociate immediately.

The accumulation of acetylcholine through its decreased metabolism augments the competition for the nicotinic receptor between acetylcholine and the non-depolarising relaxant. Less relaxant will be bound if more acetylcholine is present. This enhances the diffusion of non-depolarising relaxants away from the biophase into the blood, and speeds up the recovery from the blockade.

In the presence of anticholinesterase the residence time of acetylcholine can be prolonged, with repeated occupation of acetylcholine receptors, leading to reopening of the ion channels.[80] As more channels are present in the open state, there is an increased risk of channel blockade by other compounds.[81] The abundant quantity of acetylcholine present may also result in an increased occupancy of prejunctional acetylcholine receptors; as a result the release of acetylcholine may be diminished upon subsequent nerve stimulation.[82]

The effect of the anticholinesterases is not only restricted to inhibition of acetylcholinesterase, but also includes prejunctional acetylcholine releasing effects, and some direct effects on the postjunctional receptor.[83 84] Large concentrations may occlude acetylcholine operated ion channels.[85] All these effects contribute to the relaxant reversing effects of the anticholinesterases. With neostigmine these additional effects are stronger than with pyridostigmine or edrophonium,[86] although edrophonium has a more pronounced prejunctional effect than neostigmine and pyridostigmine.[87 88]

The anticholinesterases have minimal passage through the blood–brain barrier and thus, contrary to physostigmine, central nervous system effects upon their administration are seldom observed. The quaternary anticholinesterases are water soluble, and excreted mainly via the kidneys.

In addition, suxamethonium phase II block can be reversed by administration of anticholinesterases. This is not, however, the case if fading in train-of-four response occurs after suxamethonium administration in patients with acetylcholinesterase deficiency.[90]

Aminopyridines—The aminopyridines increase prejunctional acetylcholine release via prolongation of potassium currents.[91]

4-Aminopyridine is a weak and slow reversal agent which, however, also reverses the blockade induced by a number of antibiotics.[15 92] Furthermore, it potentiates neostigmine and pyridostigmine, but not edrophonium.[93 94] As 4-aminopyridine is a tertiary amine, it passes the blood–brain barrier and causes central nervous system effects. In clinical studies, 4-aminopyridine had a relatively weak effect which, in the dosages used, only partly reversed the non-depolarising blockade. The compound seems to be of value in the treatment of the Eaton–Lambert syndrome.[95]

2,4-Diaminopyridine and 3,4-diaminopyridine are more potent and more polar compounds. They therefore cross the blood–brain barrier to a lesser extent, having more specific peripheral effects.[96] These compounds and some of their analogues are currently being investigated.

Acetaminopyridine-*N*-oxide is another more polar derivative, which is also more potent than 4-aminopyridine.[97]

Miscellaneous reversing agents—Germine monoacetate[98] is able to antagonise both depolarising and non-depolarising neuromuscular blockade. The mechanism seems to be a direct effect on the muscle fibre.[99] Although its efficacy has been demonstrated in animal studies,[98 100] the compound has not been routinely used in the clinic. In cats the compound was able to reverse muscle relaxation from dantrolene.[101]

Galanthamine is a tertiary amine with a weaker but longer effect than neostigmine.[102] The drug binds to both the anionic and the ester sites of cholinesterase. It has, however, central nervous system effects and is unpredictable in its reversing effects.[103]

Pharmacodynamic profile of the anticholinesterases

Edrophonium has the weakest anticholinesterase effect, followed by pyridostigmine, with neostigmine being the most potent. The onset of action after administration of equipotent dosages is more rapid with edrophonium (1–2 min), followed by neostigmine (7–11 min), and finally pyridostigmine (15 min); the duration of action is, however, longest with pyridostigmine, followed by neostigmine, and then edrophonium.[104 105] The duration of action of the anticholinesterases, when administered at equipotent dosages, is clinically similar and ranges from 1 to 2 hours.[104 106]

The dose of anticholinesterase required to reverse a block is dependent on the degree of neuromuscular blockade, on the type of relaxant, and on the anticholinesterase administered.[107–110] It has, for example, been demonstrated in the rat hemidiaphragm preparation that less neostigmine is needed to reverse a benzylisoquinoline (tubocurarine, metocurine, atracurium, doxacurium, mivacurium) neuromuscular blockade than a steroidal (pancuronium, pipecuronium, vecuronium, rocuronium) blockade. Not all anticholinesterases are as effective in reversing each individual muscle relaxant. They may prolong the duration of suxamethonium induced blockade.[111] It has been noticed that there is a marked sensitivity for atracurium when this is administered 30 minutes after an anticholinesterase.[112] When edrophonium is administered during profound neuromuscular blockade induced by atracurium, the antagonism is not sustained as it is with more superficial blockade. With neostigmine the reversal is more persistent.[113]

In clinical practice it is difficult to take all these factors into consideration. Therefore an initial dose of the reversal agent should be administered, the recovery measured, and, if needed, a supplemental dose of the agent administered. In general a dose of 0·06 mg/kg neostigmine seems to be adequate.[114 115] For edrophonium the dose is 1·0 mg/kg;[116] the pyridostigmine dose is 0·3 mg/kg. The potency of the anticholinesterases thus relates as neostigmine : pyridostigmine : edrophonium = 1 : 1/5 : 1/12.

In elderly patients the duration of effect of neostigmine and pyridostigmine is significantly increased (table 8.2), similar to the effect of most non-depolarising relaxants.[117] The effect of edrophonium is not, however, prolonged,[118] and correlates with a different pharmacokinetic behaviour in elderly people.[119] As a result of larger initial volume of distribution in elderly people a larger dose is needed to produce the same effect.[117]

In one study elderly patients needed 0·031 mg/kg neostigmine versus 0·019 mg/kg in younger patients.[119] The plasma concentration needed for a given effect is thus no different in younger and elderly patients. Although, for edrophonium, such an effect on the pharmacodynamics could not be demonstrated, the clearance was decreased and the elimination half life prolonged in elderly patients.[120] The initial volume of distribution is, however, not changed.[121] Based on the results of these studies perhaps edrophonium should not be used in elderly patients. Although high dosages of edrophonium were considered adequate for the reversal of neuro-

Table 8.2 Dose and duration of action of anticholinesterase drugs in young and elderly patients[117]

Anticholinesterase	Dose (mg/kg)	Duration (min)	
		Elderly patients	Younger patients
Edrophonium	1	2·2	1·3
Neostigmine	0·07	32	11
Pyridostigmine	0·14	35	14

muscular blockade, it has now become clear that it is an unreliable antagonist for long acting relaxants, even in moderate degrees of blockade.[122]

There is no difference in the dose requirement for edrophonium in infants, children, and adults. With neostigmine infants need less than adults; children need about half the adult dose, whereas elderly people need a higher dose.

It must be remembered that anticholinesterases activate the acetylcholine receptor so that more receptors are present in the so called open state. Thus channel blockade from other drugs (for example, some antibiotics) is more likely to occur when these drugs are administered after reversal with anticholinesterases. It is also well known that anticholinesterases themselves may induce neuromuscular blockade.[123] This occurs particularly after repeated administration of anticholinesterases, not only when there is a resultant overdose, but also if a normal dose is given to reverse a superficial blockade.[124] It is probable that this occurs most frequently with the intermediate and short acting drugs such as atracurium and vecuronium.[125] For this reason, anticholinesterases should be administered only in low doses in case of residual blockade, and after evaluation of the degree of blockade upon nerve stimulation.

Anticholinesterases, with the exception of edrophonium,[126] inhibit not only true cholinesterase, but also plasma cholinesterase.[111] Therefore after administration, a more pronounced and prolonged effect of suxamethonium must be anticipated.[127] This is more pronounced with pyridostigmine than with neostigmine.[111] Mivacurium is broken down by plasma cholinesterase,[128] so its metabolism may be inhibited by administration of anticholinesterases, although at the same time there is a reversal of the blockade by an increase in acetylcholine concentration (acetylcholinesterase inhibition). It has been demonstrated, however, that mivacurium in vitro and in vivo is adequately antagonised by neostigmine.[129 130] This has been confirmed in humans.[131] As edrophonium is a weaker plasma cholinesterase inhibitor than neostigmine, and as it does not inhibit plasma cholinesterase, this compound could, at least theoretically, be a better reversal agent for mivacurium induced neuromuscular block.[131]

Should non-depolarising relaxants be routinely reversed?

Many anaesthetists recommend routine administration of an anticholinesterase (neostigmine, pyridostigmine, edrophonium) at the end of anaesthesia using a non-depolarising relaxant. It has, however, been proved that such routine administration of an anticholinesterase is not a guarantee for adequate reversal of the blockade, if the transmission is not monitored at the same time. This would imply that reversal should always be done guided by such monitoring. If, however, there is adequate recovery (train-of-four ratio > 0.7) on monitoring, administration of anticholinesterase is no longer necessary, and can even be harmful because anticholinesterases can cause neuromuscular blockade.[133] Anticholinesterases exert side effects: they increase the amount of acetylcholine at all receptor sites (nicotinic and muscarinic). At the muscarinic receptor the increased acetylcholine causes a number of unwanted effects, the signs being bradycardia, excessive secretions from salivary and bronchial glands, and bronchial and intestinal smooth muscle contractions. The adverse effects are dose dependent, and are most pronounced with neostigmine and least with edrophonium.[106] Atropine, and especially glycopyrrolate, prevent many of the cardiovascular effects of the anticholinesterases,[134] although it is unable to prevent the intestinal effects.[135] Anticholinesterases can also cause bronchoconstriction.

Administration of anticholinesterases carries the risk of induction of a central cholinergic syndrome. It is characterised by delayed recovery, restlessness, and agitation; frequently hypertension, tachycardia, mydriasis, and urinary retention are also seen. At repeated dosages of anticholinesterases, neuromuscular block may occur from transient depolarisation of the receptors, and blockade of channels in an open confirmation.[136]

The anticholinesterases have strong muscarinic effects on the gastrointestinal tract. For neostigmine, at least in one study, it has been demonstrated that it increases the incidence of nausea and vomiting in the immediate postoperative period.[137] Others have also found this effect.[138] In the same study it was also indicated that suxamethonium seems to be related to a higher incidence of nausea and vomiting than non-depolarising relaxants. Other investigators, however, found a decrease in the incidence of nausea and vomiting after reversal of neuromuscular blockade.[139] This was confirmed later for neostigmine.[140]

In patients with hemiplegia the afflicted side is more sensitive to the reversal of a non-depolarising blockade with anticholinesterases than the non-afflicted side.[141]

Pharmacokinetics of anticholinesterases

The pharmacokinetic behaviour of all three clinically used anti-cholinesterases is similar. After a peak plasma concentration is reached immediately following intravenous administration, there is a rapid decline in concentration over 5–10 minutes, corresponding to the redistribution phase. Thereafter, a slower decrease in plasma concentration is seen during the elimination phase. The volume of distribution ranges from $0 \cdot 7$–$1 \cdot 4$ l/kg, the elimination half life rate is 60–120 min and the clearance is 8–16 ml/kg per min (table 8.3).[121 142 143] In patients with renal failure the clearance is significantly decreased, and the elimination half lives prolonged. The elimination of edrophonium and neostigmine is decreased in elderly patients.[120]

In the published data on the pharmacokinetics of the anticholinesterases, there is a large spread. They all have a large and variable volume of distribution (table 8.3). Neostigmine and its breakdown products are predominantly excreted via the kidneys, so its effect is prolonged in renal

Table 8.3   Pharmacokinetic data on anticholinesterases

Anticholinesterase	VD_{ss} (l/kg)	Clearance (l/kg per h)	$T_{\frac{1}{2}\alpha}$ (min)	$T_{\frac{1}{2}\beta}$ (min)
Neostigmine	0·1–1·1	0·2–1·0	3·6–12·0	24·2–80
Pyridostigmine	0·5–1·7	0·3–1·0	0·8–8·4	46·4–112
Edrophonium	1·1	0·56	1·2–0·7	30–110

The data are given as rounded figures, and are purely illustrative.
VD_{ss}, volume distribution between central and peripheral compartments.

failure. Elimination of neostigmine in paediatric patients is faster than in adults, but elimination is slower in elderly patients.[116 144] Neostigmine is mainly eliminated through the kidney, and pyridostigmine is largely metabolised in the liver, but also extensively excreted through the kidneys.

The effect of some pathophysiological states on the effect of anticholinesterases

The effect of temperature

Hypothermia facilitates neuromuscular transmission at the electro-chemical level, but compromises mechanical contractility.[145] It has been demonstrated in vitro that non-depolarising muscle relaxants result in a statistically significant, but probably clinically irrelevant, deeper neuro-muscular blockade during hypothermia.[146] In clinical studies with atracurium an increase in potency and longer duration of action have been found.[147] This has also been found for pancuronium, vecuronium, and alcuronium.[148 149] Upon rewarming of the patent the various values return to normal (see chapter 7). The effect of anticholinesterase, however, remains the same.[150] This means that it is more difficult to reverse a neuromuscular blockade during hypothermia.

The effect of renal function

Renal failure prolongs the effect of most non-depolarising muscle relaxants (see chapter 7), which may cause a higher incidence of residual curarisation in these patients.[151] It has, however, been demonstrated that, in patients with renal failure, the plasma clearance of neostigmine is de-creased, and the elimination half life prolonged, because neostigmine is excreted 50% unchanged by the kidneys (table 8.4).[152] Neostigmine is

Table 8.4   Pharmacokinetic data on the anticholinesterases neostigmine, pyridostigmine, and edrophonium in renal failure

Anticholinesterase	VD_{ss} (l/kg) Normal	Renal failure	Cl (l/kh per h) Normal	Renal failure	$T_{\frac{1}{2}\alpha}$ (min) Normal	Renal failure	$T_{\frac{1}{2}\beta}$ (hours) Normal	Renal failure
Neostigmine	0·7	1·6	0·55	0·47	3·4	2·5	1·20	3·02
Pyridostigmine	1·1	1·0	0·52	0·13	6·8	3·9	1·87	6·32
Edrophonium	1·1	0·7	0·58	0·16	7·2	–	1·93	3·43

The data are given as rounded figures, and are purely illustrative.

excreted 50% unchanged in the urine, and further metabolised, mainly into 3-hydroxyphenyltrimethyl-ammonium.

Renal excretion is by glomerular filtration and tubular excretion, so recurarisation is unlikely to occur from the short effect of neostigmine. Edrophonium is 70% excreted in the urine. With pyridostigmine and edrophonium the clearance is also decreased in renal failure.[121 143]

Pyridostigmine is excreted 80% unchanged in the urine, and for the rest mainly metabolised into 3-hydroxy-N-methylpyridinium which is rapidly glucuronidated.

The effect of acid–base balance and potassium levels

From animal studies it can be concluded that, in hypokalaemia, more neostigmine is needed to reverse a pancuronium induced neuromuscular blockade.[153] These results probably also apply to other non-depolarising relaxants.

Respiratory acidosis and metabolic alkalosis prevent the antagonistic effect of neostigmine in cats.[154 155] In other studies it has, however, been demonstrated that antagonism with neostigmine is not affected by respiratory acidosis or alkalosis.[156]

A number of factors exist that have an effect on the choice for a particular anticholinesterase, and its dose. With the current relaxants, it is impossible to reverse a deep neuromuscular blockade (high relaxant concentration in the biophase). Therefore, the rate of spontaneous recovery should be considered when reversing a blockade.[157] However, the shorter acting the muscle relaxant, the easier it is to reverse a blockade.[109] At deeper blocks neostigmine is more effective than the other anticholinesterases.[158] Gallamine is slowly antagonised by neostigmine compared with pancuronium or tubocurarine. Atracurium and vecuronium need lower doses of neostigmine, and are antagonised more quickly than tubocurarine and pancuronium.[159] If reversal is applied during inhalational anaesthesia, higher dosages of the anticholinesterases are needed;[160] recovery is also slower.[161]

The effect of neostigmine and pyridostigmine is potentiated by 4-aminopyridine,[93] which is also able to reverse antibiotic induced neuromuscular blockade.[162]

Closed loop continuous neuromuscular blockade

For a constant and stable drug effect (steady state), a constant plasma concentration of that drug is a prerequisite. With intermittent doses, the plasma concentration will rise and decay, parallel to the administration of a bolus dose. Administration of a drug by continuous infusion leads, however, to a constant concentration and a stable effect. Therefore during anaesthesia more and more drugs are administered in this way.

As it is important that adjustments to the degree of effect are made rapidly, it must be easy to control the drug. High level of controllability demands a rapid onset, a short duration, and a rapid recovery of action. In the case of the muscle relaxants, this can be translated into short elimination half life and fast plasma clearance. A fast plasma clearance is reached by rapid redistribution, rapid metabolism, or rapid excretion. Suxamethonium is an example of a drug with rapid metabolism; vecuronium and atracurium are drugs with rapid redistribution and secondary metabolism; gallamine is dependent mainly on renal excretion. Drugs with a long duration of action are likely to accumulate, which therefore leads to prolonged duration of action when administered by infusion. The amount of drug that must be infused into an individual patient for maintenance of neuromuscular blockade depends on a variety of factors, including patient's weight and length, the pharmacokinetic characteristics of the relaxant, the presence of concurrent diseases, and the simultaneous use of other drugs (see chapter 7).

If the rate of drug delivery is equal to its plasma clearance, a steady state concentration can be reached. Such an infusion rate equals the desired plasma concentration times the clearance. It will, however, take an infusion five to seven times the elimination half life to reach a steady state. This time can be decreased by first administering a bolus dose equal to the desired plasma concentration times the volume of distribution, and starting the infusion immediately thereafter. As with bolus administration, the effect of continuous infusions of relaxants depends on the simultaneously administered anaesthetic agent. Continuous administration of relaxants can lead to a number of adverse effects, some of which are described in chapter 7.

As a result of these adverse effects, and because of the interindividual variability in effect, a periodic evaluation of neuromuscular transmission should be practised. A check on the train-of-four count or fade every one or two hours can easily be carried out during continuous infusion of relaxants, and in the intensive care unit. In the operating room continuous monitoring of neuromuscular transmission with the same parameters is possible. The aim should be to keep one response to train-of-four stimulation available. With prolonged infusion of relaxants that are metabolised, an interaction between these metabolites and the maternal compound can occur. It is also possible that the derivatives accumulate, resulting in substantial neuromuscular blockade, as has been indicated for vecuronium. The metabolites of pancuronium are unlikely to have a similar effect.[163]

Continuous infusion is not only feasible in adults, but also in children. With infusion it is possible to develop closed loop systems with feedback between response and infusion rate.

Computer controlled closed loop systems have been used for continuous administration of muscle relaxants.[73 164 165] With such systems a preset degree of neuromuscular blockade can be maintained. The measurement necessary to close the loop can be done by either electromyography or mechanomyography (contraction force or accelerometry). When infusion is started, a loading dose should be administered to obtain a rapid blockade, and then continuous infusion should start. The rate of infusion should be determined by measurement of the degree of blockade. This indicates that some overshoot and undershoot will be present, depending on the time constant of the particular relaxant administered. The shorter the time constant, that is, the more rapid the onset, and the shorter the duration, the better the performance of the closed loop system, and the smaller the overshoot and the undershoot. Versatile systems for closed loop administration of atracurium and vecuronium have been developed.[166] Rocuronium has also been administered by continuous infusion in a closed loop feedback control system.[167] Such closed loop systems are operated in the following circumstances.

- Proportional—in which the controller gain is uniformly proportional to the input (change in infusion speed)
- Integral—acts with increasing response to an error signal
- Derivative—anticipates the trend of the error signal, and thus applies a correcting action ahead of this error (on–off control).

Others have developed systems that hold pharmacokinetic algorithms to reach a desired plasma concentration.[168] In these systems there is on the whole no feedback from the degree of neuromuscular blockade, and thus accumulation, and so a prolonged effect may occur in individual cases.

Infusion is also possible without a closed loop system. After a bolus dose of the relaxant continuous infusion is started at a particular rate. When the drugs are administered in the intensive care unit, a lower dose is usually sufficient to reach adequate muscle relaxation.

1 Beecher HK, Todd DP. A study of the deaths associated with anesthesia and surgery. *Ann Surg* 1985;**140**:2–34.
2 Vervloet D. Allergy to muscle relaxants and related compounds. *Clin Allergy* 1985;**15**: 501–8.
3 Shorten GD. Postoperative residual curarisation: incidence, aetiology and associated morbidity. *Anaesth Intens Care* 1993;**21**:782–9.
4 Pedersen T, Viby-Mogensen J, Eliasen K, Ringsted C, Henriksen E. A one year prospective study of postoperative pulmonary complications after neuromuscular blockade by pancuronium and atracurium. *Anesthesiology* 1988;**69**:A902.
5 Andersen BN, Madsen JV, Schurizer BA, Juhl B. Residual curarization: a comparative study of atracurium and pancuronium. *Acta Anaesthesiol Scand* 1988;**32**:79–81.
6 Bevan DR, Smith CE, Donati F. Postoperative neuromuscular blockade: a comparison between atracurium, vecuronium and pancuronium. *Anesthesiology* 1988;**69**:272–6.
7 Brull SJ, Ehrenwerth J, Cronelly NR, Silverman DG. Assessment of residual curarization using low-current stimulation. *Can J Anaesth* 1991;**38**:164–8.
8 Moller JT, Wittrup M, Johansen SH. Hypoxemia in the postanesthesia care unit: An observer study. *Anesthesiology* 1990;**73**:890–5.
9 Beemer GH, Rozental P. Postoperative neuromuscular function. *Anaesth Intens Care* 1986;**38**:41–5.
10 Viby-Mogensen J, Jørgensen BC, Ørding H. Residual curarization in the recovery room. *Anesthesiology* 1981;**47**:491–9.
11 Lennmarken C, Löfström JB. Partial curarization in the postoperative period. *Acta Anaesthesiol Scand* 1984;**28**:260–2.
12 Pedersen T, Eliasen K, Henriksen E. A prospective study of risk factors and cardiopulmonary complications associated with anaesthesia and surgery: risk indicators of cardiopulmonary morbidity. *Acta Anaesthesiol Scand* 1990;**34**:144–55.
13 Katz RL. Neuromuscular effects of d-tubocurarine, edrophonium and neostigmine in man. *Anesthesiology* 1967;**28**:327–36.
14 Matteo RS, Spector S, Horowitz PE. Relation of serum d-tubocurarine concentration and neuromuscular blockade in man. *Anesthesiology* 1974;**41**:440–3.

15 Booij LHDJ, Miller RD, Crul JF. Neostigmine and 4-aminopyridine antagonism of lincomycin–pancuronium neuromuscular blockade in man. *Anesth Analg* 1978;57: 316–21.

16 Sokoll MD, Gergis SD. Antibiotics and neuromuscular function. *Anesthesiology* 1981;55:148–59.

17 Bevan DR, Donati F, Kopman AF. Reversal of neuromuscular blockade. *Anesthesiology* 1992;77:785–805.

18 Pavlin EG, Holle RH, Schoene RB. Recovery of airway protection compared with ventilation in humans after paralysis with curare. *Anesthesiology* 1989;70:381–5.

19 O'Connor M, Russell WJ. Muscle strength following anaesthesia with atracurium and pancuronium. *Anaesth Intens Care* 1988;16:255–9.

20 Viby-Mogensen J, Jensen NH, Engbaek J, Ording H, Skovgaard LT, Chraemmer-Jorgensen B. Tactile and visual evaluation of the response to train-of-four nerve stimulation. *Anesthesiology* 1985;63:440–3.

21 Thomas P, Worthlet L, Russel W. How useful is visual and tactile accessment of neuromuscular blockade using a peripheral nerve stimulator? *Anesth Analg* 1984;12:68.

22 Ali HH, Kitz RJ. Evaluation of recovery from nondepolarizing neuromuscular block, using a digtal neuromuscular transmission analyzer: preliminary report. *Anesth Analg* 1973;52:740–4.

23 Brull SJ, Silverman DG. Visual and tactile assessment of neuromuscular fade. *Anesth Analg* 1993;77:352–5.

24 Drenck NE, Ueda N, Olsen NV, *et al.* Manual evaluation of residual curarization using double burst stimulation: A comparison with train-of-four. *Anesthesiology* 1989;70: 578–81.

25 Engbaek J, Skovgaard LT, Friis B, Kann T, Viby-Mogensen J. Monitoring of the neuromuscular transmission by electromyography (I). Stability and temperature dependence of evoked EMG response compared to mechanical twitch recordings in the cat. *Acta Anaesthesiol Scand* 1992;36:495–504.

26 Kopman AF. The effect of resting muscle tension on the dose–effect relationship of d-tubocurarine: does preload influence the evoked EMG. *Anesthesiology* 1988; 69:1003–5.

27 Kopman AF. The relationship of evoked electromyographic and mechanical responses following atracurium in humans. *Anesthesiology* 1985;65:208–11.

28 Engbaek J, Roed J. Differential effect of pancuronium at the adductor pollicis, the first dorsal interosseous and the hypothenar muscles. An electromyographic and mechano-myographic dose–response study. *Acta Anaesthesiol Scand* 1992;36:664–9.

29 Katz RL. Electromyographic and mechanical effects of suxamethonium and tubocurarine on twitch, tetanic and post-tetanic responses. *Br J Anaesth* 1973;45:849.

30 Harper NJN, Bradshaw EG, Healy TEJ. Evoked electromyographic and mechanical responses of the adductor pollicis compared during the onset of neuromuscular blockade by atracurium or alcuronium, and during antagonism by neostigmine. *Br J Anaesth* 1986;58:1278–84.

31 Engbaek J, Ostergaard D, Viby-Mogensen J, Skovgaard LT. Clinical recovery and train-of-four ratio measured mechanically and electromyographically following atracurium. *Anesthesiology* 1989;71:391–5.

32 Harper NJN, Martlew R, Strang T, Wallace M. Monitoring neuromuscular block by acceleromyography: a comparison of the Mini-accelerograph with the Myograph 2000. *Br J Anaesth* 1994;72:411–14.

33 Smith DC, Booth JV. Influence of muscle temperature and forearm position on evoked electromyography in the hand. *Br J Anaesth* 1994;72:407–10.

34 Helbo-Hansen H, Bang U, Nielsen H, Skovgaard LT. The accuracy of train-of-four monitoring at varying stimulating currents. *Anesthesiology* 1992;76:199–203.

35 Kopman AF, Lawson D. Milliamperage requirements for supramaximal stimulation of the ulnar nerve with surface electrodes. *Anesthesiology* 1984;61:83–5.

36 Connelly N, Silverman D, O'Connor TZ, Brull SJ. Subjective response to train-of-four and double burst stimulation in awake patients. *Anesth Analg* 1990;70:650–3.

37 Kopman AF. A safe surface electrode for peripheral nerve stimulation. *Anesthesiology* 1976;44:343–4.

38 Gissen AJ, Katz RL. Twitch, tetanus and post tetanic potentiation as indices of nerve–muscle block in man. *Anesthesiology* 1969;30:481–7.

39 Ali HH, Utting JE, Gray C. Stimulus frequency in the detection of neuromuscular block in humans. *Br J Anaesth* 1970;**42**:967–78.

40 Brull SJ, Ehrenwerth J, Silverman DG. Stimulation with submaximal current for train-of-four monitoring. *Anesthesiology* 1990;**72**:629–32.

41 Paton WDM, Waud DR. The margin of safety of neuromuscular transmission. *J Physiol* 1967;**191**:59–90.

42 Bowman WC. Prejunctional and postjunctional cholinoceptors at the neuromuscular junction. *Anesth Analg* 1980;**59**:935.

43 Meretoja OA, Taivainen T, Brandon BW, Wirtavuori K. Frequency of train-of-four stimulation influences neuromuscular response. *Br J Anaesth* 1994;**72**:686–7.

44 Lee CM. Train-of-four quantitation of competitive neuromuscular block. *Anesth Analg* 1975;**54**:649–53.

45 Brand JB, Cullen DJ, Wilson NE, Ali HH. Spontaneous recovery from nondepolarizing neuromuscular blockade: correlation between clinical and evoked responses. *Anesth Analg* 1977;**56**:55–8.

46 Dupuis JY, Martin R, Tetrault JP. Clinical, electrical and mechanical correlations during recovery from neuromuscular blockade with vecuronium. *Can J Anaesth* 1990; **37**:192–6.

47 O'Hara DA, Fragen RJ, Shanks CA. Reappearance of the train-of-four after neuromuscular blockade induced with tubocurarine, vecuronium or atracurium. *Br J Anaesth* 1986;**58**:1296–9.

48 Pearce AC, Casson WR, Jones M. Factors affecting train-of-four fade. *Br J Anaesth* 1985;**57**:602–6.

49 Engbaek J, Ostergaard D, Viby-Mogensen J. Double burst stimulation (DBS): a new pattern of nerve stimulation to identify residual neuromuscular block. *Br J Anaesth* 1989;**62**:274–8.

50 Brull SJ, Silverman DG. Visual assessment of train-of-four and double-burst-induced fade at submaximal stimulating currents. *Anesth Analg* 1991;**73**:627–32.

51 Stanec A, Heyduk J, Stanec G, Orkin LR. Tetanic fade and post-tetanic tension in the absence of neuromuscular blocking agents in anesthetized man. *Anesth Analg* 1978;**57**:102–7.

52 Viby-Mogensen J, Howardy-Hansen P, Chraemmer-Jorgensen B, Ording H, Engbaek J, Nielsen A. Post-tetanic count (PTC): A new method of evaluating an intense non-depolarizing neuromuscular blockade. *Anesthesiology* 1981;**55**:458–62.

53 Gwinnutt CL, Meakin G. Use of the post-tetanic count to monitor recovery from intense neuromuscular blockade in children. *Br J Anaesth* 1988;**61**:547–50.

54 Howardy-Hansen P, Viby-Mogensen J, Gottschau A, Skovgaard LT, Chraemmer-Jorgensen B, Engbaek J. Tactile evaluation of posttetanic count (PTC). *Anesthesiology* 1984;**60**:372–4.

55 Brull SJ, Silvermann DG. Tetanus-induced changes in apparent recovery after bolus doses of atracurium and vecuronium. *Anesthesiology* 1992;**77**:642–5.

56 Eriksson LI, Lennmarken C, Staun P, Viby-Mogensen J. Use of post-tetanic count in assessment of a repetitive vecuronium-induced neuromuscular block. *Br J Anaesth* 1990;**65**:487–93.

57 Debaene B, Meistelman C, Beaussier M, Lienhart A. Visual estimation of train-of-four responses at the orbicularis oculi and posttetanic count at the adductor pollicis during intense neuromuscular block. *Anesth Analg* 1994;**78**:697–700.

58 Saitoh Y, Toyooka H, Amaha K. Recoveries of post-tetanic twitch and train-of-four responses after administration of vecuronium with different inhalation anaesthetics and neuroleptanaesthesia. *Br J Anaesth* 1993;**70**:402–4.

59 Brull SJ, Connelly NR, O'Connor TZ, Silverman DG. Effect of tetanus on subsequent neuromuscular monitoring in patients receiving vecuronium. *Anesthesiology* 1991;**74**: 64–70.

60 Stiffel P, Hameroff SR, Blitt CD, Cork RC. Variability in assessment of neuromuscular blockade. *Anesthesiology* 1980;**52**:436–7.

61 Caffrey RR, Warren ML, Becker KE. Neuromuscular blockade monitoring comparing the orbicularis oculi and adductor pollicis muscles. *Anesthesiology* 1986;**65**:95–7.

62 Donati F, Meiselman C, Plaud B. Vecuronium neuromuscular blockade at the adductor muscles of the larynx and the adductor pollicis. *Anesthesiology* 1991;**74**:833.

63 Lebrault C, Chauvin M, Guirimand F, Duvaldestin P. Relative potency of vecuronium on the diaphragm and the adductor pollicis. *Br J Anaesth* 1989;**63**:389–92.

64 Smith C, Donati F, Bevan D. Differential effects of pancuronium on masseter and adductor pollicis muscles in humans. *Anesthesiology* 1989;**71**:57–61.

65 Foldes FF, Monte AP, Brunn HM, Wolfson B. Studies with muscle relaxants in unanesthetized subjects. *Anesthesiology* 1961;**22**:230–6.

66 Gal TJ, Smith TC. Partial paralysis with d-tubocurarine and the ventilatory response to CO_2: An example of respiratory sparing? *Anesthesiology* 1976;**45**:22–8.

67 Donati F, Antzaka C, Bevan DR. Potency of pancuronium at the diaphragm and the adductor pollicis muscle in man. *Anesthesiology* 1986;**65**:1–5.

68 De Troyer A, Bastenier J, Delhez L. Function of respiratory muscles during partial curarization in humans. *J Appl Physiol* 1980;**49**:1049–56.

69 Pansard J-L, Chauvin M, Lebrault C, Gauneau P, Duvaldestin P. Effect of an intubating dose of succinylcholine and atracurium on the diaphragm and the adductor pollicis muscle in humans. *Anesthesiology* 1987;**67**:326–30.

70 Donati F, Meistelman C, Plaud B. Vecuronium neuromuscular blockade at the adductor muscles of the larynx and adductor pollicis. *Anesthesiology* 1991;**74**:833–7.

71 Bragg P, Fisher DM, Donati F, Meistelman C, Lau M, Sheiner LB. Comparison of twitch depression of the adductor pollicis and the respiratory muscles. *Anesthesiology* 1994;**80**:310–19.

72 Heier T, Caldwell JE, Sessler DI, Kitts JB, Miller RD. The relationship between adductor pollicis twitch tension and core, skin, and muscle temperature during nitrous oxide isoflurane anesthesia in humans. *Anesthesiology* 1989;**71**:381–4.

73 De Vries JW, Ros HH, Booij LHDJ. Infusion of vecuronium controlled by a closed-loop system. *Br J Anaesth* 1986;**58**:100–3.

74 Thornberry EA, Mazumdar B. The effect of changes in arm temperature on neuromuscular monitoring in the presence of atracurium blockade. *Anaesthesia* 1988;**43**:447–9.

75 Pal J. Physostigmin ein gegengift des Curare. *Zeitblatt de Physiologie* 1900;**14**:255–8.

76 Aeschlimann J, Reinert M. Pharmacological action of some analogues of physostigmine. *J Pharmacol Expl Ther* 1931;**43**:413–44.

77 DeLaPorte S, Vallette FM, Grassi J, Koenig J. Presynaptic or postsynaptic origins of acetylcholinesterase at neuromuscular junctions? An immunological study in heterologous nerve–muscle cultures. *Develop Biol* 1986;**116**:96–7.

78 Gisiger V, Stephensa H. Acetylcholinesterase content in both motor nerve and muscle is correlated with twitch properties. *Neurosci Lett* 1982;**31**:301–5.

79 Wilson IB, Harrison MA. Turnover number of acetylcholinesterase. *J Biol Chem* 1964;**236**:2292–5.

80 Taylor P, Schumacher M, Maulet Y, Newton M. A molecular perspective on the polymorphism of acetylcholinesterase. *Trends Pharmaceut Sci* 1986;**7**:321–3.

81 Dryer F. Acetylcholine receptor. *Br J Anaesth* 1982;**54**:115–30.

82 Wilson DF. Influence of presynaptic receptors on neuromuscular transmission in rat. *Am J Physiol (Cell Physiol)* 1982;**242**:C366–70.

83 Deanna A, Scuka N. Time course of neostigmine: action on the endplate response. *Neuroscience* 1990;**118**:82–4.

84 Gwilt M, Wray D. The effect of chronic neostigmine treatment on channel properties at the rat neuromuscular junction. *Br J Pharmacol* 1986;**88**:25–31.

85 Wachtel RE. Comparison of anticholinesterases and their effects on acetylcholine-activated ion channels. *Anesthesiology* 1990;**72**:496–503.

86 Braga MFM, Rowan EG, Harvey AL, Bowman WC. Prejunctional action of neostigmine on mouse neuromuscular preparations. *Br J Anaesth* 1993;**70**:405–10.

87 Blaber LC. The mechanism of the facilitatory action of edrophonium in cat skeletal muscle. *Br J Pharmacol* 1972;**46**:498.

88 Donati F, Ferguson A, Bevan DR. Twitch depression and train-of-four ratio after antagonism of pancuronium with edrophonium, neostigmine or pyridostigmine. *Anesth Analg* 1983;**62**:314.

89 Futter FE, Donati F, Sadikok AS, Bevan DR. Neostigmine antagonism of succinylcholine phase II block: a comparison with pancuronium. *Can Anaesth Soc J* 1983;**30**:575–80.

90 Bevan DR, Donati F. Succinylcholine apnoea: attempted reversal with anticholineterases. *Can Anaesth Soc J* 1983;**30**:536–9.

91 Soni N, Kam P. 4-Aminopyridine: A review. *Anaesth Intens Care* 1983;**10**:120–6.

92 Booij LHDJ, van der Pol F, Crul JF, Miller RD. Antagonism of Org NC45 neuromuscular

blockade by neostigmine, pyridostigmine and 4-aminopyridine. *Anesth Analg* 1980; **59**:31–4.

93 Miller RD, Booij LHDJ, Agoston S, Crul JF. 4-Aminopyridine potentiates neostigmine in man. *Anesthesiology* 1979;**50**:416–20.

94 Miller RD, Denissen PAF, van der Pol F, Aogston S, Booij LHDJ, Crul FJ. Potentation of neostigmine and pyridostigmine by 4-aminopyridine in the rat. *J Pharm Pharmacol* 1978;**30**:699–702.

95 Agoston S, van Weerden T, Westra P, Broekert A. Effects of 4-aminopyridine in Eaton–Lambert syndrome. *Br J Anaesth* 1978;**50**:383–5.

96 Biessels PTM, Agoston S, Horn AS. Comparison of the pharmacological actions of some new 4-aminopyridine derivatives. *Eur J Pharmacol* 1984;**106**:319–25.

97 Amaki Y, Kobayashi K, Kibayashi C. In vitro neuromuscular effect of acetaminopyridine-*N*-oxide. *Anesthesiology* 1980;**53**:S283.

98 Detwiler PB. The effects of germine-3-acetate on neuromuscular transmission. *J Pharmacol Expl Ther* 1972;**180**:244–54.

99 Brennan JL, Jones SF, McLeod JG. Effect of germine acetates on neuromuscular transmission. *J Neurol Sci* 1971;**13**:321–31.

100 Hyashi H, Yonemura K, Slimoji K. Antagonism of neuromuscular block by germine mono acetate. *Anesthesiology* 1973;**38**:145–52.

101 Lee C, Au E, Durant NN, Katz RL. Germine monoacetate counteracts dantrolene sodium. *Anesthesiology* 1980;**53**:S278.

102 Westra P, van Thiel MSJ, Vermeer GA. Pharmacokinetics of galanthamine (a long-acting anticholinesterase drug) in anaesthetized patients. *Br J Anaesth* 1986;**58**:1303–7.

103 Baraka A, Cozanitis D. Galanthamine versus neostigmine for reversal of non-depolarising neuromuscular block in man. *Anesth Analg* 1973;**52**:832.

104 Miller RD, VanNyhuis LS, Eger EI, Vitez TS, Way WL. Comparative times to peak effect and durations of action of neostigmine and pyridostigmine. *Anesthesiology* 1974; **41**:27–33.

105 Ferguson A, Egerszegi P, Bevan DR. Neostigmine, pyridostigmine, and edrophonium as antagonists of pancuronium. *Anesthesiology* 1980;**53**:390–4.

106 Cronnelly R, Morris RB, Miller RD. Edrophonium: duration of action and atropine requirement in humans during halothane anesthesia. *Anesthesiology* 1982;**57**:261–6.

107 Miller RD, Larson Jr CP, Way WI. Comparative antagonism of d-tubocurarine-, gallamine-, and pancuronium-induced neuromuscular blockade by neostigmine. *Anesthesiology* 1972;**37**:503–9.

108 Rup SM, McChristian JW, Miller RD. Neostigmine antagonises a profound neuromuscular blockade more rapidly than edrophonium. *Anesthesiology* 1984;**61**:A297.

109 Beemer GH, Bjorksten AR, Dawson PJ, Dawson RJ, Heenan BJ, Robertson BA. Determinants of the reversal time of competitive neuromuscular block by anticholinesterases. *Br J Anaesth* 1991;**66**:469–75.

110 Donati F, Lahoud J, McCready D, Bevan DR. Neostigmine, pyridostigmine and edrophonium as antagonists of deep pancuronium blockade. *Can J Anaesth* 1987; **34**:589–93.

111 Sunew KY, Hicks RG. Effects of neostigmine and pyridostigmine on duration of succinylcholine action and pseudocholinesterase activity. *Anesthesiology* 1978;**49**:188–91.

112 Shorten GD, Ali HH. Atracurium after an anticholinesterase. Does prior reversal with edrophonium or neostigmine influence the response to atracurium? *Anaesthesia* 1993;**48**:524–6.

113 Astley BA, Hughes R, Payne JP. Antagonism of atracurium-induced neuromuscular blockade by neostigmine or edrophonium. *Br J Anaesth* 1986;**58**:1290–5.

114 Goldhill DR, Embree PB, Ali HH, Savarese JJ. Reversal of pancuronium. Neuromuscular and cardiovascular effects of a mixture of neostigmine and glycopyrronium. *Anaesthesia* 1988;**43**:443–6.

115 Harper NJN, Wallace M, Hall IA. Optimum dose of neostigmine at two levels of atracurium-induced neurmuscular block. *Br J Anaesth* 1994;**72**:82–5.

116 Breen PJ, Doherty WG, Donati F, Bevan DR. The potencies of edrophonium and neostigmine as antagonists of pancuronium. *Anaesthesia* 1985;**40**:844–7.

117 Young WL, Matteo RS, Ornstein E. Duration of action of neostigmine and pyridostigmine in the elderly. *Anesth Analg* 1988;**67**:775–8.

118 Cook DR, Chakravorti S, Brandom BW, Stiller RLK. Effects of neostigmine,

edrophonium and succinylcholine on the in vitro metabolism of mivacurium: clinical correlates. *Anesthesiology* 1992;77:A433.

119 McCarthy GJ, Cooper AR, Stanley JC, Mirakhur RK. Onset and duration of action of vecuronium in the elderly: comparison with adults. *Br J Anaesth* 1992;69:281–3.

120 Matteo RS, Young WL, Ornstein E, Schwartz AE, Silverberg PA, Diaz J. Pharmacokinetics and pharmacodynamics of edrophonium in elderly surgical patients. *Anesth Analg* 1990;71:334–9.

121 Morris RB, Cronelly R, Miller RD, Stanski DR, Fahey MR. Pharmacokinetics of edrophonium and neostigmine when antagonizing d-tubocurarine neuromuscular blockade in man. *Anesthesiology* 1981;54:399–402.

122 Shorten GD, Ali HH, Goudsouzian BG. Neostigmine and edrophonium antagonism of moderate neuromuscular block induced by pancuronium or tubocurarine. *Br J Anaesth* 1993;70:160–2.

123 Payne JP, Hughes R, Al Azami S. Neuromuscular blockade by neostigmine in anaesthetized man. *Br J Anaesth* 1980;52:69–75.

124 Goldhill DR, Wainwright AP, Stuart CS, Flynn PJ. Neostigmine after spontaneous recovery from neuromuscular blockade. Effect on depth of blockade monitored with train-of-four and tetanic stimuli. *Anaesthesia* 1989;44:293–9.

125 Astley BA, Katz RL, Payne JP. Electrical and mechanical responses after neuromuscular blockade with vecuronium, and subsequent antagonism with neostigmine or edrophonium. *Br J Anaesth* 1987;59:983–8.

126 Mirakhur RK. Edrophonium and plasma cholinesterase activity. *Can Anaesth Soc J* 1986;33:588–90.

127 Valdrighi JB, Fleming NW, Smith BK, Smith GL, White DA. Effects of cholinesterase inhibitors on the neuromuscular blocking action of suxamethonium. *Br J Anaesth* 1994;72:237–9.

128 Cook DR, Stiller RL, Weakly JN, Chakravorti S, Brandom BW, Welch RM. In vitro metabolism of mivacurium chloride (BW B1090U) and succinylcholine. *Anesth Analg* 1989;68:452–6.

129 Cook DR, Chakravorti S, Brandom BW, Stiller RL. Effects of neostigmine, edrophonium and succinylcholine on the in vitro metabolism of mivacurium: clinical correlates. *Anesthesiology* 1992;77:A948.

130 Fleming NW, Lewis BK. Cholinesterase inhibitors do not prolong neuromuscular block produced by mivacurium. *Br J Anaesth* 1994;73:241–3.

131 Naguib M, Abdulatif M, Al-Chamdi A, Hamo I, Nouheid R. Dose–response relationship for edrophonium and neostigmine antagonism of mivacurium-induced neuromuscular block. *Br J Anaesth* 1993;71:709–14.

132 Mirakhur RK. Edrophonium and plasma cholinesterase activity. *Can Anaesth Soc J* 1986;33:588–90.

133 Payne JP, Hughes R, Al Azawi S. Neuromuscular blockade by neostigmine in anaesthetized man. *Br J Anaesth* 1980;52:69–76.

134 Mirakhur RK, Dundee JW. Glycopyrrolate: Pharmacology and clinical use. *Anaesthesia* 1983;38:1195–204.

135 Child CS. Prevention of neostigmine-induced colonic activity. A comparison of atropine and glycopyrronium. *Anaesthesia* 1984;39:1083–5.

136 Maselli RA, Leung C. Analysis of anticholinesterase-induced neuromuscular transmission failure. *Muscle Nerve* 1993;16:548–53.

137 Ding Y, Fredman B, White PF. Use of mivacurium during laparoscopic surgery: effect of reversal drugs on postoperative recovery. *Anesth Analg* 1994;78:450–4.

138 King MJ, Milazkiewicz R, Carli F, Deacock AR. Influence of neostigmine on postoperative vomiting. *Br J Anaesth* 1988;61:403–6.

139 Janhunen L, Tammisto T. Post-operative vomiting after different methods of general anaesthesia. *Ann Chir Gynaecol Fenniae* 1972;61:152–9.

140 Boeke AJ, De Lange JJ, van Druenen B, Langemeijer JJM. Effect of antagonizing residual neuromuscular block by neostigmine and atropine on postoperative vomiting. *Br J Anaesth* 1994;72:654–6.

141 Iwasaki H, Hamiki A, Omote K, Omote T, Takahashi T. Response differences of paretic and healthy extremities to pancuronium and neostigmine in hemiplegic patients. *Anesth Analg* 1985;64:864–6.

142 Cronelly R, Stanski DR, Miller RD, Sheiner LB. Pyridostigmine kinetics with and without renal function. *Clin Pharmacol Ther* 1980;28:78–81.

185

143 Morris RB, Cronnelly R, Miller RD, Stanski DR, Fahey MR. Pharmacokinetics of edrophonium in anephric and renal transplant patients. *Br J Anaesth* 1981;**53**:1311–14.

144 Fisher DM, Cronnelly R, Miller RD, Sharma M. The neuromuscular pharmacology of neostigmine in infants and children. *Anesthesiology* 1981;**59**:220–5.

145 Buzello W, Pollmaecher T, Schluermann D, Urbanyi B. The influence of hypothermic cardiopulmonary bypass on neuromuscular transmission in the absence of muscle relaxants. *Anesthesiology* 1986;**64**:279–81.

146 Farrell L, Dempsey MJ, Waud BE, Waud DR. Temperature and potency of d-tubocurarine and pancuronium in vitro. *Anesth Analg* 1981;**60**:18–20.

147 Diefenbach C, Abel M, Buzello W. Greater neuromuscular blocking potency of atracurium during hypothermic than during normothermic cardiopulmonary bypass. *Anesth Analg* 1992;**75**:675–8.

148 Buzello W, Schluermann D, Schindler M, Spillner G. Hypothermic cardiopulmonary bypass and neuromuscular blockade by pancuronium and vecuronium. *Anesthesiology* 1985;**62**:201–4.

149 Buzello W, Schluermann D, Schindler M, Spillner G. Unequal effects of cardiopulmonary bypass-induced hypothermia on neuromuscular blockade from constant infusion of alcuronium, pancuronium and vecuronium. *Anesthesiology* 1987;**66**:842–7.

151 Miller RD, Cullen DJ. Renal failure and postoperative respiratory failure: recurarization. *Br J Anaesth* 1976;**48**:253–6.

152 Cronnelly R, Stanski DR, Miller RD, Sheiner LB, Sohn YJ. Renal function, and the pharmacokinetics of neostigmine in anesthetized man. *Anesthesiology* 1979;**51**:222–6.

153 Miller RD, Roderick LL. Diuretic-induced hypokalaemia, pancuronium neuromuscular blockade and its antagonism by neostigmine. *Br J Anaesth* 1978;**50**:541–4.

154 Miller RD, Van Nyhuis LS, Eger EI, II, Way WL. The effect of acid–base balance on neostigmine antagonism of d-tubocurarine-induced neuromuscular blockade. *Anesthesiology* 1975;**42**:377–83.

155 Miller RD, Roderick LL. Acid–base balance and neostigmine antagonism of pancuronium neuromuscular blockade. *Br J Anaesth* 1978;**50**:317–24.

156 Aziz L, Ono K, Ohta Y, Morita K, Hirakawa M. The effect of CO_2-induced acid-base changes on the potencies of muscle relaxants and antagonism of neuromuscular block by neostigmine in rat in vitro. *Anesth Analg* 1994;**78**:322–7.

157 Engbaek J, Ostergaard D, Skovgaard LT, Viby-Mogensen J. Reversal of intense neuromuscular blockade following infusion of atracurium. *Anesthesiology* 1990;**72**:803–6.

158 Caldwell JE, Robertson EN, Baird WLM. Antagonism of profound neuromuscular blockade induced by vecuronium or atracurium. Comparison of neostigmine and edrophonium. *Br J Anaesth* 1986;**58**:1285–9.

159 Bevan DR, Donati F, Kopman AF. Reversal of neuromuscular blockade. *Anesthesiology* 1992;**77**:785–805.

160 Booij LHDJ, Crul JF, van der Pol F. The influence of halothane and enflurane on the reversibility of an Org NC45 neuromuscular blockade in cats. *Anaesth Intensivther Notfallmed* 1982;**17**:78–80.

161 Deslisle S, Bevan DR. Impaired neostigmine antagonism of pancuronium during enflurane anaesthesia in man. *Br J Anaesth* 1982;**54**:441–5.

162 Booij LHDJ, Miller RD, Jones MJW, Stanski DR. Antagonism of pancuronium and its metabolites by neostigmine in cats. *Anesth Analg* 1979;**58**:483–6.

163 Miller RD, Agoston S, Booij LHDJ, Kersten US, Crul JF, Ham J. The comparative potency and pharmacokinetics of pancuronium and its metabolites in anesthetized man. *J Pharmacol Expl Ther* 1978;**207**:539–43.

164 Ritchie G, Ebert JP, Jannett TC, Kissin I, Sheppard LC. A microcomputer based controller for neuromuscular block during surgery. *Ann Biomed Eng* 1985;**13**:3–15.

165 O'Hara DA, Derbyshire GJ, Overdyk FJ, Bogen DK, Marshall BE. Closed-loop infusion of atracurium with four different anesthetic techniques. *Anesthesiology* 1991;**74**:258–63.

166 Assef SJ, Lennon RL, Jones KA, Burke MJ, Behrens TL. A versatile, computer-controlled, closed-loop system for continuous infusion of muscle relaxants. *Mayo Clin Proc* 1993;**68**:1074–80.

167 Olkkola KT, Tammisto T. Quantifying the interaction of rocuronium (Org 9426) with etomidate, fentanyl, midazolam, propofol, thiopental, and isoflurane using closed-loop feedback control of rocuronium infusion. *Anesth Analg* 1994;**78**:687–90.

168 Olkkola KT, Schwilden H, Appfelstaedt C. Model-based adaptive coded-loop feedback control of atracurium-induced neuromuscular blockade. *Acta Anaesthesiol Scand* 1991;**35**:420–3.

Index